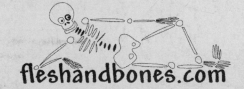

OBSTETRICS ILLUSTRATED

Commissioning Editor: Ellen Green
Project Development Manager: Janice Urquhart
Project Manager: Nancy Arnott
Designer: Erik Bigland
Page Layout: Jim Hope

OBSTETRICS ILLUSTRATED

KEVIN P. HANRETTY MD MRCOG

Consultant Obstetrician and Gynaecologist, The Queen Mother's Hospital, Glasgow;
Honorary Clinical Senior Lecturer, University of Glasgow, Glasgow, UK

Illustrated by

IAN RAMSDEN

Formerly Head of Medical Illustration Unit, University of Glasgow, Glasgow, UK

ROBIN CALLANDER FFPh FMAA AIMBI

Medical Illustrator, Formerly Director of Medical Illustrations, University of Glasgow, UK

SIXTH EDITION

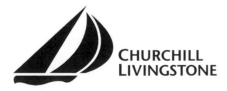

CHURCHILL
LIVINGSTONE

EDINBURGH LONDON NEW YORK OXFORD PHILADELPHIA ST LOUIS SYDNEY TORONTO 2003

CHURCHILL LIVINGSTONE
An imprint of Elsevier Science Limited

First published 1969
Second edition 1974
Third edition 1980
Fourth edition 1989
Fifth edition 1997
Sixth edition 2003

ISBN 0 443 07267 1
International edition ISBN 0 443 07268 X

British Library Cataloguing in Publication Data
A catalogue record for this book is available from the British Library

Library of Congress Cataloging in Publication Data
A catalog record for this book is available from the Library of Congress

Notice
Medical knowledge is constantly changing. Standard safety precautions must be followed,
but as new research and clinical experience broaden our knowledge, changes in treatment and
drug therapy may become necessary or appropriate. Readers are advised to check the most
current product information provided by the manufacturer of each drug to be administered to
verify the recommended dose, the method and duration of administration, and contraindications.
It is the responsibility of the practitioner, relying on experience and knowledge of the patient,
to determine dosages and the best treatment for each individual patient. Neither the Publisher
nor the author assumes any liability for any injury and/or damage to persons or property
arising from this publication.
The Publisher

PREFACE

This is the first edition of this book of the new millennium and Kevin Hanretty continues as author with Ian Ramsden as medical artist.

Many of the changes in this edition reflect the illustrated nature of the book. Textual alterations reflect changes of emphasis in clinical practice. These relate chiefly to two areas: ironically, the return of infection, bacterial as well as viral, as a source of danger to mother and her unborn child and secondly, to conditions previously only seen in developing countries but which are now seen throughout the world due to changes in migration patterns. We hope therefore that this text would remain of value to all of those involved in the care of pregnant women.

As previously Dr Tom Turner, neonatal paediatrician, Mrs Dorothy Sorley, obstetric physiotherapist and Mrs Anne Mackenzie, parenthood and breastfeeding counsellor, have continued to advise on areas of their specific expertise. We all hope that pregnancy will be a normal process with a happy outcome, however, obstetrics remains a beguiling specialty in which normality can quickly turn to crisis. We hope this text might contribute to the management of complicated pregnancies in order to achieve the aim of the safe birth of a healthy baby to a healthy mother.

K. H.

CONTENTS

CONTENTS

GLOSSARY OF ABBREVIATIONS

A&E	Accident and Emergency department		HBV	Hepatitis B Virus
AFE	Amniotic fluid embolism		HCG	Human Chorionic Gonadotrophin
APH	Antepartum haemorrhage		HDU	High-dependency unit
ARDS	Acute respiratory distress syndrome		HELLP	Haemolysis, elevated liver enzymes, low platelets
ARM	Artificial rupture of membranes		HIV	Human immunodeficiency syndrome
BhCG	Beta human chorionic gonadotrophin		ICU	Intensive Care Unit
BMI	Body mass index		IUGR	Intra-uterine growth restriction
BP	Blood pressure		IVF	In vitro fertilisation
bpm	Beats per minute		IV	Intravenous
CEMD	Confidential Enquiries into Maternal Death		LCFD	Low cavity forceps delivery
CS	Caesarean section		LUSCS	Lower uterine segment caesarean section
CTG	Cardiotocograph		MCFD	Mid cavity forceps delivery
CT	Computed tomography		MDR(UK)1	Maternal Death Report Form for the United
CVP	Central venous pressure			Kingdom
CVS	Chorion Villus Sampling			(from October 1995)
D&C	Dilatation and curettage		MRI	Magnetic resonance imaging
DIC	Disseminated intravascular coagulation		MSAFP	Maternal serum alphafetoprotein
DVT	Deep vein thrombosis		NND	Neonatal death
ECMO	Extra-corporeal membrane oxygenation		PMR	Perinatal mortality rate
ECV	External cephalic version		PND	Prenatal diagnosis
ERCP	Evacuation of retained products of conception		PND	Postnatal depression
			PPH	Postpartum haemorrhage
GBS	Group B streptococcus		SB	Stillbirth
GP	General practitioner		SFD	Small for dates
Hb	Haemoglobin concentration		TSH	Thyroid Stimulating
Hb SC	Haemoglobin sickle cell			Hormone

THE WEB AND OBSTETRICS

The availability of the internet throughout the world makes valuable information accessible to countries with both limited facilities and poor access to library resources.

It is important to identify the difference between high quality world wide web sites and sites which are full of biased information. Try to determine that any sites you access are evidence based.

Remember that sites which are evidence based may still have links to sites which are not.

The following is a variety of sites which may be of value. The contents are neither endorsed nor guaranteed by the author but reflect a spectrum of what is available for 'discerning' web browsers.

American College of Obstetricians and Gynecologists
http://www.acog.com/

Commission for Health Improvement (UK)
http://www.chi.nhs.uk/

The Fetal Medicine Foundation
http://www.fetalmedicine.com/

General Medical Council (UK)
http://www.gmcc-uk.org/

The International Federation of Gynecology and Obstetrics
http://www.figo.org/

National Institute for Clinical Excellence
http://www.nice.org.uk/

Obstetric Anaesthetists' Association
http://www.oaa-anaes.ac.uk/home.htm

Pubmed: a service of the National Library of Medicine
http://www.ncbi.nlm.nih.gov/entrez/query.fcgi

The Royal College of Midwives
http://www.rcm.org.uk/

Royal College of Obstetricians and Gynaecologists
http:www.rcog.org.uk/

Scottish intercollegiate guidelines network.
http://www.sign.ac.uk/index.html

United states Library of Medicine
http://www.nlm.nih.gov/

West Midlands Perinatal Institute
http://www.wmpi.net/main.htm

Women's Health Information
http://www.womens-health.co.uk/

The author welcomes comment or (ideally constructive) criticism at
kevin.hanretty@yorkhill.nhs.scot.uk

CHAPTER 1

PHYSIOLOGY OF REPRODUCTION

OVULATION

The processes leading to ovulation, fertilisation, and implantation of the fertilised ovum are complex and still incompletely understood. Ovulation results from an interplay between the hypothalamus, pituitary, ovary and endometrium. The ovary has two roles: the first is the endocrine function of producing oestrogen and progesterone to prepare the endometrium to receive the fertilised ovum. The second, which is intrinsically related, is gametogenesis and ovulation.

OVULATION

Development of the ovarian follicle occurs in response to stimulation from the pituitary gland.

The hypothalamus and pituitary are intimately associated. Together they regulate ovarian structure and function throughout the menstrual cycle.

The hypothalamus produces Gonadotrophin Releasing Hormone (GnRH) in a pulsatile fashion and this in turn stimulates production of the gonadotrophins Follicle Stimulating Hormone (FSH) and Luteinising Hormone (LH).

PITUITARY CONTROL OF OVARY

The ovarian changes are controlled mainly by the anterior pituitary which produces three principal hormones: Follicle Stimulating Hormone (FSH) stimulates follicular growth. Luteinising Hormone (LH) stimulates ovulation and causes luteinisation of granulosa cells after escape of the ovum. Prolactin is also produced by the anterior pituitary.

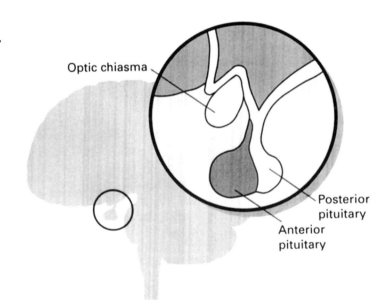

Optic chiasma

Posterior pituitary

Anterior pituitary

OVULATION AND MENSTRUATION

PITUITARY CONTROL OF OVARY (CONTINUED)

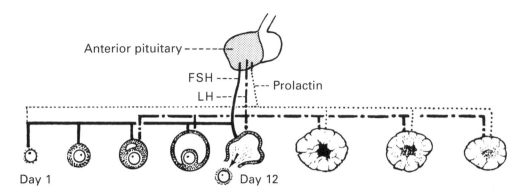

At the end of the menstrual cycle oestrogen levels are low. Low oestrogen levels stimulate production of FSH by the pituitary. FSH in turn acts upon the ovary to stimulate growth of ovarian follicles. The increasing levels of oestrogen produced by the developing follicles act on the pituitary to reduce FSH levels by the process of *negative feedback*. In the majority of cycles only one follicle, the so-called *dominant follicle*, is sufficiently large and has a greater density of FSH receptors to respond to the lower FSH levels and develops to the stage of ovulation. Non-identical twinning results when more than one follicle proceeds to ovulation. Oestrogen levels continue to rise. In the mid-cycle the nature of the ovarian control of pituitary function changes. Increasing oestrogen levels are required to produce a *positive feedback* mechanism which causes a surge in FSH and LH levels. This surge evokes ovulation. LH acts to increase local production of prostaglandins and proteolytic enzymes to allow oocyte extrusion. LH is responsible for the development of the corpus luteum which produces progesterone.

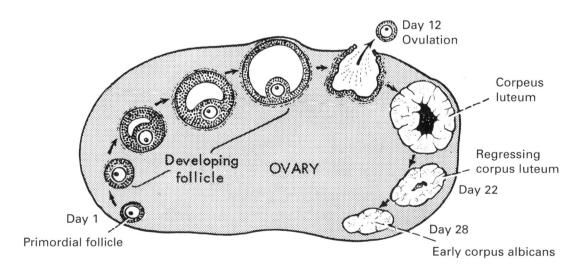

MENSTRUATION

These alterations in oestrogen and progesterone levels are responsible for the dramatic changes in the endometrium throughout the ovarian cycle. At the completion of the menstrual period the endometrium is only one to two millimetres thick. Under the influence of increasing levels of oestrogen this increases until by day 12 of the cycle the endometrium is 10 to 12 mm thick. This growth results from an increase in epithelial and stromal cells of the superficial layer of endometrium. This **Proliferative Phase** is characterised by an increase in oestrogen receptor content and increase in size of the endometrial glands.

As ovulation approaches, the progesterone receptor content increases. Within two days of ovulation the effect of ovarian production of progesterone becomes apparent as the endometrium enters the **Secretory Phase** of the cycle. During this phase the mitotic activity in the epithelium ceases and the glands become dilated and tortuous. The blood vessels become more coiled. Glycogen accumulation in the endometrium reaches a peak under the combined influence of oestrogen and progesterone. These processes prepare the endometrium for embedding of the embryo. If fertilisation does not occur then progesterone and oestrogen levels decline and menstruation occurs.

ENDOMETRIAL CHANGES

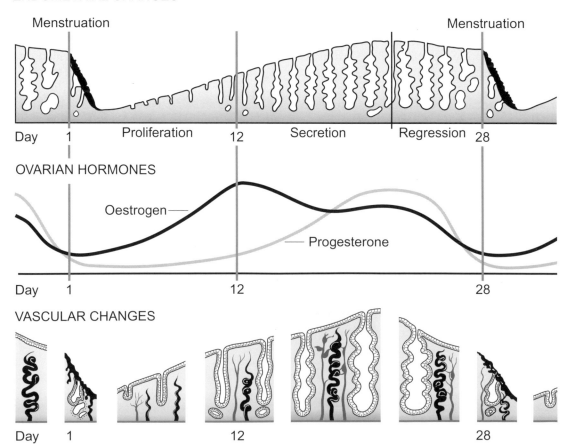

FERTILISATION

Fertilisation, if it occurs, takes place in the fallopian tube. The zygote divides repeatedly to form a solid sphere of cells as it passes down the fallopian tube and into the uterine cavity. The developing embryo begins to differentiate into the tissue which will become the fetus and that which will form the placenta and fetal membranes. The primitive precursor of the chorionic membrane produces Human Chorionic Gonadotrophin (HCG). HCG has a biological action very similar to LH and takes over its luteinising function.

For the first fourteen days after fertilisation uterine growth and the development of the decidua (the endometrium of pregnancy) are dictated by the corpus luteum under the influence of the pituitary. Thereafter the pituitary LH levels are reduced in response to the increasing levels of HCG.

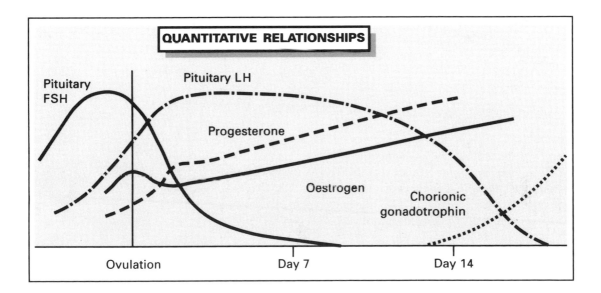

Under the influence of chorionic gonadotrophin the corpus luteum continues to grow and to secrete ovarian steroids for the maintenance of uterine growth. HCG levels reach a peak around 10 to 12 weeks and thereafter decline to a lower constant level throughout pregnancy. The response to this reduction is a decrease in ovarian oestrogen and progestogen output. As the ovarian contribution to maintaining the pregnancy declines, the placenta increases steroid production. Placental steroid production is impressive and analogues of both hypothalamic and pituitary hormones are produced. The capacity to produce these hormones increases as the early placenta develops.

DEVELOPMENT OF THE EMBRYO

The differentiation of the embryo itself into those tissues which will become the fetus and those which will form the placenta occurs soon after fertilisation; the fertilised ovum divides repeatedly as it travels through the fallopian tube. When the resulting mass of cells, the morula, reaches the endometrial cavity an eccentric space develops resulting in the formation of a hollow sphere with a mound of cells on one aspect of the inner surface. This mass of cells is called the inner cell mass.

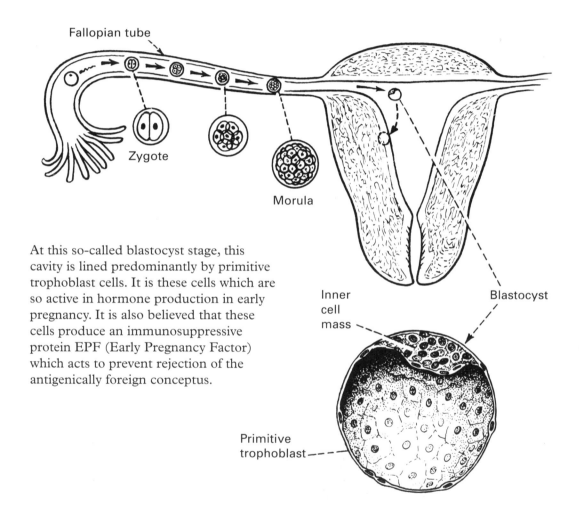

Fallopian tube

Zygote

Morula

At this so-called blastocyst stage, this cavity is lined predominantly by primitive trophoblast cells. It is these cells which are so active in hormone production in early pregnancy. It is also believed that these cells produce an immunosuppressive protein EPF (Early Pregnancy Factor) which acts to prevent rejection of the antigenically foreign conceptus.

Inner cell mass

Blastocyst

Primitive trophoblast

DEVELOPMENT OF THE EMBRYO

At this stage implantation is required for the zygote to obtain sufficient oxygen and nutrition. The inner cell mass develops into an ectodermal layer and endodermal layer. A mesodermal layer develops between these and grows outwards to form the extra-embryonic mesoderm. Two cavities appear around this stage, the yolk sac and the amniotic cavity. The amniotic sac is derived from ectoderm and the yolk sac from the endoderm. At this stage the amniotic cavity is very much smaller.

The two cavities, covered by mesoderm, move into the middle of the blastocyst cavity. A mesodermal stalk appears which will eventually form the umbilical cord. The embryonic area, comprising the ectoderm, endoderm and interposed mesoderm will become the fetus.

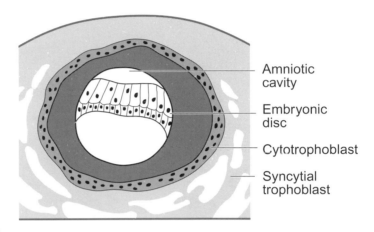

As development and growth continue the amniotic cavity enlarges to reach the wall of the blastocyst. In doing this, part of the yolk sac becomes enclosed within the embryo whilst the remainder forms a vestigial tube applied to the mesodermal stalk.

Blood vessels develop in the embryonic mesoderm and in the mesoderm of the trophoblast. Extension of these vessels along the connecting stalk results in the formation of the two arteries and single vein of the umbilical cord.

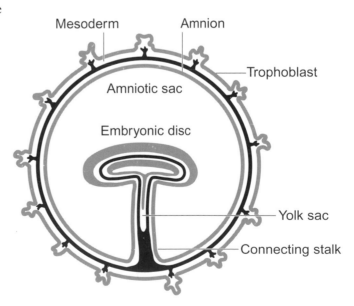

DEVELOPMENT OF THE EMBRYO

Within the embryo the vessels at the cephalic end differentiate to form the heart. Fetal blood formation occurs within the primitive blood vessels of the trophoblast and developing fetus. Interchange of nutrients and respiratory gases is facilitated by the formation of this fetotrophoblastic circulation. The formation and differentiation of the haemopoietic vascular system occurs between the third and fourth weeks of pregnancy. Following development of this rudimentary circulation further development of the fetus can proceed.

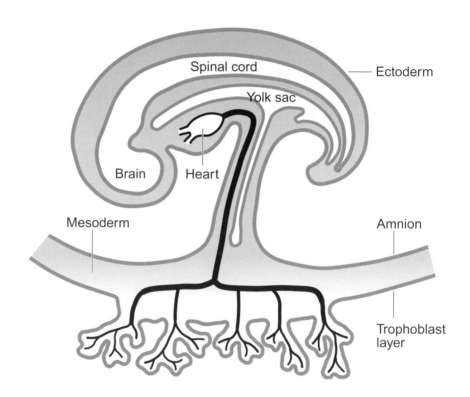

Structures derived from Primary Layers

Ectoderm	Skin appendages	Mesoderm	Bone and cartilage
	Nervous system		Muscle
	Glandular structures		Connective tissue
			Serous linings
Endoderm	Gastro-intestinal tract		Cardiovascular system
	Liver and biliary tract		Kidneys and most of
	Pancreas		the non-gonadal
	Respiratory tract		genital tract
	Gonadal germ cells		

PLACENTAL DEVELOPMENT AND PHYSIOLOGY

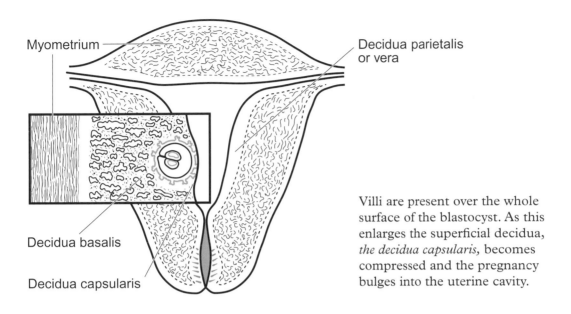

Myometrium

Decidua parietalis or vera

Decidua basalis

Decidua capsularis

Villi are present over the whole surface of the blastocyst. As this enlarges the superficial decidua, *the decidua capsularis,* becomes compressed and the pregnancy bulges into the uterine cavity.

The compression of the decidua capsularis gradually cuts off the circulation through it. This results in atrophy and disappearance of the villi in association with it. The surface of the blastocyst becomes smooth and this portion of the chorion is known as the chorion laeve. At the opposite pole of the blastocyst the villi proliferate and enlarge and this is known as the chorion frondosum. The connecting stalk of the embryo is attached to the wall of the blastocyst at this point. Ultimately, with the expansion of the blastocyst, the decidua capsularis comes in contact with the decidua vera and the uterine cavity is obliterated.

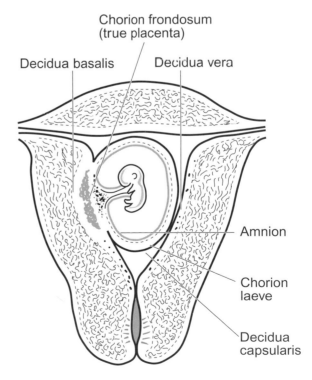

Chorion frondosum (true placenta)

Decidua basalis

Decidua vera

Amnion

Chorion laeve

Decidua capsularis

PLACENTAL DEVELOPMENT AND PHYSIOLOGY

The primitive trophoblast of the chorion frondosum invades the decidua. In this process the glands and stroma are destroyed but the small maternal vessels dilate to form sinusoids. The trophoblast develops a cellular layer, the cytotrophoblast and a syncytial layer, the syncytiotrophoblast. Fetal vessels surrounded by cytotrophoblast grow down into the syncytiotrophoblast. This structure, the chorionic villus, is bathed in maternal blood. As pregnancy advances the villus structure becomes more complex and the true villi divide repeatedly to form complex tree-like structures in which branches of the umbilical vessels form vascular cascades closely related to the surface trophoblast epithelium. The majority of branches of the true villi, called terminal villi, float freely in the maternal blood facilitating transfer of nutrients and waste products. Some villi attach to maternal tissue and are termed anchoring villi.

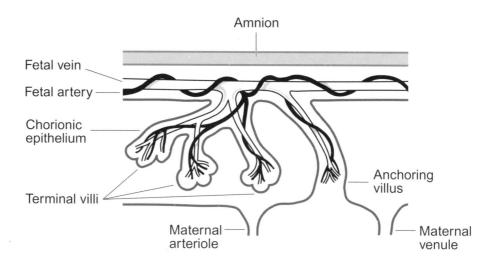

The structure and relationships of the terminal villi are more readily appreciated when examined in cross section.

As pregnancy advances the relationship of the trophoblast and maternal vasculature become more intimate. Trophoblast migrates into the maternal spiral arteries from the intervillous space.

Villous structure

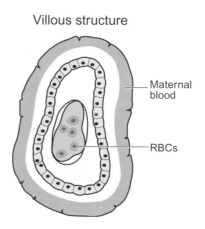

PLACENTAL DEVELOPMENT AND PHYSIOLOGY

This so-called 'physiological change' results in dilatation of the maternal arteries throughout the inner one third of the myometrium. The result of this is conversion of the uteroplacental blood supply into a low resistance–high flow vascular bed which is necessary for fetal growth and development.

Failure of this trophoblast invasion is associated with a number of later pregnancy complications including pregnancy induced hypertension and intra-uterine growth restriction.

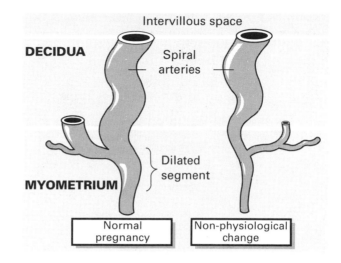

Placental transfer of nutrients, waste products, hormones and gases increases with advancing gestation as the structures between the maternal and fetal circulations become thinner. There is no direct connection between the two circulations and this 'placental barrier' in later pregnancy is the site of microvilli of syncytiotrophoblast, which increase the available surface area for nutrient transfer. Further, the syncytiotrophoblast and fetal mesoderm are reduced in thickness and the villus vessels dilate.

The fully formed placenta is a red discoid structure approximately 2 to 3 cm in thickness at the insertion of the umbilical cord. The average weight at term is around 500 g.

The umbilical cord, containing the two umbilical arteries and the single umbilical vein normally attaches to the placenta near its centre. Usually they immediately divide to provide a very rich blood supply on the fetal side, which, coupled with the maternal blood in the intervillous spaces, gives it its colour.

The two arteries and single vein of the umbilical circulation lie in a supporting myxomatous tissue derived from the mesoderm and termed 'Wharton's Jelly'. This jelly acts as a buffer, attenuating any pressure on the vessels, resisting occlusion and preventing kinking of the cord.

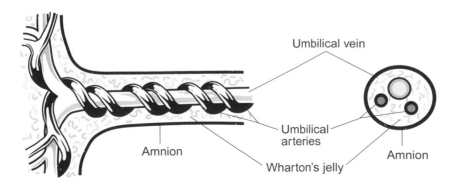

PLACENTAL FUNCTION

It is now clear that the function of the placenta is not merely the transport of nutrients and respiratory gases. The endocrine functions of the placenta are beginning to be unravelled.

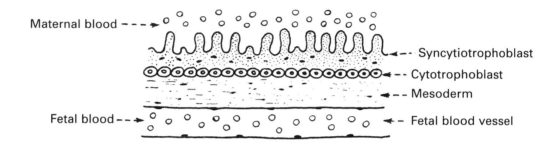

a) **Respiratory Function.** The anatomy of the fetal and maternal blood supply to the placenta ensures efficient transport of oxygen and carbon dioxide, chiefly by diffusion. The difference in oxygen dissociation characteristics of fetal blood from maternal blood further enhances fetal oxygen uptake.

b) **Excretory Function.** Little is known of the excretory functions of the human placenta but it is known that placental transfer of molecules like urea is linked to lipid solubility.

c) **Nutritional.** Since the permeability of the placenta to glucose is much greater than would be expected from its lipid solubility it is now known that there is a specific transport mechanism for glucose. This is known to be an integral membrane protein.

Three separate mechanisms exist for amino acids though the acidic acids are only poorly transported.

Lipids transfer only slowly. Placental transfer of free fatty acids is inversely related to the length of the carbon chain. Cholesterol is transported by endocytosis into the trophoblast.

PLACENTAL FUNCTION

d) Endocrine Function. A large number of hormones are produced by the placenta. These include hormones analogous to adult hypothalamic and pituitary hormones and steroid hormones.

A variety of other products are produced by the placenta. Many of these are glycoproteins such as Pregnancy Associated Proteins A to D, Pregnancy Specific Glycoprotein (SP1) and Placental Protein 5 (PP5). The functions of these are being clarified but remain uncertain in human pregnancy.

Hormone	Properties
Human Chorionic Somatomammotropin (HCS)	Similar to growth hormone and prolactin
Human Chorionic Gonadotrophin (HCG)	Stimulates adrenal and placental steroidogenesis. Analogous to LH
Human Chorionic Thyrotropin (HCT)	Analogous to Thyrotropin.
Corticotrophin Releasing Hormone (CRH)	As in adult.
Oestrogen	Complex. Stimulates uterine blood flow and growth.
Progestogens	Enables implantation and relaxes smooth muscle.
Adrenocorticoids	Induction of fetal enzyme systems and fetal maturity

Some products of placental and fetal metabolism may be used to screen for fetal disease. Measurement of alphafetoprotein, produced by the fetal liver, gut and yolk sac, may be used to screen for a number of anatomical abnormalities. Together with measurement of maternal serum HCG the risk of the fetus having a trisomy may also be calculated. This will be discussed later (see Chapter 6).

DEVELOPMENT OF THE MEMBRANES

The membranes are derived from the amnion and the chorion laeve, which is that part of the trophoblast which atrophies as the blastocyst expands.

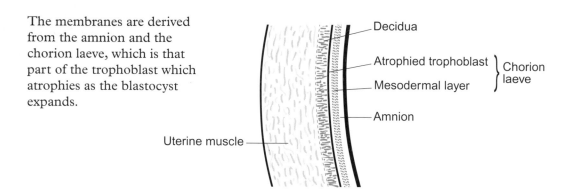

THE AMNIOTIC FLUID

The amniotic fluid cavity is a metabolically active compartment and is a remarkably dynamic site of fluid volume changes. The normal amniotic fluid volume increases from around 250 ml at 16 weeks gestation to 800 ml around 38 weeks. Thereafter the volume decreases towards and beyond term.

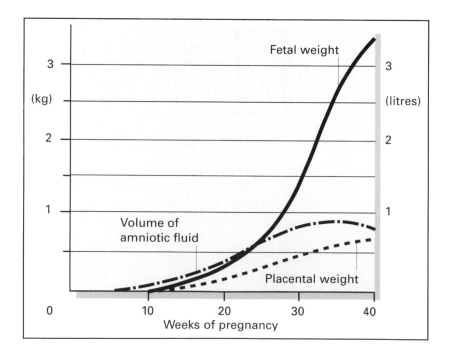

At term the circulation time allowing complete changeover of amniotic fluid is around three hours. The amniotic fluid is composed of fluid output from the kidneys which, being fetal urine, is hypotonic, and lung fluid secretion. Absorption is by fetal swallowing, removal at the amniotic–chorionic interface and at the intervillous space.

CHAPTER 2

FETAL AND MATERNAL PHYSIOLOGY

DIFFERENTIATION OF FETAL TISSUE

The development of the fetus relies on the differentiation of primitive tissues into physiological systems, their complete development and their maturation. Thus, the differentiation of part of the mesoderm to form primitive lungs is established around week 5. The formation of lung structure is established between 24 and 28 weeks. The physiological maturation, requiring production by pneumocytes of surfactant may occur later than this and is dependent in turn on maturation of the endocrine system.

The effect of drugs on fetal development is heavily dependent therefore on the gestation at the time of administration as well as the actual potential for teratogenicity of the agent concerned. This will be discussed later.

ORGAN	DIFFERENTIATION	COMPLETE FORMATION
Spinal cord	3–4 weeks	20 weeks
Brain	3	28
Eyes	3	20–24
Olfactory apparatus	4–5	8
Auditory apparatus	3–4	24–28
Respiratory system	5	24–28
Heart	3	6
Gastro-intestinal system	3	24
Liver	3–4	12
Renal system	4–5	12
Genital system	5	7
Face	3–4	8
Limbs	4–5	8

Fetal Cardiovascular Development

The respiratory function of the placenta requires that oxygenated blood be returned via the umbilical vein and into the fetal circulation. The changes which then occur at birth are dramatic.

Oxygenated blood from the placenta returns to the fetus via the umbilical vein. This vessel penetrates the liver and gives off small branches to that organ. Most of the blood is directed via the ductus venosus into the inferior vena cava which is carrying the returning non-oxygenated blood from the lower limbs, kidneys, liver etc. There is only partial mixing of the two streams and most of the oxygenated blood is directed to the crista dividens at the upper end of the inferior vena cava through the foramen ovale into the left atrium and thence to the left ventricle and aorta.

CARDIOVASCULAR SYSTEM

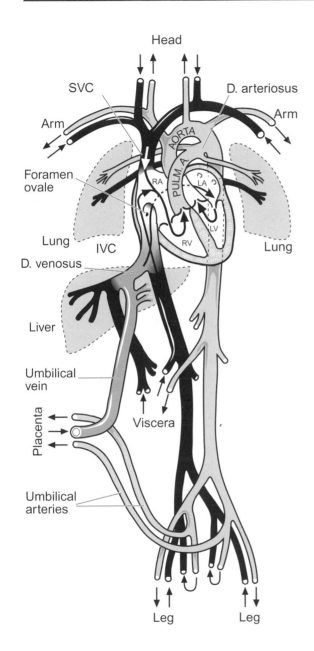

This relatively well oxygenated blood supplies the head and upper extremities. The remainder of the blood from the superior vena cava mixes with that of the inferior vena cava, passes to the right ventricle and thence to the pulmonary artery. A small amount of blood goes to the lungs. Most of it passes on via the ductus arteriosus into the aorta beyond the vessels supplying the head and upper extremities. Thereafter it passes down the aorta to supply the viscera and lower limbs. Little blood actually goes to the lower limbs. Most at this level passes into the umbilical arteries which arise as branches of the right and left internal iliac arteries. At birth the umbilical vessels contract. Breathing helps to create a negative thoracic pressure thus sucking more blood from the pulmonary artery into the lungs and diverting it from the ductus arteriosus which gradually closes. The foramen ovale is a valvular opening, the valve functioning from right to left. The left atrial pressure rises and closes this valve.

The greatest volume of cardiac output from both ventricles, around 40%, goes to the placenta. The organ which receives the greatest flow is the brain which receives about 13%.

The autonomic nervous system is the principal control mechanism for fetal heart rate, stroke volume and blood pressure. In the first half of pregnancy control is chiefly by the sympathetic system. In the second half the parasympathetic system becomes increasingly dominant. It is this development which explains the reduction in fetal heart rate with advancing gestation.

FETAL HAEMATOLOGY

The fetus is hypoxic relative to the maternal oxygen state yet does not become acidotic. There are three factors accounting for this: fetal haemoglobin concentration is high, around 180 g/l, the cardiac output is greater, and finally, the oxygen affinity of fetal haemoglobin is greater. Fetal haemoglobin is comprised of two α and two γ chains. The presence of γ chains increases oxygen affinity beyond that of adult haemoglobin so that for a given oxygen tension in the blood a greater percentage oxygen saturation is obtained. This is seen in comparisons of the oxygen dissociation curves for fetal and maternal haemoglobin.

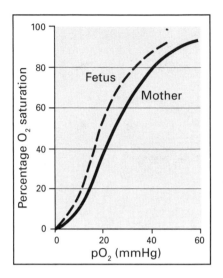

FETAL LUNG DEVELOPMENT

The placenta is the organ of respiration for the fetus but adaptation to extra-uterine life requires that the lungs go through four recognised phases of development. The last of these, the terminal sac period, is when alveolar development occurs from 24 weeks gestation to term. Fetal breathing movements are established even before this and are required for proper anatomical development of the lungs. Absence of fetal breathing movements in later pregnancy may be a sign of fetal acidosis and its identification can be used to assess fetal well being. This will be discussed later.

During this time development of pneumocytes occurs and production of surface acting phospholipids is established. These components of surfactant are required to enable lung function to occur post-natally. Surfactant deficiency, a consequence of prematurity, causes respiratory distress syndrome in the newborn and is the greatest determinant of outcome in babies born preterm.

MATERNAL PHYSIOLOGY

Enormous physiological changes occur throughout pregnancy and may not be clinically obvious. Thus, alterations in metabolic rate are more apparent than, for example, changes in the renin angiotensin system.

Nevertheless the alterations in the physiology require changes in energy consumption and use.

The energy demands of pregnancy derive from:

a) **Basic physiological processes** such as respiration, circulation, digestion, secretion, thermoregulation, growth and repair. These account for 66% of the total energy requirements in the non-pregnant female and amount to 1440 kcal/day. It is these processes which undergo greatest increase in pregnancy due to the demands of the fetus and placenta, uterus, breast growth etc.

b) **Activities of daily living.** These account for 17% of the total energy use in the nonpregnant state, approximately 360 kcal/day. Advancing pregnancy usually entails some reduction in activity though there is great individual variation in this.

c) **Work.** The requirements associated with work differ with occupation but comprise around 10% for most women or 150–200 kcal/day. This contribution to energy requirements generally reduces with advancing gestation, notably in the third trimester.

d) Specific dynamic action of food. Metabolism appears to be stimulated by food intake and comprises around 7% of the total or 150 kcal/day. This should be met by increased consumption during pregnancy.

Overall there is a 14% increase in energy requirement during pregnancy.

During lactation a further increase is required for milk production and the total requirements will be in the region of 3000 kcal/day.

WEIGHT INCREASE

These metabolic changes, accompanied by fetal growth, result in an increase in weight of around 25% of the non-pregnant weight: approximately 12.5 kg in the average woman. There is marked variation in normal women but the main increase occurs in the second half of pregnancy and is usually around 0.5 kg per week. Towards term the rate of gain diminishes and weight may fall after 40 weeks.

The increase is due to the growth of the conceptus, enlargement of maternal organs, maternal storage of fat and protein and increase in maternal blood volume and interstitial fluid.

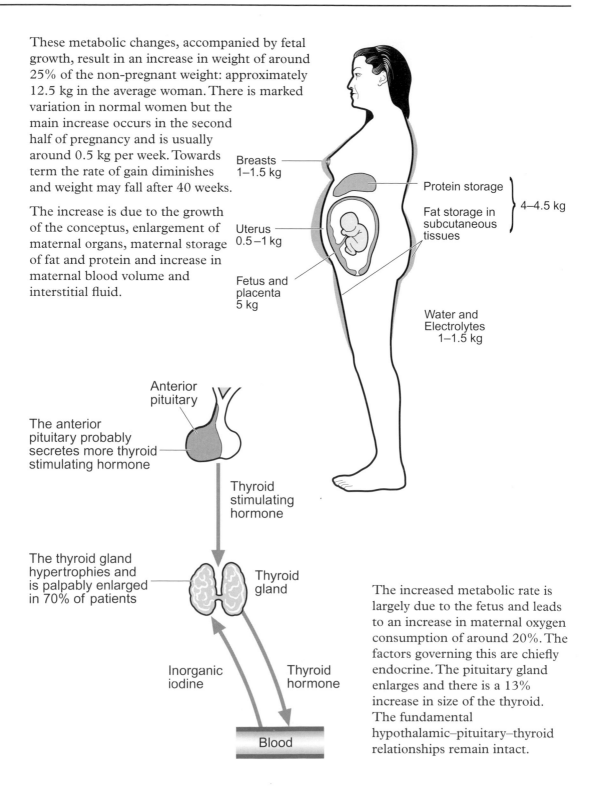

Breasts
1–1.5 kg

Protein storage

Fat storage in subcutaneous tissues

4–4.5 kg

Uterus
0.5–1 kg

Fetus and placenta
5 kg

Water and Electrolytes
1–1.5 kg

Anterior pituitary

The anterior pituitary probably secretes more thyroid stimulating hormone

Thyroid stimulating hormone

The thyroid gland hypertrophies and is palpably enlarged in 70% of patients

Thyroid gland

Inorganic iodine

Thyroid hormone

Blood

The increased metabolic rate is largely due to the fetus and leads to an increase in maternal oxygen consumption of around 20%. The factors governing this are chiefly endocrine. The pituitary gland enlarges and there is a 13% increase in size of the thyroid. The fundamental hypothalamic–pituitary–thyroid relationships remain intact.

CARBOHYDRATE METABOLISM

In the non-pregnant state ingested glucose is dealt with in four ways. Under the influence of insulin it may be deposited in the liver as glycogen. Some escapes into the general circulation and a proportion of this is metabolised directly by the tissues: some is converted to depot fat and a further portion is stored as muscle glycogen again with the aid of insulin.

The blood sugar is maintained between 4.5 and 5.5 mmol/litre (80–100 mg/dl). Sugar which passes out in the renal glomerular filtrate is never in excess of the amount which can be reabsorbed by the tubules, and none appears in the urine.

A marked alteration in carbohydrate metabolism occurs in pregnancy.

There is a demand on the part of the fetus for an easily convertible source of energy. At the same time there is a need to store energy for future demands such as lactation and the steadily increasing growth of the pregnancy and also to provide a more steady source of energy in the form of a high energy fuel. This the maternal body achieves by storage of fat. The major component of the diet is carbohydrate based and this requires to be redirected to satisfy the above requirements. The first noticeable change occurs in the blood sugar and this can be demonstrated by giving a glucose load as in an oral glucose tolerance test. It can be seen from this that the blood sugar, after a meal, remains high thus facilitating placental transfer.

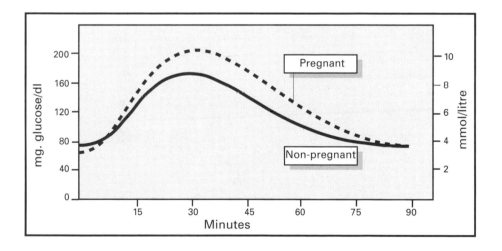

Pregnancy is said to be diabetogenic and this is associated with reduced tissue sensitivity to insulin.

Sensitivity to the actions of insulin may be reduced in tissues by up to 80 per cent. This effect is in part due to an increase in specific antagonists to insulin. The most important of these is Human Placental Lactogen (HPL).

21

CARBOHYDRATE METABOLISM

With the increased steroid levels produced by the placenta less glycogen is deposited in the liver and muscles. Higher circulating levels of blood sugar mean that more glucose is available to the fetus.

The effect of fasting is pronounced in pregnancy and even an overnight fast of 12 hours will result in hypoglycaemia and increased production of beta hydroxybutyric acid and acetoacetic acid, the ketone bodies.

Glucose levels are lower in the fetus and transport across the placenta is by a carrier mediated mechanism which gives a greater rate of transfer than simple diffusion.

High glucose levels in the renal circulation together with an increased glomerular filtration rate give rise to glycosuria which, as a result, is commonly seen in pregnancy.

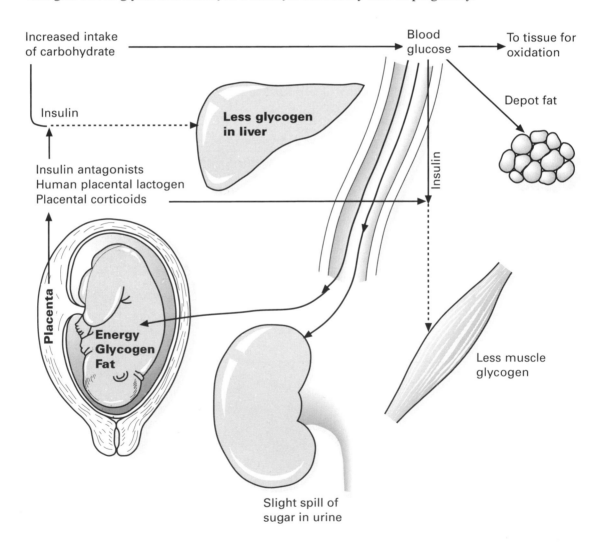

PROTEIN METABOLISM

The overall picture is one of positive nitrogen balance. There is on average a 20% increase in dietary protein intake. On average 500 g of protein have been retained by the end of pregnancy. Half of this is accounted for by maternal gain and the rest by the fetus and placenta.

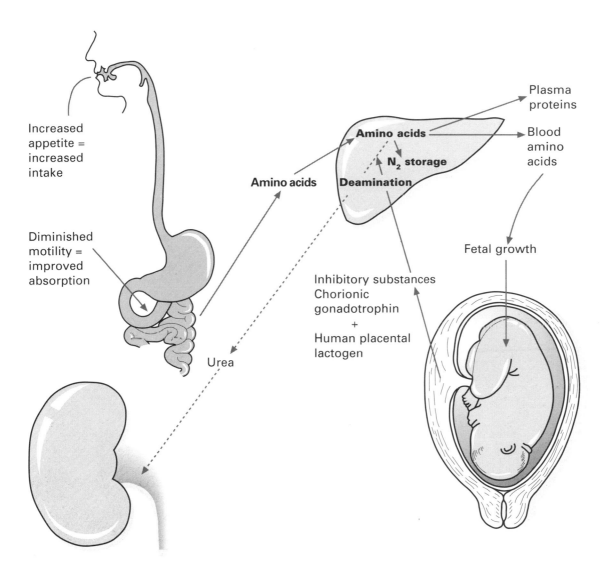

Increased appetite = increased intake

Diminished motility = improved absorption

Amino acids

Urea

Amino acids

N₂ storage

Deamination

Plasma proteins

Blood amino acids

Fetal growth

Inhibitory substances Chorionic gonadotrophin + Human placental lactogen

Both chorionic gonadotrophin and the placental lactogen tend to reduce the deamination process. As a result, blood and urine urea are reduced.

23

FAT METABOLISM

Fat is the major form of stored energy during pregnancy. By 30 weeks some 4 kg are stored. Most of this is in the form of depot fat in the abdominal wall, back and thighs. A modest amount is stored in the breast.

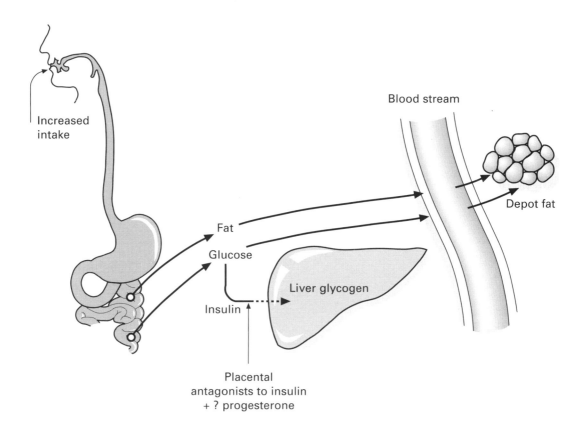

Three points may be made in relation to fat metabolism.
1. The total metabolism and demand for energy are increased in pregnancy.
2. Glycogen stores are diminished and therefore energy obtained directly from carbohydrate will be reduced.
3. Although blood fat is greatly increased only a moderate amount is laid down in fat stores.

RESPIRATORY CHANGES

Physical changes in the respiratory system begin early in pregnancy and are responsible for the improvements in gaseous exchange.

The respiratory rate is unchanged and the elevation of the diaphragm decreases the volume of the lungs at rest, but the tidal volume is increased by up to 40% leading to an increase in minute ventilation from 7.25 litres to 10.5 litres.

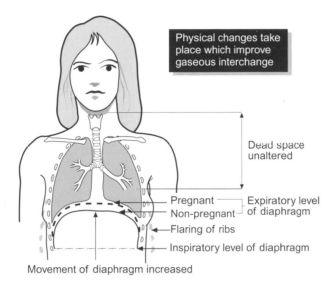

Physical changes take place which improve gaseous interchange

Dead space unaltered

Pregnant
Non-pregnant — Expiratory level of diaphragm

Flaring of ribs

Inspiratory level of diaphragm

Movement of diaphragm increased

Fetal plasma carbon dioxide tension exceeds that of maternal plasma and therefore passes easily into maternal blood. Despite this, due to the pulmonary hyperventilation, the concentration of carbon dioxide in maternal plasma is reduced by around 8% compared with nonpregnant levels.

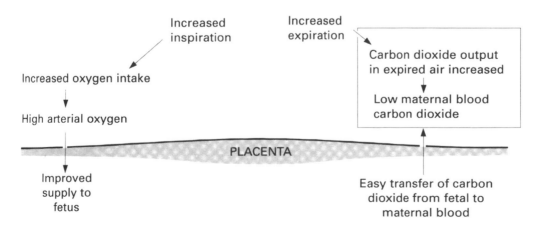

Increased inspiration

Increased expiration

Increased oxygen intake

Carbon dioxide output in expired air increased

High arterial oxygen

Low maternal blood carbon dioxide

PLACENTA

Improved supply to fetus

Easy transfer of carbon dioxide from fetal to maternal blood

CARDIOVASCULAR PHYSIOLOGY

Cardiac output increases dramatically in pregnancy. The average increase is from 4.5 l/minute to 6.0 l/minute. The greatest increase is seen within the first trimester although further rises lead to a peak at around twenty-four weeks. This increase results from an increase in both heart rate and stroke volume.

Heart rate increases from 70 bpm in the non-pregnant state to 78 bpm at twenty weeks gestation with a peak of around 85 bpm in late pregnancy. Stroke volume increases from 64 ml to 70 ml in mid-pregnancy. Stroke volume actually reduces towards term and the increase in cardiac output is maintained by the increase in heart rate.

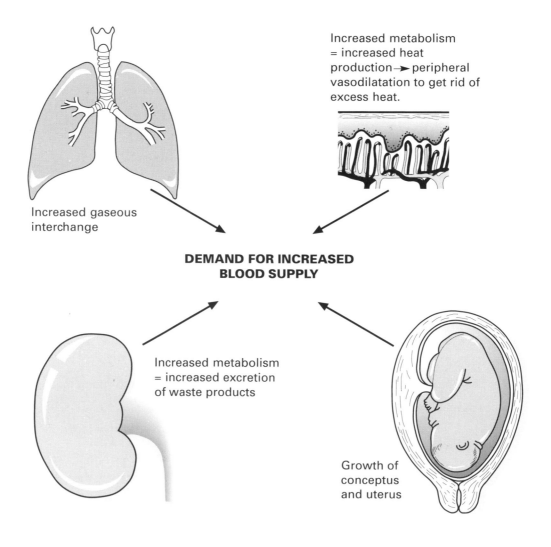

Increased gaseous interchange

Increased metabolism = increased heat production → peripheral vasodilatation to get rid of excess heat.

DEMAND FOR INCREASED BLOOD SUPPLY

Increased metabolism = increased excretion of waste products

Growth of conceptus and uterus

CARDIOVASCULAR PHYSIOLOGY

Reduced pulmonary vascular resistance results in a 40% increase in pulmonary blood flow. Renal blood flow increases by 35% and uterine blood flow by around 250%. Blood volume and organ perfusion increase.

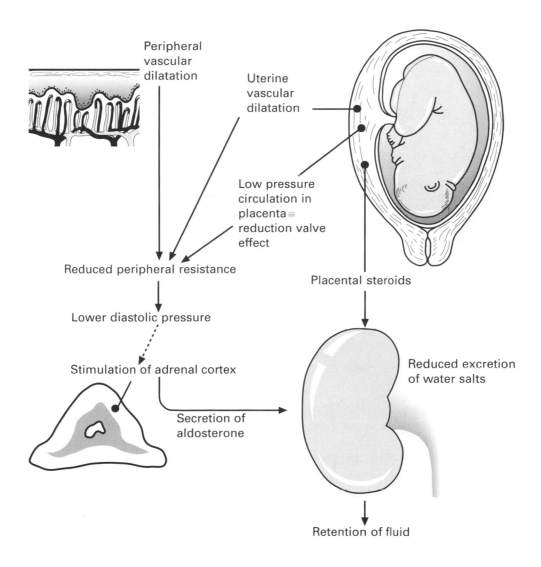

BLOOD VOLUME CHANGES

In the non-pregnant state 70% of body weight is water. Of this 5% is intravascular. Intracellular fluid makes up about 70% and the remainder is interstitial fluid.

In pregnancy intracellular water is unchanged but both blood and interstitial fluid are increased.

Plasma volume increases at a greater rate than red cell mass and protein levels resulting in a reduction in blood viscosity.

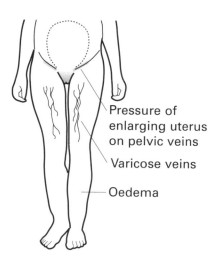

Pressure of enlarging uterus on pelvic veins

Varicose veins

Oedema

LOCAL VASCULAR CHANGES

Local changes are most apparent in the lower limbs and are due to pressure exerted by the enlarging uterus on the pelvic veins. Since one third of the total circulating blood is distributed to the lower limbs the increased venous pressure may produce varicosities and oedema of the vulva and legs. These changes are most marked during the daytime due to the upright posture. They tend to be reversed at night when the woman retires to bed: oedema fluid is reabsorbed, venous return increased and renal output rises, resulting in nocturnal frequency. If the patient adopts the supine position, however, the uterine pressure on the veins increases and this may lead to reduced venous return to the heart. This in turn leads to a reduction in cardiac output.

As extreme example of this occurs when the uterus compresses the vena cava and reduces cardiac output to the point where the mother feels faint and may become unconscious. A sensation of nausea also occurs and vomiting may result. This condition, SUPINE HYPOTENSION SYNDROME, should be borne in mind when examining women in late pregnancy.

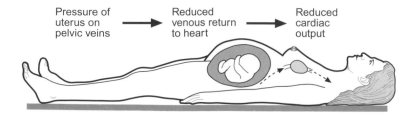

Pressure of uterus on pelvic veins → Reduced venous return to heart → Reduced cardiac output

HAEMATOLOGICAL CHANGES

The change in blood values such as haemoglobin content is the result of demands of the growing pregnancy modified by the increase in plasma volume.

This represents an increase in red cell mass of 18%. The plasma volume increases by 40–45%. Thus there is a reduction in the red cell count per millilitre from 4.5 million to around 3.8 million. Towards term as the plasma volume diminishes the red cell count rises slightly. Similarly the haematocrit falls during pregnancy with a slight rise at term.

Packed Cell Volume (per cent)

Non-pregnant	40–42
20 weeks pregnant	39
30 weeks pregnant	38
40 weeks pregnant	40

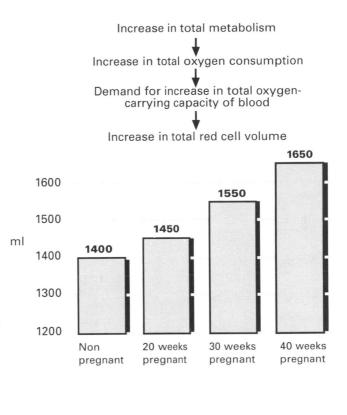

Increase in total metabolism
↓
Increase in total oxygen consumption
↓
Demand for increase in total oxygen-carrying capacity of blood
↓
Increase in total red cell volume

Changes in haemoglobin run parallel with those in red cells. The mean cell haemoglobin concentration in the non-pregnant is 34 per cent, that is, each 100 ml of red cells contain 34 g of haemoglobin. This does not alter in pregnancy, therefore, as with the total red cell volume, the total haemoglobin rises throughout pregnancy.

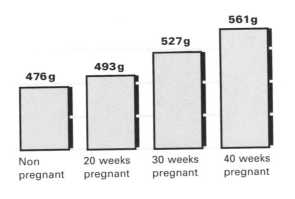

This is a total increase of 85 g, equivalent to 18%

HAEMATOLOGICAL CHANGES

The increasing plasma volume, however, produces an apparent reduction in haemoglobin. The haemoglobin concentration falls throughout pregnancy until the last four weeks when there might be a slight rise. The fall is apparent by the 12th week of pregnancy and the minimum value is reached at 32 weeks.

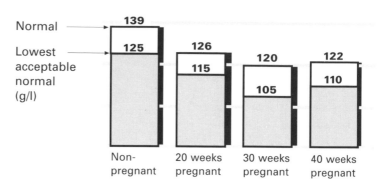

It will be seen from this that no single value can be taken as normal throughout pregnancy. This is important when diagnosing anaemia. At 30 weeks a haemoglobin reading of 105 g/l is normal but the same value at 20 weeks indicates anaemia.

Leukocytes
There is a marked increase in white cells during pregnancy from 7×10^9/litre in the non-pregnant to 10.5×10^9/litre in late pregnancy. The increase is almost entirely due to an increase in neutrophil polymorphonuclear cells. The white cell count may rise markedly during labour.

Platelets
Platelets decline progressively through pregnancy. The mean value in early pregnancy is 275 000/mm³ to 260 000/mm³ beyond 35 weeks. Mean platelet size increases slightly and the lifespan of platelets is shortened.

Coagulation System
Pregnancy is said to be a hypercoagulable state. Fibrinogen and Factors VII to X rise progressively. Factors II, V and XI to XIII are unaltered or slightly lower. It seems likely that the increased risk of thrombo-embolism associated with pregnancy results more from venous stasis and vessel wall injury than changes in the coagulation factors themselves.

GASTRO-INTESTINAL TRACT

Changes in the gastro-intestinal tract are chiefly the result of relaxation of smooth muscle. This effect is induced by the high progesterone levels of pregnancy.

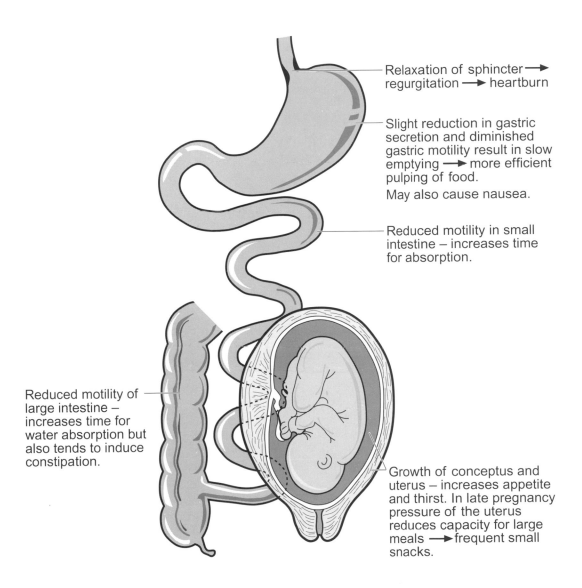

Relaxation of sphincter ⟶ regurgitation ⟶ heartburn

Slight reduction in gastric secretion and diminished gastric motility result in slow emptying ⟶ more efficient pulping of food.
May also cause nausea.

Reduced motility in small intestine – increases time for absorption.

Reduced motility of large intestine – increases time for water absorption but also tends to induce constipation.

Growth of conceptus and uterus – increases appetite and thirst. In late pregnancy pressure of the uterus reduces capacity for large meals ⟶ frequent small snacks.

RENAL SYSTEM

Frequency of micturition is a common symptom of early pregnancy and again at term. This is due to changes in pelvic anatomy and is a feature of 'normal' pregnancy.

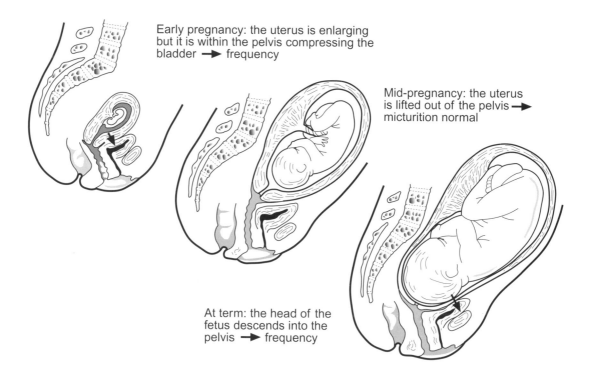

Early pregnancy: the uterus is enlarging but it is within the pelvis compressing the bladder ➜ frequency

Mid-pregnancy: the uterus is lifted out of the pelvis ➜ micturition normal

At term: the head of the fetus descends into the pelvis ➜ frequency

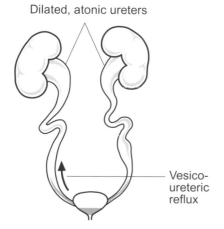

Dilated, atonic ureters

Vesico-ureteric reflux

Striking anatomical changes are seen in the kidneys and ureters. A degree of hydronephrosis and hydro-ureter exist. These result from loss of smooth muscle tone due to progesterone, aggravated by mechanical pressure from the uterus at the pelvic brim. Vesico-ureteric reflux is also increased. These changes predispose to urinary tract infection. The appearances improve in the latter part of pregnancy as the uterus grows above the pelvic brim and rising oestrogen levels cause hypertrophy of the ureteric muscle.

RENAL SYSTEM

Urinary output on a normal fluid intake tends to be slightly diminished. This seems paradoxical in view of the increased renal blood flow. However there is an increase in tubular reabsorption of water and electrolytes.

Glycosuria occurs commonly because the increased glomerular filtration rate presents the tubules with a sugar load which cannot be completely reabsorbed.

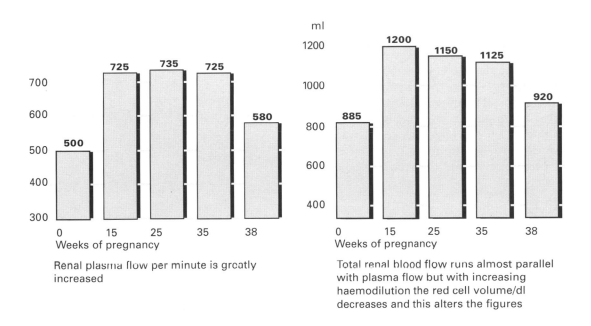

Renal plasma flow per minute is greatly increased

Total renal blood flow runs almost parallel with plasma flow but with increasing haemodilution the red cell volume/dl decreases and this alters the figures

As a result the amount of fluid filtered off the plasma through the renal glomeruli is similarly increased and 100 extra litres of fluid pass into the renal tubules each day. Despite this the urinary output is diminished. Obviously there must be an increased tubular reabsorption. It is estimated that extracellular water is increased by 6 to 7 litres during pregnancy. Along with this water, sodium and other electrolytes are reabsorbed by the tubules to maintain body osmolarity. Under test the pregnant patient excretes only 80% of the total found in the urine of non-pregnant subjects.

The mechanism whereby this is achieved is not yet known, but it is thought that the increased amounts of aldosterone, progesterone and oestrogen are responsible.

Glycosuria of mild degree occurs in 35–50% of all pregnant women. Increased glomerular filtration leads to more sugar reaching the tubules than can be reabsorbed. Glycosuria occurs therefore with lower blood sugar levels than in the non-pregnant, the so-called lowered renal threshold.

REPRODUCTIVE SYSTEM

Breasts

Each breast is made up of 15–20 glandular lobules separated by fat. The glands lead into tubules and then into ducts which open onto the nipple. The breasts increase in size in pregnancy due to proliferation of the glands and ducts under the influence of oestrogen and progesterone. The secretion of colostrum may begin in the first trimester and continues to term.

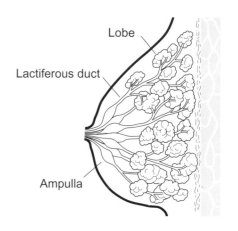

Body of Uterus

Under the influence of oestrogen the uterus grows by hyperplasia and hypertrophy of its muscle fibres. Its weight increases from the non-pregnant level of 50 g up to 1000 g. The lower segment is formed from the isthmus, the area between the uterine cavity and the endocervical epithelium.

Cervix

The cervix softens due to increased vascularity, and changes in its connective tissue, due mainly it seems to oestrogen. There is increased secretion from its glands and the mucus becomes thickened thus forming a protective plug, the so-called operculum, in the cervical os.

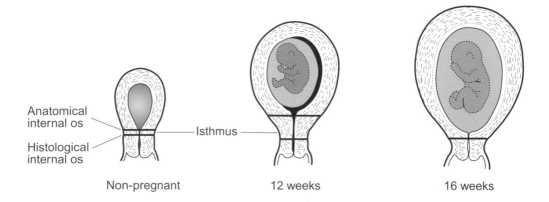

Vagina and Pelvic Floor

The changes of increased vascularity, muscular hypertrophy and softening of connective tissues are seen, allowing distension of the vagina at birth.

Pelvic Ligaments

There is softening of the ligaments of the pelvic joints, presumably due to oestrogen. The effect is to make the pelvis more mobile and increase its capacity.

ENDOCRINE CHANGES IN PREGNANCY

The following is a summary of the changes in maternal and placental hormones in pregnancy and their supposed effects.

Progesterone is produced by the corpus luteum in the first few weeks of pregnancy. Thereafter it is derived from the placenta. Levels rise steadily during pregnancy with, it has been suggested, a fall towards term. Output reaches a maximum of at least 250 mg per day.

Possible actions:
1. Reduces smooth muscle tone — stomach motility diminishes — may induce nausea. Colonic activity reduced — delayed emptying — increased water reabsorption — constipation.
Reduced uterine tone — diminished uterine activity — reduced bladder and ureteric tone — stasis of urine.
2. Reduces vascular tone — diastolic pressure reduced — venous dilatation.
3. Raises temperature.
4. Increases fat storage.
5. Induces over-breathing — alveolar and arterial carbon dioxide tension reduced.
6. Induces development of breasts.

Oestrogens. In early pregnancy the source is the ovary. Later oestrone and oestradiol are probably produced by the placenta and are increased a hundredfold. Oestriol, however, is a product of the interaction of the placenta and the fetal adrenals and is increased one thousandfold. The output of oestrogens reaches a maximum of at least 30 to 40 mg per day. Oestriol accounts for 85% of this total. Levels increase up to term.
Possible actions:
1. Induce growth of uterus and control its function.
2. Responsible, together with progesterone, for the development of the breasts.
3. Alter the chemical constitution of connective tissue, making it more pliable — stretching of cervix possible, joint capsules relax, pelvic joints mobile.
4. Cause water retention.
5. May reduce sodium excretion.

Cortisol. The maternal adrenals are the sole source in early pregnancy but later considerable quantities are thought to be produced by the placenta. Some 25 mg are produced each day. Much of this is protein bound and therefore may not be generally active.

Possible actions:
1. Increases blood sugar.
2. Modifies antibody activity.

Aldosterone is almost certainly wholly derived from the maternal adrenals. The amounts produced during pregnancy are much increased. It promotes the retention of sodium and water.

Renin. Plasma renin activity is five to ten times that in the non-pregnant state. Likewise angiotensinogen levels are increased although in normal pregnancy women show a reduced sensitivity to the hypertensive effects of angiotensin.

ENDOCRINE CHANGES IN PREGNANCY

Human chorionic gonadotrophin (HCG) is produced by the trophoblast and peak levels are reached before 16 weeks of gestation. From 18 weeks onwards, levels remain relatively constant. Apart from the early maintenance of the corpus luteum, the physiological role of HCG remains unclear. It appears to have a thyrotrophic action and to initiate testosterone secretion from the Leydig cells.

Human placental lactogen (HPL). Levels of HPL (or chorionic somatomammotrophin) rise steadily with the growth of the placenta throughout pregnancy. It is lactogenic and antagonistic to insulin.

Relaxin is a hormone produced by the corpus luteum. It can be detected throughout pregnancy but highest levels are in the first trimester. Its physiological role is uncertain but it has been used clinically in cervical ripening.

Pituitary hormones. Maternal FSH and LH levels are suppressed during pregnancy but prolactin levels rise throughout. Lactation does not start, however, until delivery when high prolactin levels persist in association with falling oestrogen levels.

CHAPTER 3

OBSTETRICAL ANATOMY

PELVIC ORGANS

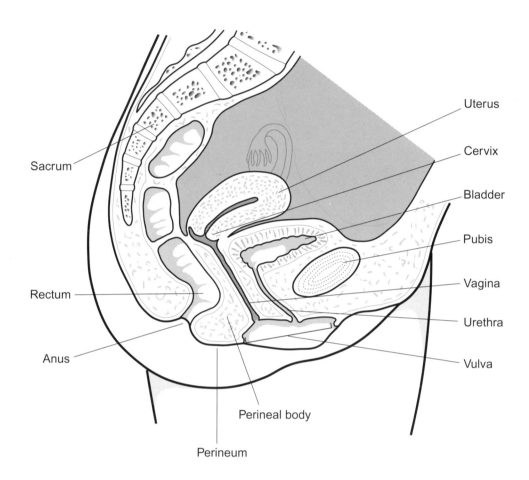

Sacrum

Uterus

Cervix

Bladder

Pubis

Rectum

Vagina

Urethra

Anus

Vulva

Perineal body

Perineum

VULVA

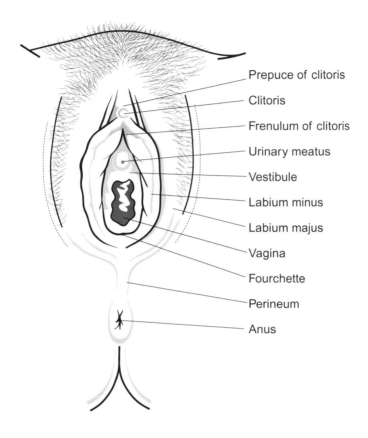

- Prepuce of clitoris
- Clitoris
- Frenulum of clitoris
- Urinary meatus
- Vestibule
- Labium minus
- Labium majus
- Vagina
- Fourchette
- Perineum
- Anus

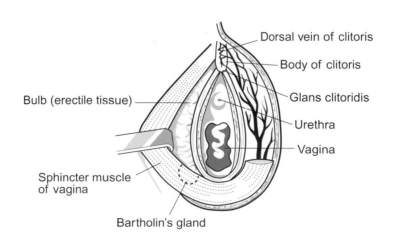

- Dorsal vein of clitoris
- Body of clitoris
- Glans clitoridis
- Urethra
- Vagina
- Bulb (erectile tissue)
- Sphincter muscle of vagina
- Bartholin's gland

PELVIC FLOOR

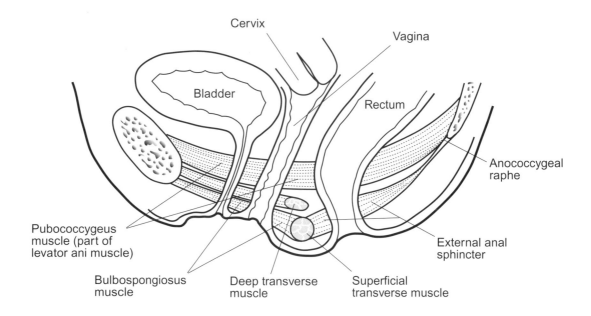

Cervix

Vagina

Bladder

Rectum

Anococcygeal raphe

Pubococcygeus muscle (part of levator ani muscle)

External anal sphincter

Bulbospongiosus muscle

Deep transverse muscle

Superficial transverse muscle

SOFT TISSUES OF THE OBSTETRIC PELVIS (Schematic)

A muscular basin with an opening below at the front. The muscular tissues are supported by and enclosed in the pelvic bones.

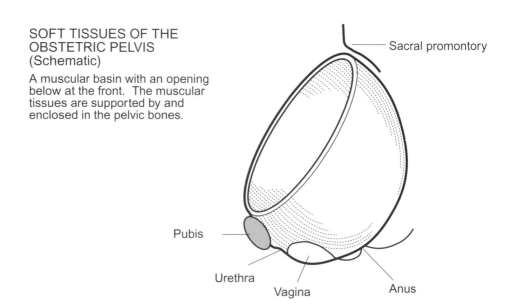

Sacral promontory

Pubis

Urethra

Vagina

Anus

PELVIC FLOOR

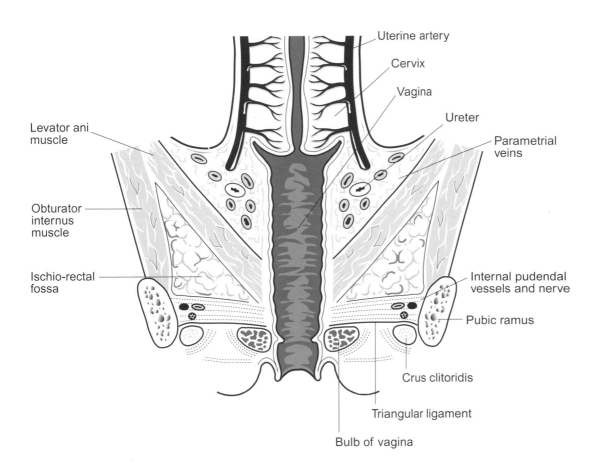

Uterine artery

Cervix

Vagina

Ureter

Parametrial veins

Levator ani muscle

Obturator internus muscle

Ischio-rectal fossa

Internal pudendal vessels and nerve

Pubic ramus

Crus clitoridis

Triangular ligament

Bulb of vagina

ISCHIORECTAL FOSSA

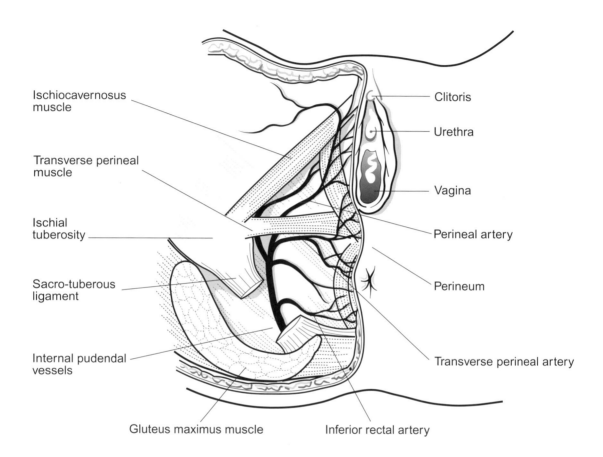

Ischiocavernosus muscle

Transverse perineal muscle

Ischial tuberosity

Sacro-tuberous ligament

Internal pudendal vessels

Clitoris

Urethra

Vagina

Perineal artery

Perineum

Transverse perineal artery

Gluteus maximus muscle

Inferior rectal artery

ISCHIORECTAL FOSSA

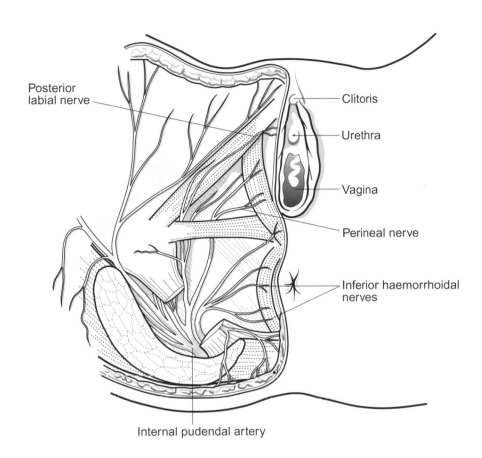

Posterior
labial nerve

Clitoris

Urethra

Vagina

Perineal nerve

Inferior haemorrhoidal
nerves

Internal pudendal artery

PERINEUM

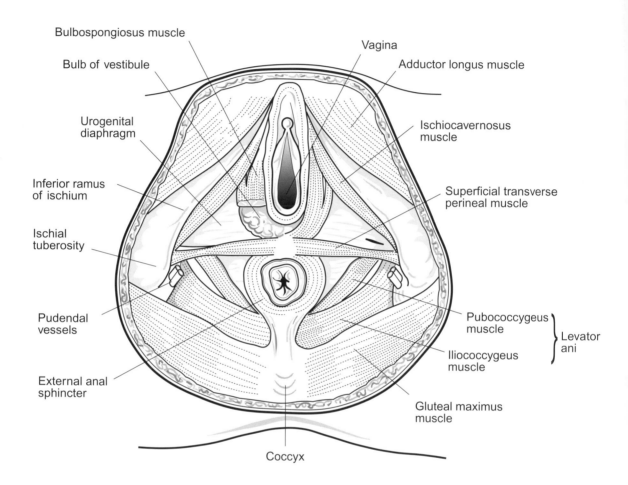

Bulbospongiosus muscle

Bulb of vestibule

Urogenital diaphragm

Inferior ramus of ischium

Ischial tuberosity

Pudendal vessels

External anal sphincter

Vagina

Adductor longus muscle

Ischiocavernosus muscle

Superficial transverse perineal muscle

Pubococcygeus muscle

Iliococcygeus muscle

Levator ani

Gluteal maximus muscle

Coccyx

PELVIC BLOOD SUPPLY

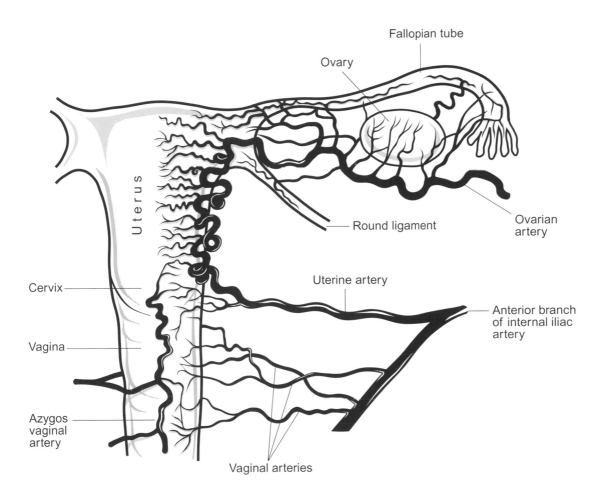

Note coiling of vessels to allow stretching as uterus grows in pregnancy.

PELVIC SYMPATHETIC NERVES

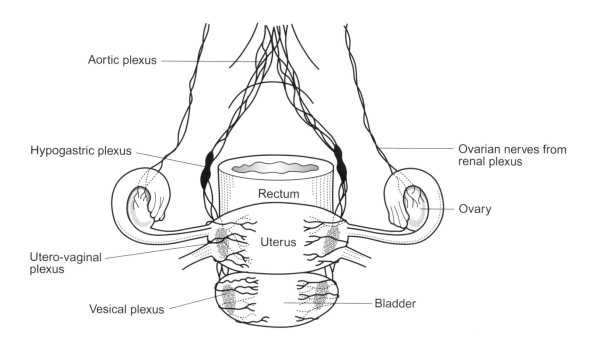

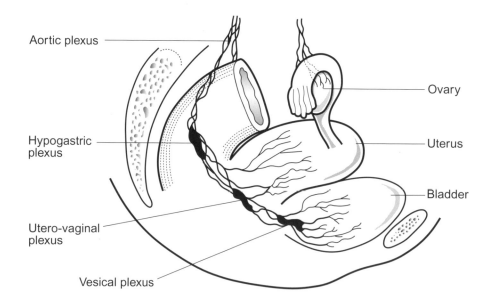

SUPPORTS OF UTERUS

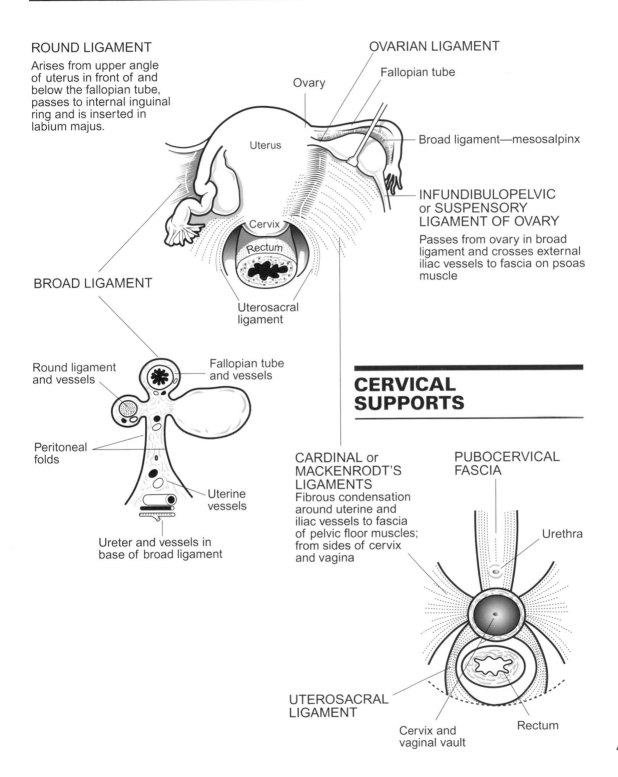

ROUND LIGAMENT

Arises from upper angle of uterus in front of and below the fallopian tube, passes to internal inguinal ring and is inserted in labium majus.

Ovary

Uterus

Cervix

Rectum

BROAD LIGAMENT

Round ligament and vessels

Fallopian tube and vessels

Peritoneal folds

Uterine vessels

Ureter and vessels in base of broad ligament

Uterosacral ligament

OVARIAN LIGAMENT

Fallopian tube

Broad ligament—mesosalpinx

INFUNDIBULOPELVIC or SUSPENSORY LIGAMENT OF OVARY

Passes from ovary in broad ligament and crosses external iliac vessels to fascia on psoas muscle

CERVICAL SUPPORTS

CARDINAL or MACKENRODT'S LIGAMENTS

Fibrous condensation around uterine and iliac vessels to fascia of pelvic floor muscles; from sides of cervix and vagina

PUBOCERVICAL FASCIA

Urethra

UTEROSACRAL LIGAMENT

Cervix and vaginal vault

Rectum

BONY PELVIS — SAGITTAL VIEW

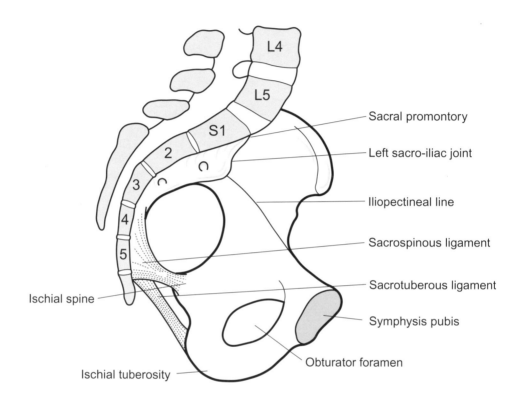

BONY PELVIS — BRIM

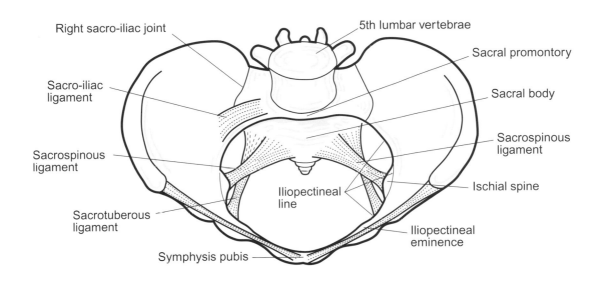

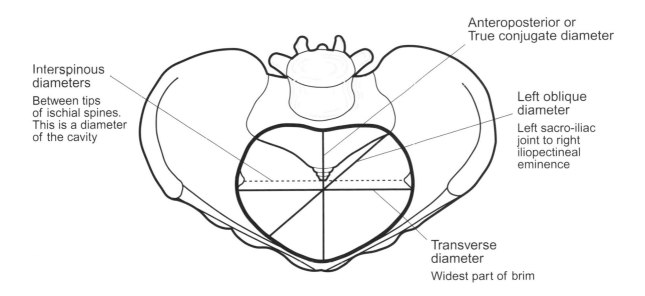

The Plane of the Brim is bounded

anteriorly by the Pubis,
laterally by the Iliopectineal lines,
posteriorly by the Alae and Promontory of the Sacrum.

BONY PELVIS — CAVITY

The Pelvic Cavity is bounded
    Above by the Plane of the Brim,
    Below by the Plane of the Outlet,
    Posteriorly by the Sacrum,
    Laterally by the Sacrosciatic ligaments
        and Ischial bones and
    Anteriorly by Obturator Foramina,
        Ascending Rami of Ischia and Pubis.

Plane of mid cavity or plane of greatest pelvic diameters

Mid pubis to junction of second and third sacral vertebrae

Plane of least pelvic diameters

Symphysis pubis through ischial spines to end of sacrum

Note that pelvic outlet plane is in two parts angled to each other

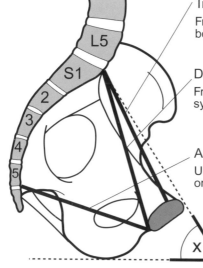

True conjugate of brim

From sacral promontory to upper and inner border of symphysis pubis

Diagonal conjugate diameter of brim

From sacral promontory to under border of symphysis pubis

Antero-posterior diameter of outlet

Under body of symphysis pubis to end of sacrum or coccyx if fused

Inclination of pelvic brim 50°– 60° (usually 55°)

BONY PELVIS — OUTLET

The Plane of the Outlet is bounded
   Anteriorly by Pubic Arch,
   Laterally by Great Sacrosciatic Ligaments
     and Ischial Tuberosities,
   Posteriorly by Tip of Coccyx if fused or
     to End of Sacrum.

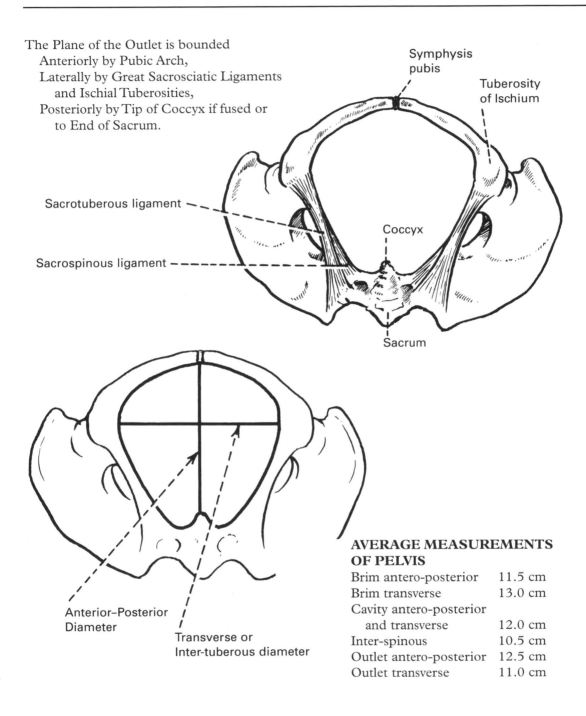

AVERAGE MEASUREMENTS OF PELVIS

Brim antero-posterior	11.5 cm
Brim transverse	13.0 cm
Cavity antero-posterior and transverse	12.0 cm
Inter-spinous	10.5 cm
Outlet antero-posterior	12.5 cm
Outlet transverse	11.0 cm

If the pelvic diameters are abnormally small the pelvis is said to be 'contracted'.

PELVIC TYPES

Four types of pelvis are described — Gynaecoid (50%), Anthropoid (25%), Android (20%), Platypelloid or Flat (5%). In many cases the pelvis is of mixed type.

GYNAECOID
or female type

ANTHROPOID
or ape type

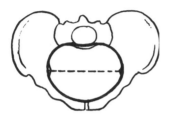

The brim is a transverse ellipse – almost like a circle.

The brim is an A.P. ellipse (= Gynaecoid turned round 90°)

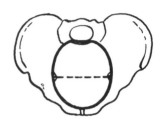

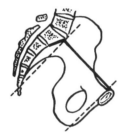

The transverse diameter (widest part of brim) and the available transverse diameter (at mid-point of antero-posterior diameter of brim) coincide in the gynaecoid and anthropoid pelves. The hind pelvis is the area behind the transverse diameter and the fore pelvis the area in front. These areas are roughly equal in both the gynaecoid and anthropoid pelves.

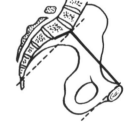

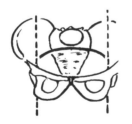

The delivery of the fetal head through these types of pelves has equal mechanical problems at all levels, i.e. if it is easy at brim it should be easy in cavity and outlet.

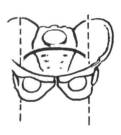

PELVIC TYPES

ANDROID
or male type

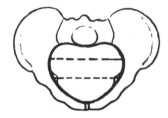

Brim is roughly triangular. Trans. diameter near sacrum. 'Available trans.' diameter is shortened.

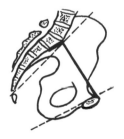

The area of the hind pelvis is reduced and shallow. Area of the fore pelvis is reduced and narrowed at front.

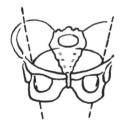

The delivery of a fetal head through this pelvis gives increasing problems the further it descends.

PLATYPELLOID
type

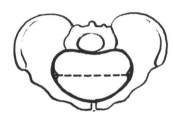

Brim is kidney shaped. Trans. and 'available trans.' diameters coincide.

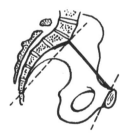

The hind pelvis is shallow and the area reduced. Fore pelvis is shallow and the area reduced.

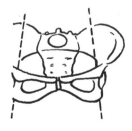

The delivery of a fetal head through this pelvis meets problems at the brim but thereafter the difficulties decrease with descent.

FETAL SKULL

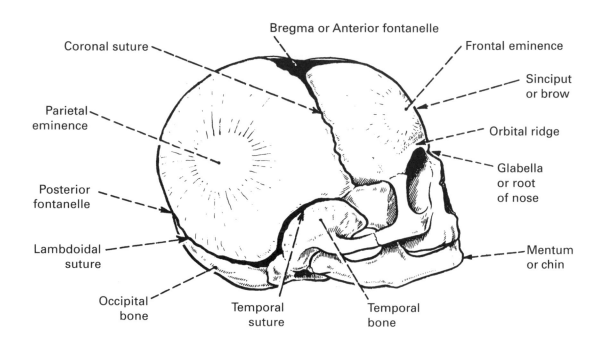

Bregma or Anterior fontanelle

Coronal suture

Frontal eminence

Sinciput or brow

Parietal eminence

Orbital ridge

Glabella or root of nose

Posterior fontanelle

Lambdoidal suture

Mentum or chin

Occipital bone

Temporal suture

Temporal bone

(Diameters)

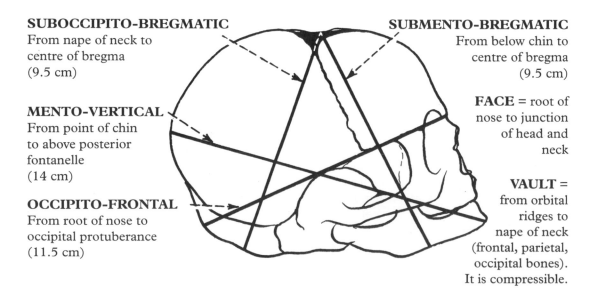

SUBOCCIPITO-BREGMATIC
From nape of neck to centre of bregma
(9.5 cm)

SUBMENTO-BREGMATIC
From below chin to centre of bregma
(9.5 cm)

MENTO-VERTICAL
From point of chin to above posterior fontanelle
(14 cm)

FACE = root of nose to junction of head and neck

OCCIPITO-FRONTAL
From root of nose to occipital protuberance
(11.5 cm)

VAULT = from orbital ridges to nape of neck (frontal, parietal, occipital bones). It is compressible.

(Measurements shown in brackets.)

FETAL SKULL

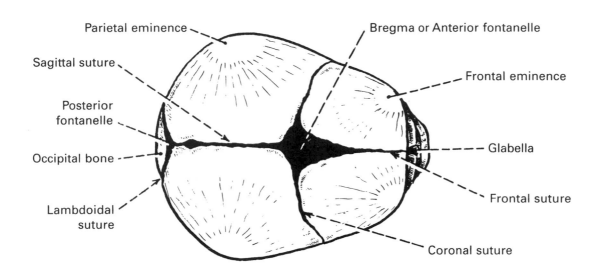

The **VERTEX** is the area bounded by the anterior and posterior fontanelles and the parietal eminences.

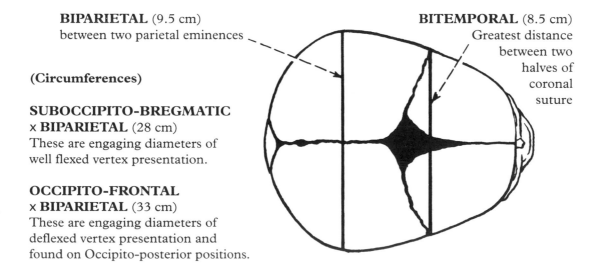

BIPARIETAL (9.5 cm)
between two parietal eminences

(Circumferences)

SUBOCCIPITO-BREGMATIC
x **BIPARIETAL** (28 cm)
These are engaging diameters of well flexed vertex presentation.

OCCIPITO-FRONTAL
x **BIPARIETAL** (33 cm)
These are engaging diameters of deflexed vertex presentation and found on Occipito-posterior positions.

BITEMPORAL (8.5 cm)
Greatest distance between two halves of coronal suture

MENTO-VERTICAL x **BIPARIETAL** (35.5 cm)
This is the largest circumference of the head and is found in Brow presentation.

CHAPTER 4

DIAGNOSIS OF PREGNANCY

SYMPTOMS AND SIGNS

Amenorrhoea

An overdue menstrual period remains, for most women with a regular menstrual cycle, the first suggestion of pregnancy.

Pregnancy is the commonest cause of amenorrhoea but other causes such as disturbances in the hypothalamic–pituitary–ovarian axis or recent use of the contraceptive pill may be responsible.

Occasionally a women may continue to bleed in early pregnancy around the time of suppressed menstruation. This is usually called decidual bleeding and may, in theory, continue until about 12 weeks when the decidua capsularis fuses with the decidua vera (see Chapter 1).

Nausea or sickness

Many women suffer some gastric upset in the early months of pregnancy, from nausea and anorexia to repeated vomiting, especially in the morning. The cause is unknown and raised levels of both oestrogen and human chorionic gonadotrophin (HCG) in the circulation have been blamed. Gastric motility is reduced, and in early pregnancy, the lower oesophageal sphincter is relaxed.

Bladder symptoms

Increased frequency of micturition in the second and third months is due to a combination of increased vascularity and pressure from the enlarging uterus. Near term, frequency may again appear due mainly to pressure of the fetal head on the bladder.

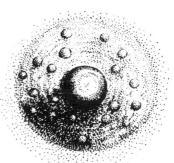

The breast at 8 weeks

Breast changes

The earliest symptoms and signs — increased vascularity and a sensation of heaviness, almost of pain — appear at 6 weeks. By 8 weeks the nipple and surrounding area — the primary areola — have become more pigmented. Montgomery's tubercles — sebaceous glands which become more prominent as raised pink-red nodules on the areola.

By 16 weeks a clear fluid (colostrum) is secreted and may be expressed. By 20 weeks the secondary areola — a mottled effect due to further pigmentation — has become prominent.

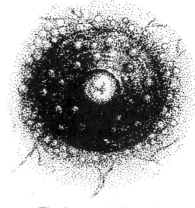

The breast at 16 weeks

SYMPTOMS AND SIGNS

Uterine changes

Although no longer commonly undertaken, uterine enlargement may be detected on bimanual examination at seven to eight weeks.

PALPABLE UTERINE ENLARGEMENT

At 7 weeks the uterus is the size of a large hen's egg.
At 10 weeks it is the size of an orange.
At 12 weeks it is the size of a grapefruit.

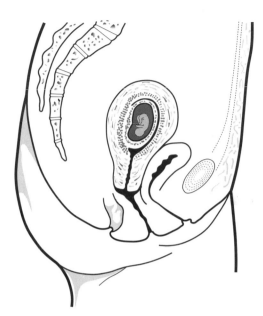

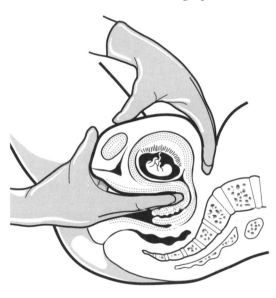

Cervical and uterine softening and a bluish discoloration of the cervix, due to increased vascularity, may be apparent but these signs are not invariable. The uterus is palpable abdominally by 12 weeks and the mother may be aware of an increase in abdominal size by 16 weeks. The fundal height increases progressively until near term. It is an uncertain guide to gestational age of the fetus, however, because of factors such as liquor volume, obesity and muscle tone. A reduction in fundal height ('lightening') may occur at the end of pregnancy when the presenting part of the fetus descends as the lower segment and cervix prepare for labour.

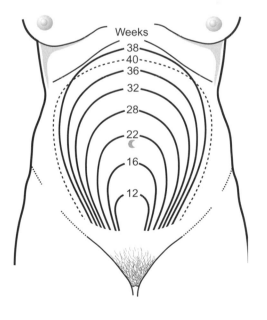

Weeks
38
40
36
32
28
22
16
12

SYMPTOMS AND SIGNS

AWARENESS OF FETAL MOVEMENT ('QUICKENING')
This may be felt by the mother at 16–18 weeks in parous women and two to three weeks later in a primigravida.

PALPABLE UTERINE CONTRACTIONS
The uterus undergoes irregular, painless contractions from the 9th to 10th week onward. These may become palpable by the 20th week on abdominal examination. They are known as Braxton Hicks' contractions and they become more frequent as pregnancy advances.

AUSCULTATION OF THE FETAL HEART
The fetal heart may be heard with a fetal stethoscope (Pinard) pressed on the abdomen, over the back of the fetus, from about 24–26 weeks.

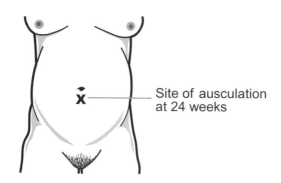

Site of ausculation at 24 weeks

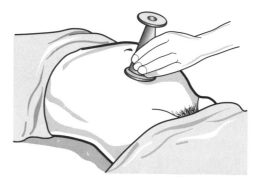

The rate varies between 120 and 140/minute and the rhythm should be regular.

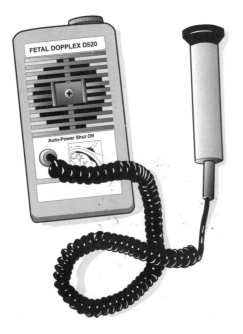

Using small, highly portable fetal heart detectors, which rely on Doppler ultrasound, fetal heart activity may be identified from 12–14 weeks. As Doppler methods detect movements within a beam of transmitted ultrasound, the sounds obtained have to be distinguished from the maternal pulse, transmitted by the aorta, and the uterine souffle, a blowing sound caused by pulsation of blood through the enlarged uterine arteries.

SYMPTOMS AND SIGNS

PALPABLE FETAL PARTS

Fetal parts, such as the head and limbs, begin to be felt from around 26 weeks.

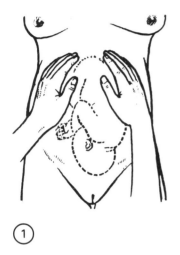 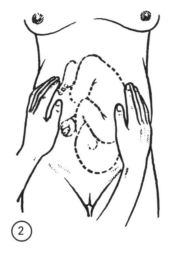 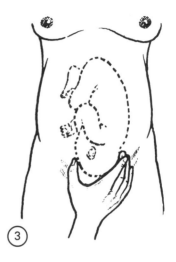

1. The fundus is palpated and its contents (here the breech) identified.

2. The hands palpate the contours of the uterus, identifying the back and thc limbs.

3. The head should be palpated, and it should be noted whether it is mobile or fixed in the pelvic brim.

SYMPTOMS AND SIGNS

SKIN CHANGES

As pregnancy proceeds, areas which are already pigmented become more so — the nipples, external genitalia and anal region. Some fresh pigmentation appears on the face (chloasma) and on the abdomen (linea nigra). These changes are thought to be due to the deposition of melanin. Melanocyte-stimulating hormone is elevated from early pregnancy.

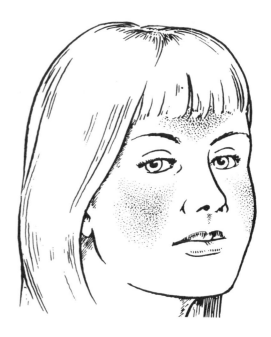

Striae gravidarum are depressed streaks on the skin of the fat areas — abdomen, breasts and thighs. After delivery they regress and persist as striae albicantes. They are due to stretching, but may also be associated with increased secretion of ACTH affecting connective tissues.

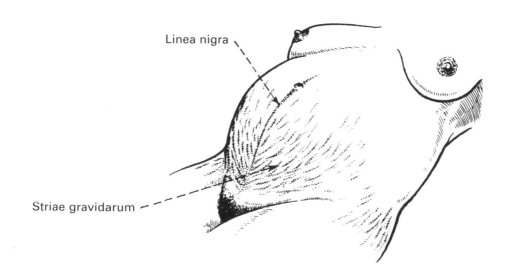

Linea nigra

Striae gravidarum

PREGNANCY TESTS

DETECTION OF HCG

By 14 days after fertilisation the chorion of the blastocyst is secreting chorionic gonadotrophin (HCG) and this can be detected in either the mother's blood or urine by the time of the first missed period. Modern pregnancy tests identify specifically the beta subunit of HCG and can detect as little as 25 IU/l HCG. They are available commercially as simple slide tests.

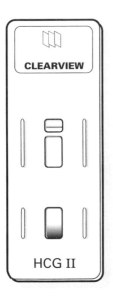

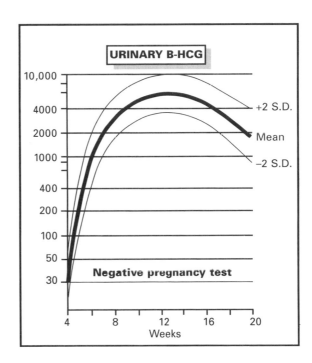

PREGNANCY TESTS

ULTRASOUND

An ultrasound scan can detect an intrauterine gestation sac after 5 to 6 weeks of amenorrhoea. Scanning by the vaginal route will identify a fetus as early as 5 weeks gestation. Trans-abdominal scanning from 7 weeks will permit measurement of the crown–rump length of the fetus. This can be measured to determine gestational age. Ultrasound is the only technique which can confirm fetal viability in early pregnancy.

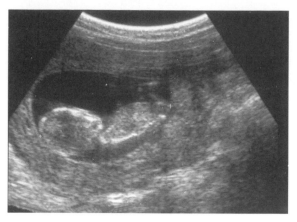

Ultrasound in early pregnancy

SYMPTOMS, SIGNS AND TESTS

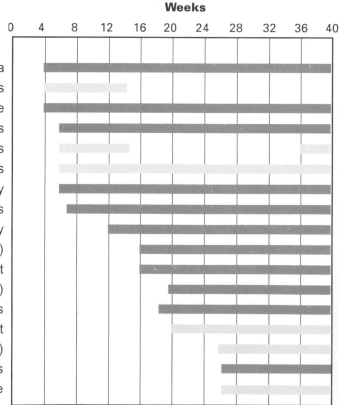

(The more useful symptoms, signs and tests are shown in the darker tint.)

CHAPTER 5

ANTENATAL CARE

PRE-PREGNANCY CARE

Good antenatal care begins before pregnancy. Even for an apparently normal, healthy couple planning a pregnancy there may be advantages in discussing this with a professional adviser. This will often be their family doctor or practice nurse but may be a family-planning doctor or community midwife. Such pre-pregnancy advice and counselling should cover:

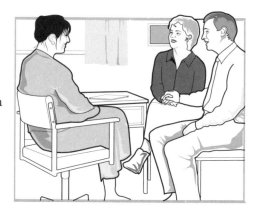

a) General health, medical and family history

Does the mother suffer from a chronic disorder (e.g. diabetes, epilepsy) and if so what is the effect of the pregnancy on that disease and the effect of the disease on the pregnancy? Is she taking any medication and would that medication be harmful to her fetus if she conceives? Are there any inherited family diseases and, if so, what is the chance of a baby being affected?

b) Obstetric history

Has there been a previous pregnancy or pregnancies? What was the outcome? Was any advice given about future pregnancies?

c) Advice on lifestyle

A good general diet is advised and it is now recommended that all women should supplement this with 400 micrograms of folic acid per day before trying to conceive and for the first 12 weeks of pregnancy. This reduces the incidence of neural tube defects in the fetus.

The adverse effects of smoking should be highlighted, particularly with regard to intra-uterine growth restriction. Alcohol should be avoided when trying to conceive and in early pregnancy although it appears safe in moderation in the second and third trimesters.

The use of illicit substances such as marijuana should be advised against. Women using drugs such as heroin and crack cocaine are unlikely to attend for pregnancy advice.

d) Discontinuation of hormonal contraception

Replacement of hormonal contraception by barrier methods before conception is often advised. This allows the return of regular ovulation and menstruation in most cases and thus facilitates the proper calculation of gestational age when pregnancy occurs. This is less important if access to early ultrasound scanning is available.

e) Baseline observations of maternal weight, blood-pressure and rubella and HIV status

These observations are important in managing potential later complications of pregnancy. Rubella vaccination can be offered to those who are not immune and fetal infection thereby be prevented.

In areas of high prevalence knowledge of the HIV status may be important. This will be discussed later.

Many hospitals now have Pre-Pregnancy Clinics where specialist advice from an obstetrician, supported, where necessary, by a clinical geneticist or a physician is available. This will allow detailed review of a previous obstetric problem, a significant family history, especially where inheritance is uncertain, or assessment of a medical disorder. Planning for pregnancy should be a feature of school health and health education programmes.

CARE IN PREGNANCY

PURPOSE

1. To maintain the best possible state of health of mother and fetus by screening for problems, actual and potential, as early as possible, and instituting appropriate management.
2. Any screening test generates anxiety and those for congenital abnormality and those for infectious disease, such as HIV, are particularly difficult in this regard. It is essential that all of those involved in antenatal care ensure adequate information and advice is made available to the woman and her partner. The woman should clearly understand the nature, purpose and implications of any such screening.

RESPONSIBILITY

This usually begins, in the United Kingdom, with the woman's general practitioner or community midwife who will discuss with her the choices of care available, i.e. the place of birth and the pattern of her antenatal supervision. This is usually shared between specialist obstetrician, family doctor and midwife but arrangements vary widely according to local circumstances. There is concern regarding the 'medicalisation' of the care of normal pregnant women.

However, good cooperation between all of those involved is essential and facilitated by patient-held records or shared care cards.

CARE IN PREGNANCY

Home delivery remains uncommon in the UK and for most women, the choice lies between a consultant unit or a GP or midwifery-led unit. Domino care (Domiciliary In Out) in which the woman is accompanied from home by her own midwife, gives birth in hospital and returns home early, is increasingly popular.

Even in consultant units, increasing numbers of clinics are held in health centres close to the community they serve, with attendance at hospital required only for birth.

Fetal problems diagnosed prenatally, such as congenital heart disease, may necessitate delivery in a specialist unit.

BOOKING VISIT

Ideally all women should be assessed early in pregnancy for the reasons noted above and to allow accurate assessment of gestational age. A plan for the conduct of the antenatal care and delivery can then be made.

A detailed history is required:

MENSTRUAL HISTORY

Date and certainty of last menstrual period (LMP).

Length and regularity of menstrual cycle.

Recent hormonal contraception use.

Calculate the expected date of delivery (EDD) by Naegele's rule — 280 days from first day of LMP. This is easily done by adding 7 days to the date of the LMP and then going forward 9 months. This rule is based on a menstrual cycle of 28 days and assumes ovulation in mid-cycle. Where the cycle is regularly greater or less than 28 days the calculation should be adjusted accordingly, e.g. add a further 7 days for a 35 day cycle and subtract a further 7 for a 21 day cycle.

MEDICAL HISTORY

Surgical, including gynaecological procedures
Anaesthetic difficulties, difficult intubation in particular
Blood transfusion, where, when and why?
Allergies
Medical disorders
Prescribed medications and drug allergies
Thrombo-embolism
Mental illness

FAMILY HISTORY

Hypertension
Diabetes in 1st degree relative
Congenital/hereditary disorders
Multiple pregnancy
Thrombo-embolism

SOCIAL HISTORY

Home and family situation
Marital status
Employment status
Alcohol
Smoking
Illicit drug use/substance abuse

BOOKING VISIT

OBSTETRIC HISTORY

Detailed enquiry is needed to identify any point which may influence management in the present pregnancy.

PREVIOUS OBSTETRIC HISTORY

| Preg No. | Date | Place | Labour and Delivery | | | | Infant | | | |
			Gest.	Onset sp/ind	Dur. Hr.	Mode of delivery	Sex	Weight	LB/SB lst week Death	Name and Unit No.
1	23/1/96	Maternity	40	S	10½	SVD	M	3.3K	LB	John
	Complications: HBP at 38 weeks						Feeding: Breast			
2										
	Spontaneous abortion—Evacuation of uterus									
3										

The patient above is described as para 1 + 1 (i.e. 1 delivery and 1 abortion). She might also be described as gravida 3 (i.e. pregnant for the third time). Note, however, that this convention does not take account of the outcome of the delivery, e.g. a woman who has had a single pregnancy ending in a live birth or a still-birth or the delivery of twins is still a para 1 + 0.

CONTRACEPTIVE HISTORY

Details of method used.
If hormonal, when was 'pill' discontinued?
Was the pregnancy planned?
Length of time trying to conceive?

RISK FACTORS

Any factor from the above list liable to increase maternal or fetal morbidity should be highlighted in the case record.

THE FIRST EXAMINATION

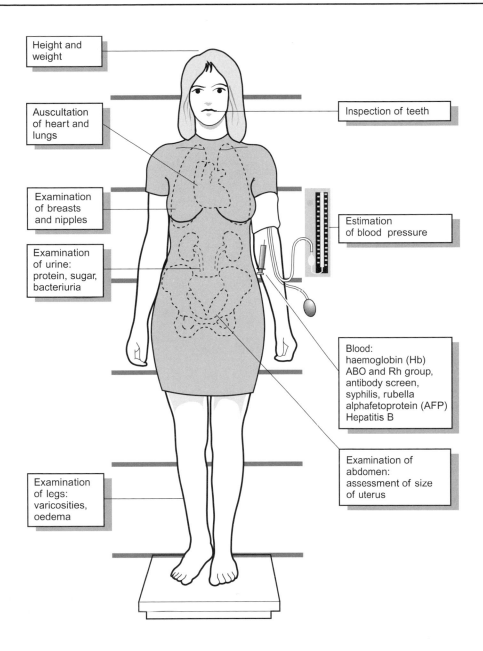

Height and weight

Inspection of teeth

Auscultation of heart and lungs

Examination of breasts and nipples

Estimation of blood pressure

Examination of urine: protein, sugar, bacteriuria

Blood:
haemoglobin (Hb)
ABO and Rh group,
antibody screen,
syphilis, rubella
alphafetoprotein (AFP)
Hepatitis B

Examination of abdomen:
assessment of size of uterus

Examination of legs: varicosities, oedema

This illustration highlights the investigations which *might* be undertaken at a booking visit. Auscultation of heart and lungs and examination of the teeth and breasts are commonly omitted in the UK on the basis that significant previous medical disorders have already been identified by the health care system. This assumption *cannot* be made for women who are migrants or refugees from many parts of the developing world and conditions such as rheumatic heart disease and significant pulmonary scarring from tuberculosis are being seen once again.

THE FIRST EXAMINATION

Many aspects of the first examination which were previously routine have been abandoned, either because they are recognised as unnecessary or as part of the 'demedicalisation' of the care of pregnant women. However, as with general physical examination, in women from the developing world and immigrants, there may still be a place for vaginal examination and cervical cytology if this has not previously been done. This is possible in the first trimester when the transformation zone remains sufficiently small.

In the majority of cases however this is not required.

An ultrasound scan has become routine in most centres and may be done as part of a first trimester screening programme for fetal abnormality (see later), or at the first visit, or as part of an anomaly screening programme later (usually between 18 and 20 weeks).

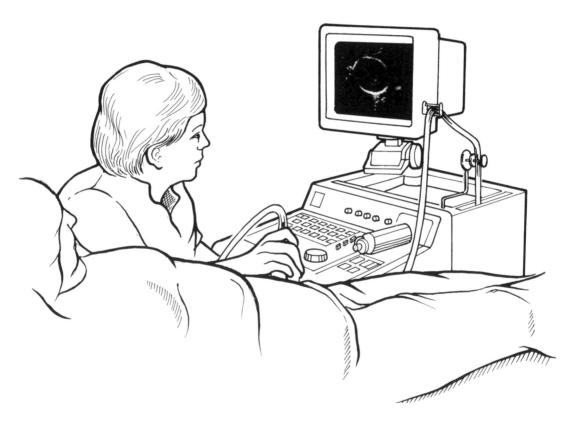

The advantages of routine early scanning are:
Confirmation of continuing pregnancy.
Exclusion, or identification, of multiple pregnancy.
Accurate identification of gestational age (upon which many obstetrical assessments and decisions are based).
Recognition of major fetal anomalies.

GENERAL RECOMMENDATIONS AT THE BOOKING VISIT

PRE-NATAL DIAGNOSIS
The facilities available for pre-natal screening and diagnosis of fetal anomalies should be explained. It should be emphasised that the mother 'opts in' to these services rather than the reverse.

The tests and procedures available are described in Chapter 6.

DIET, SMOKING AND ALCOHOL
These have already been discussed under pre-pregnancy care. A good mixed diet should supply all the pregnant woman's nutritional requirements. The routine use of iron and folic acid supplements to prevent anaemia is less common than formally. As many women, however, have poor iron reserves at the start of pregnancy, a low threshold for prescribing is sensible. A combined preparation containing 100 milligrams elemental iron and 300–350 micrograms of folic acid daily will prevent most cases of iron deficiency or megaloblastic anaemia.

EXERCISE AND WORK
Most mothers should be encouraged to see pregnancy as a healthy state and, within reason, normal activity both domestic and recreational, may be continued. Outside employment usually continues at least until the end of the second trimester. Increasingly women, especially in the professional groups, work until term. They should make efforts to ensure adequate rest.

COITUS
Normal behaviour in pregnancy encompasses continued sexual intercourse. Uncommonly, in complicated pregnancies, this may not be appropriate.

DRUGS
The mother should be advised to avoid any form of medication unless authorised by her doctor. See Chapter 7.

TEETH
A full dental check in early pregnancy should be recommended and treatment in the UK is free to pregnant women. There is no objection to the use of local anaesthesia for dental treatment.

BOWEL ACTION
Constipation is common in pregnancy and should not be a cause for concern. A diet high in fibre and fruit helps and mild laxatives may be taken if required.

SUBSEQUENT ANTENATAL EXAMINATIONS

The traditional pattern, monthly examination until 28 weeks, then fortnightly until 38 weeks and weekly thereafter has much to commend it since antenatal care remains a screening test for impaired fetal growth, malpresentation, anaemia, pre-eclampsia and other disorders. Special investigations are only used when indicated by a possible abnormality by the routine examinations.

In parous, healthy women, a less intensive pattern of antenatal care is appropriate.

BLOOD PRESSURE
This should be measured at each visit and should be 130/80 mmHg or less and not above 140/90 mmHg. Elevation above these levels demands further investigation.

URINE
The urine should be tested at each visit for protein and sugar. When protein is detected, contamination and infection should be excluded before the observation is significant. Glycosuria is common but if persistent or recurrent a glucose tolerance test is indicated.

HAEMOGLOBIN
Dietary anaemia is now less common. Haemoglobin levels should be estimated early in pregnancy and at about 30 and 36 weeks. Levels below 100 g/l are indicative of anaemia regardless of gestation.

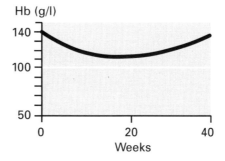

RHESUS TESTING
Rhesus negative women are identified at the booking visit. A screening test for other red cell antibodies is also carried out. This should be repeated regularly throughout the pregnancy (see Chapter 7).

ABDOMINAL EXAMINATION

Regular abdominal palpation remains an important part of antenatal care. It is the easiest and cheapest method of fetal monitoring and repeated examinations by the same observer may give a first indication of restricted fetal growth, or excessive increase in uterine size due to polyhydramnios or multiple pregnancy. Continuity of care is clearly important in this context.

DEFINITIONS

The Presentation is that part of the fetus in the lower pole of the uterus overlying the pelvic brim, e.g. cephalic, vertex, breech etc.

The Attitude is the posture of the fetus.

Flexion   Deflexion   Extension

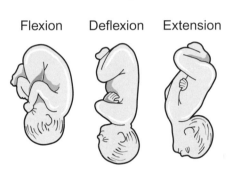

The Lie of the baby is the relation of the long axis of the fetus to the mother. Only a longitudinal lie is normal.

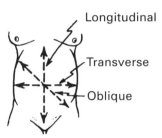

Longitudinal

Transverse

Oblique

The Position of the baby is the relationship of the presenting part to the mother's pelvis. It is conveniently expressed by referring to the position of one area of the presenting part known as the denominator.

The Pelvis is divided into eight parts for the purpose of description.

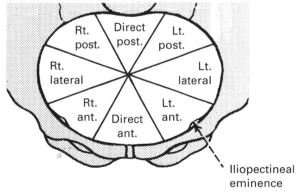

Rt. post.   Direct post.   Lt. post.

Rt. lateral   Lt. lateral

Rt. ant.   Direct ant.   Lt. ant.

Iliopectineal eminence

The Denominator is an arbitrary part of the presentation;
    occiput in vertex presentation,
    sacrum in breech presentation
    mentum in face presentation
and is used to denote the position of the presenting part with reference to the pelvis.

The denominator is in one of these segments and takes its position from it. Thus in a vertex presentation if the denominator, which is the occiput, is close to the left iliopectineal eminence, the position is described as Left Occipito-Anterior or LOA.

ABDOMINAL PALPATION

This examination must be made systematically.

Remember that the following tissue layers may interpose between your fingers and the fetal head.

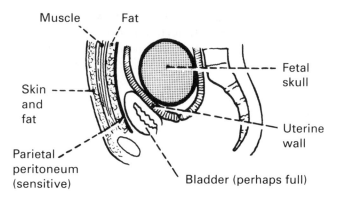

Muscle   Fat

Skin and fat

Fetal skull

Parietal peritoneum (sensitive)

Bladder (perhaps full)

Uterine wall

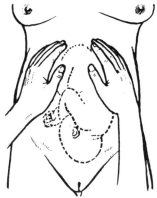

① The fundus is palpated and its contents (here the breech) identified.

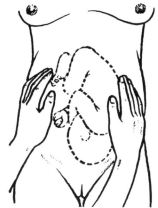

② The hands palpate the contours of the uterus, identifying the back and the limbs.

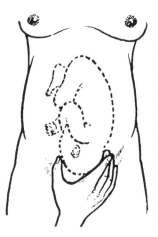

③ The head should be palpated, and note made of whether it is mobile or fixed in the brim. This technique is more commonly used by obstetricians in determining the safety of assisted vaginal delivery, than by midwives.

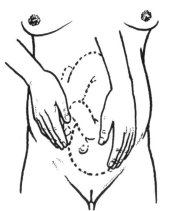

④ The examiner faces the patient's feet and gently pushes two fingers towards the pelvis. This is the best method of palpating the fetal head and determining whether it is fixed or mobile.

ABDOMINAL PALPATION

The examiner must ask, and answer, **SIX** questions

1. Is the **FUNDAL HEIGHT** consistent with the estimation of maturity?

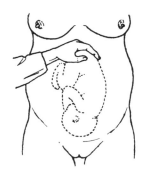

The height of the fundus in centimetres should equal approximately the weeks of gestation.

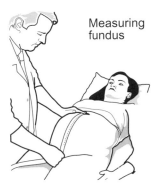

Measuring fundus

2. Is the **LIE** longitudinal? The Lie is the relation of the long axis of the fetus to the mother. Only a longitudinal lie is normal.

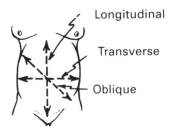

Longitudinal

Transverse

Oblique

3. What is the **PRESENTATION?** The presenting part is that part of the fetus which occupies the lower pole of the uterus. Only a cephalic presentation is normal after 32 weeks. At 30 weeks, however, up to 25% of babies present by the breech.

Breech

Cephalic

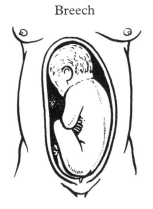

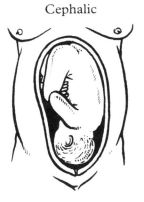

ABDOMINAL PALPATION

4. Is the **CEPHALIC PRESENTATION** a **VERTEX?**

This depends on the **ATTITUDE** of the fetus i.e. the relationship of its different parts to each other. The normal attitude is **FULL FLEXION.**

In full flexion, every fetal joint is flexed.

This gives a **VERTEX** presentation, the only normal presentation.

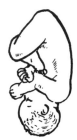

Sometimes the head may be extended.

This gives a **FACE** presentation, which is highly abnormal.

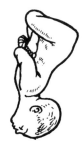

5. What is the **POSITION** of the **VERTEX?**

The position is the relationship of the presenting part to the mother's pelvis. It is conveniently expressed by referring to the position of one area of the presenting part known as the **DENOMINATOR.**

The denominator of the vertex is the OCCIPUT and there are eight recognised positions (see page 75). The lateral and anterior positions are regarded as normal as the occiput will rotate forward in labour.

If the fetus is in a posterior position (i.e. the occiput rotates towards the sacrum and the fetus faces forwards), the labour may be longer and more difficult.

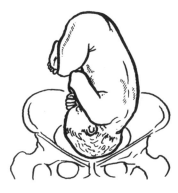

Left Occipito-Anterior (LOA)

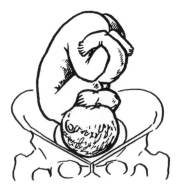

Right Occipito-Posterior (ROP)

ABDOMINAL PALPATION

6. Is the **VERTEX ENGAGED?**

Engagement means the descent of the biparietal diameter through the pelvic brim.

A convenient way to describe the amount of head above the brim is to identify the number of 'fifths' palpable. When the head is engaged 2/5 or less will be felt abdominally.

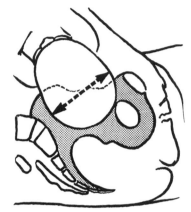

The head is 'fixed' (3/5 palpable)

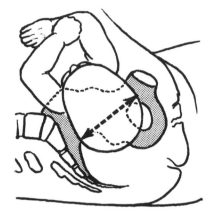

The head is 'engaged' (2/5 palpable)

Although it is discussed as a pre-labour phenomenon, engagement seldom occurs until after labour is established, and the term is often used to mean that the presenting part is 'fixed' — entering the pelvis — as opposed to 'free' or still mobile above the brim.

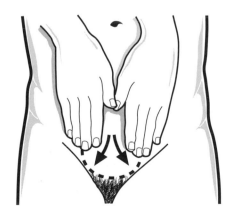

This presenting part is 'fixed'

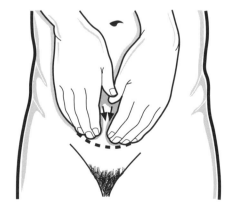

This presenting part is 'mobile'

VAGINAL EXAMINATION IN PREGNANCY

Bimanual examination is no longer a routine part of antenatal examination but is still sometimes required:

1. To assess maturity in early pregnancy.

2. To exclude suspected abnormalities such as incarcerated retroversion of the uterus or ovarian tumour.

3. To identify a presenting part which cannot be confidently identified abdominally.

4. To exclude or confirm gross degrees of contraction (in very small patients).

5. To assess the ripeness of the cervix near term.

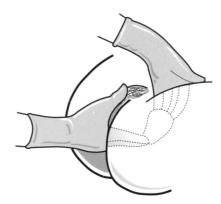

A bimanual examination in early pregnancy. Two fingers are shown in the vagina, but often one finger will give as much information as the patient will be more relaxed.

6. To assess pelvic capacity. The diagonal conjugate may be measured if the sacral promontory can be reached, in which case the pelvis is smaller than normal. The intertuberous diameter should be as wide as the normal fist. Prominence of the ischial spines and the width of the subpubic arch can be assessed. There is no doubt that some idea of the pelvic shape and size can be obtained after much practice by this palpation, but there is a wide margin of error.

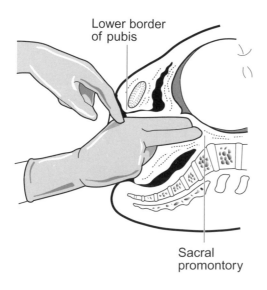

Lower border of pubis

Sacral promontory

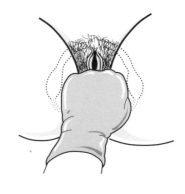

COMMON COMPLAINTS

SUBJECTIVE COMPLAINTS

Fatigue, somnolence, headache, 'blackouts', are often noticed in the early months and their cause is uncertain. Hypotension, secondary to peripheral vasodilatation, may be responsible for feelings of faintness.

MORNING SICKNESS

Nausea and vomiting are due probably to the effects of large amounts of circulating steroids, especially oestrogens or HCG and they seldom last beyond the 16th week. They can occur at any time of the day and are aggravated by cooking and fatigue.

Mild cases are treated by a light carbohydrate diet (biscuits and milk) in the morning and sometimes by anti-emetics. If the condition worsens it becomes hyperemesis gravidarum and is best treated in hospital (see Chapter 7).

CONSTIPATION

This is due principally to the relaxing effect of progesterone on smooth muscle. A bowel motion every second or third day is perfectly consistent with good health, but sometimes laxatives are required. Any of the commonly used drugs may be taken with safety.

HEARTBURN

The enlarging uterus encourages oesophageal reflux of gastric acid. Sleeping in a semi-recumbent position is helpful. Antacids or compound presentations, with alginates, can be prescribed safely.

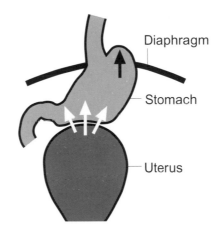

PELVIC PRESSURE

Pressure from the enlarged uterus gradually obstructs venous return and may lead to haemorrhoids and varicose veins of the legs and vulva. Support tights may be helpful for leg varicosities and suppositories are used for haemorrhoids. Nothing can be done for varicosities of the vulva beyond advising the patient to rest.

COMMON COMPLAINTS

PELVIC JOINT PAIN

This can occur because the ligaments of the pelvic joints are softened and relaxed during pregnancy by steroid induced fluid retention and the increased vascularity which occurs in all the soft tissues. The pelvis becomes less rigid which may be of some advantage in labour but movements can now take place in joints which are normally immovable and various symptoms may arise. Backache and sacro-iliac strain may occur because the softening of ligaments is aggravated by the postural change of pregnancy, a characteristic lordosis as the uterus grows.

Separation of up to 1 cm of the symphysis pubis is accepted as normal. It may go beyond this, however, and together with sacroiliac pain can be crippling. The only treatment is support, bed rest and analgesics.

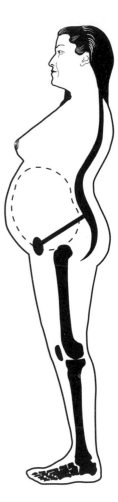

CARPAL TUNNEL SYNDROME

The median nerve is compressed in the carpal tunnel under the flexor retinaculum. Pregnant women often complain of tingling pain in the fingers, but median nerve neuropathy is uncommon. The patient complains of pain and numbness in one or both hands referred along the fingers supplied by the median nerve. It is worst on waking when the fingers feel lifeless. There is reduced pinprick sensation in the affected area but little else is found on examination. The usual treatment is to immobilise the wrist with splinting. Occasionally diuretics are employed though not of proven value. In extreme cases surgical management may be required.

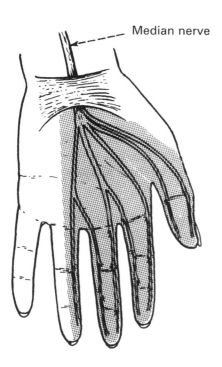

Median nerve

COMMON COMPLAINTS

VAGINAL DISCHARGE

Increased secretion of cervical mucus and the vascularity of the vagina combine to produce a fairly copious discharge in pregnancy. It should not be offensive or itchy and ordinary hygiene should be the only treatment required.

Infection with *Candida albicans*, however, is a common complication. This is encouraged by the warmth and moisture of the vulva and vagina together with the increased vaginal glycogen which favours the fungus. The complaints are of discharge and constant irritation. A swab should be taken and the characteristic plaques of yeast may be seen.

Trichomonads may also be seen.

Bacterial vaginosis is said to be commoner in pregnancy and may be associated with some cases of pre-term labour.

Treatment of candidal and trichomonal infection is by the use of clotrimazole pessaries. It may be difficult to eradicate in pregnancy but treatment is desirable to relieve symptoms and reduce the chances of infecting the fetus during its passage down the vagina.

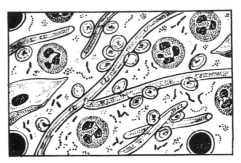

Mycelia and spores of C. albicans

OTHER ISSUES

Over recent years two main themes have developed in the modern provision of antenatal care: the first of these is recognition of mental illness during pregnancy and risk assessment of post natal depression in the antenatal period and puerperium. A high index of suspicion must be maintained by all caring for pregnant women and early recourse to mental health agencies made if there is anxiety regarding this aspect of maternal welfare.

The second issue is the recognition of the increased levels of domestic violence which may be seen in pregnancy and the puerperium. Often women will not make a complaint of any form of abuse and this makes helping them difficult. An empathic manner may enable them to express themselves and seek help but the first move must usually be made by them and this can be traumatic. Again, all of those involved in the care of pregnant women must be alert to the possibility of domestic abuse and engage with those social services which may offer aid.

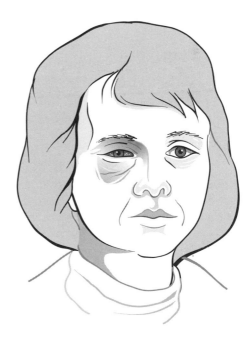

PHYSIOTHERAPY IN THE ANTENATAL PERIOD

The physiotherapist has an important role in promoting health throughout the childbearing period, and to help women adjust to both the physical and psychological changes of pregnancy and the puerperium.

ANTENATAL PREPARATION

1. EARLY PREGNANCY SESSION

Most centres offer at least one Early Pregnancy session when the interest and motivation of the women are at their highest. The physiotherapy input will include:

Back care. Postural and weight changes, bending and lifting, sitting and working positions.

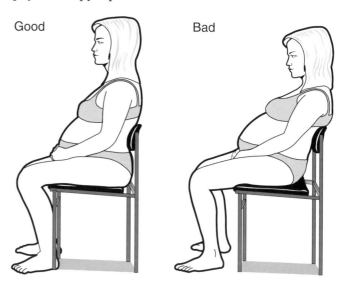

Good   Bad

Pelvic floor. Raise awareness of the pelvic floor by explaining its role and teaching correct method of contracting this muscle group.

Circulation. Changes within the cardio-vascular system will be explained. General advice will be given and exercises to stimulate circulation in the lower limbs will be demonstrated.

Exercise. There should be a discussion of the group's normal participation in exercise and sport and advice on adapting these if necessary. Information on local groups offering exercise in pregnancy can be given. Many areas now offer aqua-natal sessions, water being a particularly good medium for exercise.

Specific exercises to help maintain abdominal muscle strength, in particular Transversus Abdominis to maintain lumbo-pelvic stability and pelvic tilting which may also relieve backache.

Relaxation. The fatigue of pregnancy and the anxieties about future labour and parenthood make the introduction of relaxation techniques invaluable. The physiotherapist can support the pregnant woman by enabling her to understand the causes and effects of stress, how to recognise it in themselves and learning to control and manage it.

The most common relaxation technique used by physiotherapists is the Mitchell method of physiological relaxation.

PHYSIOTHERAPY IN THE ANTENATAL PERIOD

2. PREPARATION FOR LABOUR

The physiotherapy and parenthood education departments generally offer a series of between five and eight sessions. These provide a group for expectant mothers and supporters, where its members can feel free to discuss their fears and expectations. The interaction of the group often provides very useful peer support.

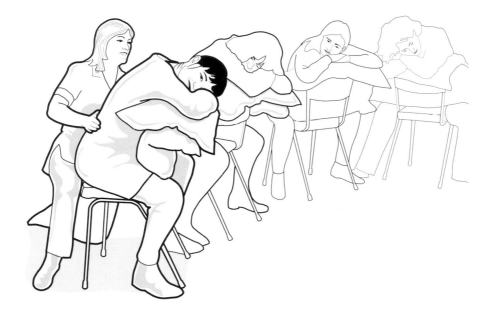

The physiotherapist aims to gradually build confidence in each woman, both in herself and in those looking after her in labour. This is achieved through knowledge, an understanding of her own reactions, and an ability to know and trust her own body.

These classes will include the anatomy and physiology of labour; coping techniques such as relaxation, massage, breathing and positioning to encourage progress and reduce the pain of labour.

Time should also be devoted antenatally to the problems that may be encountered during the puerperium and especially the importance of prophylactic back care. This can help to prevent problems developing in the weeks following childbirth when ligaments are still relatively lax, musculature is weak and the mother may be tired, from coping with the demands of a new baby.

PHYSIOTHERAPY IN THE ANTENATAL PERIOD

3. SPECIFIC REFERRALS

The hormonal effects in pregnancy and the mechanical stresses on the musculo-skeletal system of increasing weight and abdominal girth, can lead to great discomfort in pregnancy. Most women seem to experience some discomfort due to these factors at some stage of their pregnancy.

The pregnant woman should have easy access to an obstetric physiotherapist who will examine the patient and depending on that assessment will offer an appropriate treatment.

The most common referrals are for the back and pelvic girdle regions e.g. sacro-iliac dysfunction, pubic symphysis, postural backache and even the occasional disc protrusion. There is a wide variation in the severity of conditions and treatment may range from advice on daily living to mobilising or manipulative techniques.

ANTENATAL CARE SUMMARY

Improvements in the social conditions and general health of the child-bearing population are more effective in reducing the mortality and morbidity of pregnancy than any amount of antenatal care. Doctors and midwives, however, should still offer close supervision to all pregnant women by the traditional screening method, employing special tests where indicated. These are discussed in Chapter 7. The undernoted should be regarded as a basic standard of care:

1. Early assessment of the mother and identification of risk factors.
2. Confirmation of maturity by ultrasound.
3. Counselling and screening for detectable congenital and chromosomal abnormalities.
4. Regular visits shared between health professionals. Defaulting patients should be visited by a community midwife.
5. Regular examination to detect impaired fetal growth, pregnancy induced hypertension, anaemia, malpresentation and suspected disproportion.
6. An active health education programme and sessions on parenting skills.

CHAPTER 6

ASSESSMENT OF THE FETUS

FETAL MATURITY

This chapter deals with the investigations available to obstetricians to help assess the fetal condition. The techniques will be described under four headings:

1. Gestational age.
2. Identification of fetal abnormality.
3. Assessment of fetal growth.
4. Fetal wellbeing/functional maturity.

1. GESTATIONAL AGE

The traditional method of determining gestational age is from the date of the last menstrual period and clinical examination (see Chapter 5).

These methods may not be reliable:

1. LMP uncertain or forgotten.
2. Calculation depends on a 'normal' 28 day cycle.
3. The widespread use of hormonal contraception, oral and parenteral, makes ovulation unpredictable.
4. Uterine size may be difficult to determine, particularly in the patient who is obese or tense.

ULTRASOUND

Ultrasound examination, pioneered by Donald in Glasgow in the late 1950s and early 1960s, has become the cornerstone of fetal assessment. Increased resolution and portability have led to the widespread use of ultrasound equipment from the earliest stages of pregnancy through to care during labour. Further, ultrasound is the only reliable technique which can be used in early pregnancy to identify both fetal viability and multiple pregnancy.

The contribution of ultrasound to obstetric practice is so great that it is useful to summarise the uses to which ultrasound may be applied:

Routine Use: Confirmation of ongoing intra-uterine pregnancy.
Assessment of gestational age (measurement of crown–rump length, biparietal diameter, femur length).
Identification of multiple pregnancy.
Recognition of major anomalies.

Specific Uses: Threatened miscarriage (to confirm fetus is alive).
Antepartum haemorrhage (placental localisation).
Fetal growth studies (head–trunk ratio, estimated fetal weight, liquor volume, placental grade).
Assessment of high risk cases (maternal disease, elevated serum alphafetoprotein, history of anomaly).
Postpartum (retained products).

Pelvic masses.

Adjunct to Interventional Procedures: Chorion villus sampling
Amniocentesis.
Fetal blood sampling (cordocentesis).
Intra-uterine therapy e.g. intra-uterine transfusion.
Fetoscopy

FETAL MATURITY

Ultrasound in the estimation of gestational age

An ultrasound scan of the fetus in early pregnancy is the best method of determining gestational age. Accuracy is essential in the application of biochemical screening tests for fetal abnormality and, in later pregnancy, to determine that fetal growth is proceeding normally.

Measurement of the Crown–Rump Length of the fetus is the ideal before twelve weeks gestation.

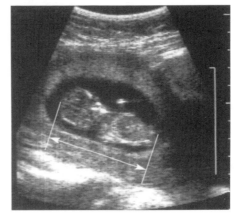

Crown–rump length measurement

Thereafter measurement of the fetal biparietal diameter, in conjunction with measurement of fetal long bones such as the femur, provides reasonable accuracy until the third trimester. The accuracy achieved depends on the observation that there is relatively little biological variation in these measurements in the first and second trimesters.

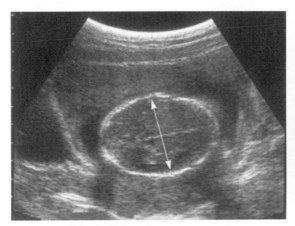

Biparietal diameter measurement

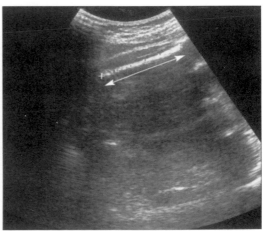

Femoral length measurement

FETAL ABNORMALITY

2. IDENTIFICATION OF FETAL ABNORMALITY

The identification of fetal abnormality is an important component of antenatal care. It is now possible to identify a large number of abnormalities. Many of these are sufficiently severe to be detectable at early gestations allowing the woman to elect for termination of the pregnancy if she wishes.

In other cases, termination may not be indicated but knowledge of the presence of the condition permits preparation of the woman, her partner and the paediatric and obstetric teams for treatment following delivery. A number of conditions may be amenable to fetal surgery but this expertise remains largely within a small number of highly specialised centres.

The term 'prenatal diagnosis' has become established to describe these diagnostic techniques.

SCREENING TESTS AND DIAGNOSTIC TESTS

It is important to distinguish between tests which are applied as screening tests and those which are diagnostic.

Screening tests are offered to a population in which there are no specific risk factors which would indicate the need for diagnostic testing. Thus a woman who had previously had a pregnancy complicated by fetal trisomy may elect to opt for diagnostic testing from the outset. The more sensitive and specific a screening test the closer it approximates a diagnostic test.

A. Screening at 11 to 14 weeks

Screening for congenital abnormality may be undertaken using biochemical assays, ultrasound or both.

Ultrasound can be used at this stage to identify structural abnormalities. Anencephaly and anterior abdominal wall defects may be seen but more subtle signs are now used, the foremost of which is measurement of nuchal translucency. In normal first trimester pregnancy a fluid filled area on the posterior surface of the neck may be seen and measured. An association between increased size of nuchal translucency (NT) and chromosomal and heart abnormalities is now well recognised. At any given maternal age the measurement of NT can be used to modify the underlying age related risk of a fetal trisomy.

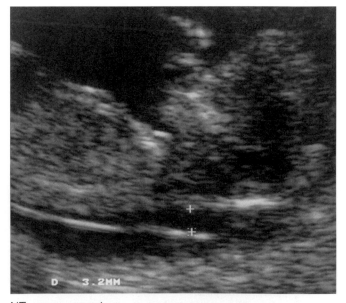

NT measurement

FETAL ABNORMALITY

The measurement of NT can be analysed in combination with biochemical markers such as Pregnancy Associated Proteins and oestriol and HCG to give a specific risk of the fetus being affected. In many centres a risk of 1:250 would be used to identify women at sufficiently high risk to merit diagnostic testing such as chorionic villus sampling or amniocentesis.

B. Screening at 15 to 21 weeks

Detailed ultrasound assessment of fetal anatomy is commonly undertaken around 18 to 20 weeks gestation but at this stage ultrasound is not of value in identifying Down's syndrome since nuchal translucency has disappeared at this stage (in the absence of associated abnormalities such as anterior abdominal wall defects such as exomphalos). Biochemical measurement of maternal serum alphafetoprotein (AFP), HCG and oestriol can be used in conjunction with maternal age, to calculate a risk for Down's syndrome, so-called triple testing. Again a high risk indicates the need for amniocentesis to obtain a fetal karyotype.

Measurement of AFP alone can be used as a screening test for a number of defects if detailed anatomy screening by ultrasound is not available. AFP is elevated in a number of conditions and, if elevated, indicates the need for further ultrasound assessment.

AFP is elevated in conditions such as:
Ancncephaly (AFP screening detects all cases)
Open neural tube defect (AFP screening detects 85–90% of cases)
Exomphalos
Gastroschisis
Placental haemangiomas
Certain fetal renal dysplasias.

AFP is also elevated in multiple pregnancies and in cases of fetomaternal bleeding as may occur with threatened miscarriage.

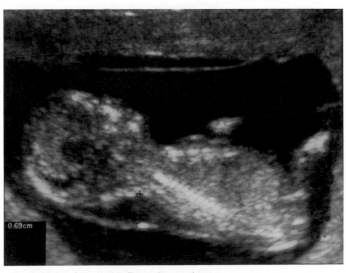

NT = 0.69 cm fetus with Down's syndrome

FETAL ABNORMALITY

Some structural anomalies are best identified by detailed ultrasound examination later in pregnancy and fetal echocardiography may be undertaken between 20 and 24 weeks.

DIAGNOSTIC TESTING

Ultrasound examination may be used to diagnose structural abnormality as the consequence of the results of a screening test, for example, an elevated MSAFP level.

When there is a question of chromosomal abnormality, invasive testing is required to obtain fetal tissue from which chromosomes can be identified for karyotyping.

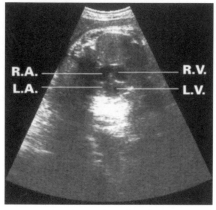

Normal for four-chamber heart

In the first trimester *Chorion Villus Sampling (CVS)* may be undertaken, using ultrasound guidance. Tissue can be obtained either transvaginally or transabdominally.

The pregnancy loss rate after CVS is 4% but this reflects the high spontaneous miscarriage rate between eight and twelve weeks. This procedure is now usually performed around eleven weeks gestation.

The more established technique of *amniocentesis,* in which amniotic fluid is removed, carries a loss rate of between one half and one per cent but requires culture of exfoliated skin cells before a karyotype can be obtained.

Fetal blood sampling offers a rapid result for karyotyping but requires considerable expertise in removing blood from the fetal umbilical vessels. This technique may also be used diagnostically in cases of rhesus disease, when blood grouping of the fetus can be performed, and therapeutically when blood transfusion into the fetal circulation is highly effective.

Biopsy needle guides

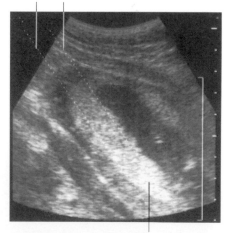

Placental tissue

Chorion villus sampling

FETAL GROWTH

3. ASSESSMENT OF FETAL GROWTH

The progress of fetal growth is observed by serial abdominal palpation and measurement of the symphysis/fundal height. This is one of the traditional 'arts' of the obstetrician, but it is important to recognise its limitations. Obesity, abdominal tenseness, the amount of amniotic fluid, the lie of the baby and the level of the presenting part can all affect observation.

The graph shows the progress of fetal growth for babies with weights between the fifth and ninety fifth centile values for the population. Babies whose weights are estimated to be below the tenth centile may be considered to be small-for-dates though some obstetricians reserve this term for babies below the fifth centile.

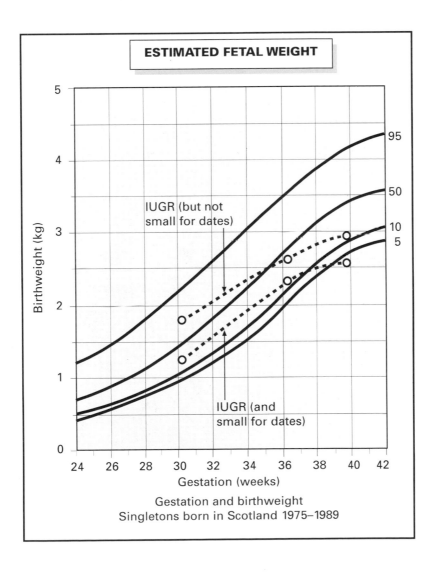

FETAL GROWTH

Traditionally obstetricians have expended most effort on the identification of the small-for-dates fetus. The reason for this effort is that a significant number of small babies have suffered from Intra-Uterine Growth Restriction (IUGR). It is important to appreciate that the terms IUGR and 'small-for-dates' are not synonymous. A fetus with IUGR is one which has not met its genetic growth potential. The small-for-dates fetus may be so constitutionally. It is logical to state also that some fetuses may have failed to reach their genetic growth potential but still be heavier than the tenth centile for weight. It is partly the recognition of the difficulty of identifying these larger babies that has led to the focus of attention being upon the small baby.

This aim is nevertheless justified by the higher perinatal mortality rate in these small babies.

IUGR may be associated with some maternal complications in pregnancy or the result of toxic insult or fetal abnormality.

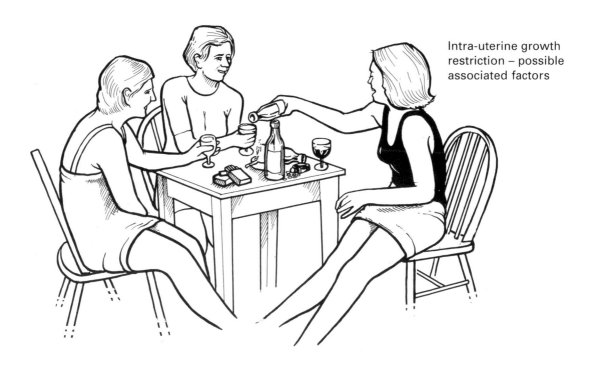

Intra-uterine growth restriction – possible associated factors

FETAL GROWTH

At present there is no ideal test to identify the IUGR fetus. Attention should be directed to those in certain groups:

Clinically suspected poor growth.
Hypertension in pregnancy (regardless of cause).
Maternal medical disorder e.g. renal disease
Antepartum haemorrhage.
Diabetes (with microvascular disease).
Multiple pregnancy.
Previous IUGR.
Previous bad obstetric outcome.
Toxins, particularly tobacco, alcohol, illicit drug use.

The only reliable assessment of fetal growth is based on ultrasound measurements of the fetus. Serial measurements of the fetal biparietal diameter, abdominal circumference, head circumference and long bones can be measured.

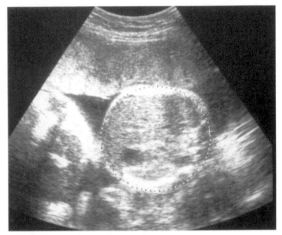

Fetal abdominal circumference

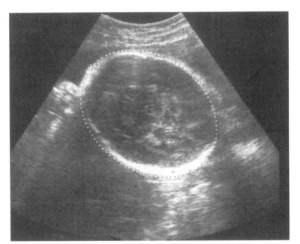

Fetal head circumference

FETAL GROWTH

Fetal weight may also be estimated using a variety of formulae based upon these measurements.

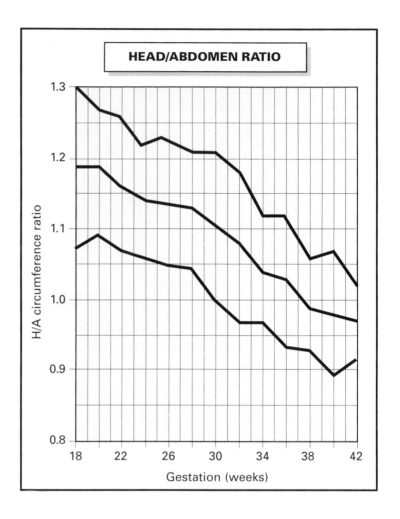

In cases of IUGR there is the phenomenon of head sparing in which blood flow to the head is maintained in preference to other organs. This results in an increase in the ratio of the circumference of the head to that of the abdomen. This increase in the head/abdomen circumference ratio is said to identify 'assymetric' growth restriction. The small fetus in which the head/abdomen circumference is normal is said to exhibit 'symmetric' growth restriction. It is likely that some of these babies are constitutionally small rather than being truly growth restricted.

FETAL WELLBEING

4. FETAL WELLBEING/FUNCTIONAL MATURITY

The fetus may die in utero from a sudden event such as premature separation of the placenta, a phenomenon called placental abruption, or cord prolapse. These cannot be predicted, but fetal death may come at the end of a process of growth restriction or placental impairment due to hypertension or maternal disease, or in pregnancies proceeding beyond 42 weeks when placental function may deteriorate.

In such circumstances the obstetrician tries to determine whether the fetus is at risk of hypoxic damage or death. Tests of fetal wellbeing are complementary to tests of fetal growth and will often be used in conjunction with them.

They are indicated:
1. Where fetal growth is already under surveillance
2. Prolonged pregnancy — more than ten days after the expected date of confinement or earlier in older mothers
3. In any mother complaining of reduced fetal movement.

A. FETAL MOVEMENT COUNT

The normal range of fetal activity falls from 90 movements in 12 hours at 32 weeks to about 50 perceived movements at term. This diminution is in part due to a change in the nature of the movement from clearly identified 'kicks' to more rolling and squirming movements.

A reduction in fetal movement has been described in cases of fetal death from hypoxia. Consequently a clear history of reduced fetal movement is an indication for further investigation.

The Cardiff 'count to ten' chart is an excellent way of recording the time taken for a mother to feel ten fetal movements. If the mother has not felt 10 movements within 12 hours she is asked to record the number of movements felt and contact the hospital. Further investigation is indicated.

Fetal movement counting is a simple, physiologically sound and inexpensive method of monitoring. Unfortunately its subjective nature means that it is not universally applicable to all mothers who may be anxious and inconsistent in recording.

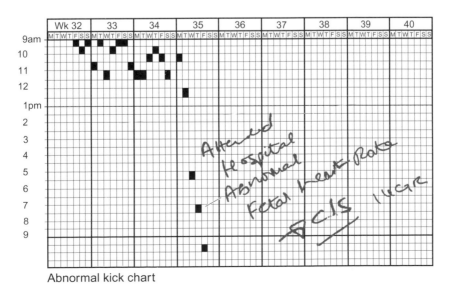

Abnormal kick chart

FETAL WELLBEING

B. FETAL BIOPHYSICAL ASSESSMENT

The Fetal Biophysical Profile is an established technique utilising ultrasound technology to visualise the fetus and Doppler ultrasound to measure the fetal heart rate.

There are five components to the biophysical profile. Each carries a score of two possible points to make a possible 'Biophysical Score' of 10 points. Four of the components, fetal breathing movements, gross body movements, fetal tone and amniotic fluid volume are assessed by conventional ultrasound to visualise the fetus and its environment.

VARIABLE	SCORE 2	SCORE 0
Fetal breathing movements (FBM)	The presence of at least 30 seconds of sustained FBM in 30 minutes of observation	Less than 30 seconds of FBM in 30 minutes
Fetal movements	Three or more gross body movements in 30 minutes of observation. Simultaneous limb and trunk movements are counted as a single movement	Two or less gross body movements in 30 minutes of observation
Fetal tone	At least one episode of motion of a limb from a position of flexion to extension and a rapid return to flexion	Fetus in a position of semi- or full-limb extension with movement. Absence of fetal movement is counted as absent tone
Fetal reactivity	The presence of two or more fetal heart rate accelerations of at least 15 bpm and lasting at least 15 seconds and associated with fetal movements in 40 minutes	No acceleration or less than two accelerations of the fetal heart rate in 40 minutes of observations
Quantitative amniotic fluid volume	A pocket of amniotic fluid that measures at least 1 cm in two perpendicular planes	Largest pocket of amniotic fluid measures <1 cm in two perpendicular planes
Maximal score	10	—
Minimal score	—	0

MANAGEMENT SCHEME BASED ON BIOPHYSICAL PROFILE SCORING	
Score	Recommended management
8–10	Repeat in 1 week. In diabetic (insulin-dependent) and postdates patients, repeat twice weekly. No indications for active interventions
4–6	If fetal pulmonary maturity assured and cervix favourable, deliver, otherwise repeat in 24 hours. If persistent score of 4 to 6, deliver if fetal pulmonary maturity certain. Otherwise treat with steroids and deliver in 48 hours
0–2	Evaluate for immediate delivery. In cases of certain pulmonary immaturity give steroids and deliver in 48 hours

The final component is fetal cardiotocography. This technique uses Doppler ultrasound to record the fetal heart rate and its response to fetal movement and uterine activity. The normal response of the fetus to movement is to increase the heart rate. This phenomenon is recorded on the cardiotocograph. An increase in heart rate over the baseline heart rate of fifteen beats per minute, and lasting for fifteen seconds or greater should be seen in healthy fetuses following movement. The absence of these *accelerations* may indicate fetal hypoxia. If a fetal heart rate trace shows two accelerations in a twenty minute period it is said to be 'reactive.' The absence of accelerations indicates a 'non-reactive' trace and requires further evaluation. Decelerations in the fetal heart rate are occasionally seen before the onset of labour and require urgent investigation. Computerised systems for interpreting cardiotocographs are now available and give an automated analysis of the recordings of fetal heart rate patterns. These may be used to determine the likelihood of fetal hypoxia though the proper application of such systems relies on the clinical judgement of the obstetrician who interprets the clinical situation and not just the heart rate trace.

A proposed scheme of management based upon the biophysical score is shown above.

FETAL WELLBEING

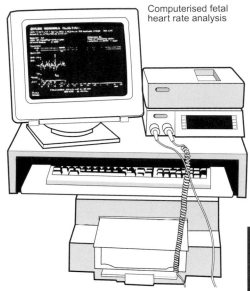

Computerised fetal
heart rate analysis

Examination of fetal blood vessels,
particularly the umbilical arteries, to
obtain flow velocity waveforms using
Doppler ultrasound, is now widely
used in fetal evaluation.

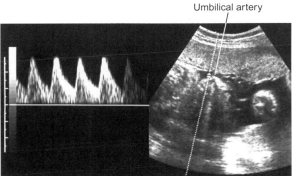

Umbilical artery

A normal flow velocity
waveform in the umbilical
artery shows continuous flow
throughout the cardiac cycle.

Normal

In pregnancies complicated by
fetal hypoxia a different pattern
is seen in which the flow
through the artery is reduced
in diastole. When there is
absence of flow at the end of
diastole the fetus is likely to be
severely compromised.

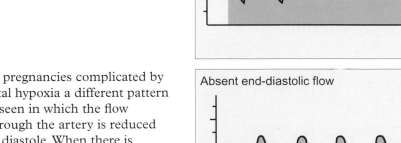

Absent end-diastolic flow

FETAL FUNCTIONAL MATURITY

When there is evidence of fetal compromise delivery may be indicated. While this may seem in the fetal interest at term there are situations in which knowledge of fetal functional maturity may be important. Neonatal Respiratory Distress Syndrome (RDS) or Hyaline Membrane Disease is a serious disorder of the premature fetus. The fetal alveoli contribute surfactants to the lung secretions. These are required for inflation of the alveoli at birth and their function thereafter. The principal components of the surfactants in the human lung are the phospholipids, Lecithin and Sphingomyelin. These phospholipids can be measured in amniotic fluid removed by amniocentesis.

The ratio of the former to the latter gives an indication of neonatal lung function. This ratio, the L/S ratio, rises with advancing gestation and likelihood of lung maturity. A ratio of 2:1 is more likely after 34 weeks gestation and suggests that RDS is unlikely.

Another phospholipid, phosphatidyl glycerol is an even more sensitive indicator. Its presence in the liquor strongly suggests fetal lung maturity and, in contrast with LS ratio, is reliable even when measured in samples obtained vaginally after spontaneous rupture of the membranes.

CHAPTER 7

DISEASES OF PREGNANCY

VOMITING IN PREGNANCY

Nausea and retching are common in the early weeks of pregnancy, sufficiently so almost to be recognised as evidence of being pregnant. Although often described as morning sickness, symptoms can occur at any time of the day. Most women cope with this readily and the problem disappears spontaneously by the end of the first trimester. Sometimes, however, drug treatment may be necessary and antihistamines such as cyclizine or a phenothiazine can be prescribed safely.

HYPEREMESIS GRAVIDARUM
Occasionally there is a progression from ordinary nausea and vomiting to the rejection of all food and drink. Unchecked this may lead to dehydration and starvation with ketosis, liver damage, jaundice, neuropathies and even death.

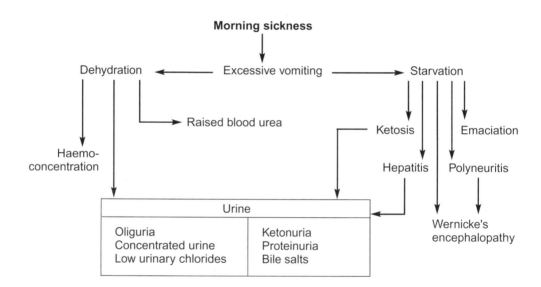

VOMITING IN PREGNANCY

The cause of vomiting in pregnancy is not clear. Alterations in serum hormone levels are often blamed but social and psychological factors also appear to play a role. Support for the first explanation comes from the fact that the condition is commoner in multiple pregnancies and in hydatidiform mole, and for the latter two, by the improvement in symptoms with hospitalisation alone.

High levels of Human Chorionic Gonadotrophin appear to elevate thyroxine levels and 60% of women with hyperemesis have biochemical or clinical hyperthyroidism.

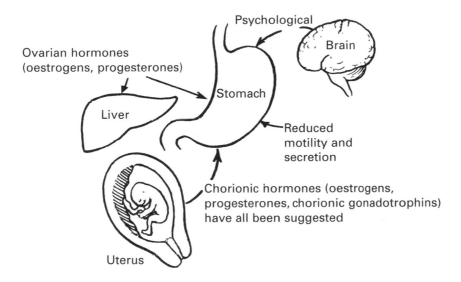

TREATMENT OF HYPEREMESIS
1. Admit to hospital.
2. Exclude other causes of vomiting such as urinary tract infection and surgical causes such as appendicitis and bowel obstruction.
3. Blood taken for haemoglobin, urea & electrolytes, glucose, liver function tests, thyroxine and TSH levels.
4. Restrict oral intake initially.
5. Intravenous fluids should be given to treat any dehydration.
6. Prepared feeds via a fine naso-gastric tube are usually effective, the volume being given ideally through a pump system delivering small volumes over time. The volume given can progressively be increased.
7. Gradual reintroduction of oral foods.
8. Pyridoxine, 25 mg three times daily by mouth may be effective in severe nausea.
9. Low dose intravenous infusions of Promethazine have been found useful in some centres.
10. Rarely, total parenteral nutrition or even termination of pregnancy may be indicated.

RHESUS INCOMPATIBILITY

Haemolytic disease of the newborn occurs when antibodies formed in the mother, in response to the introduction into her circulation of foreign antigen, cross the placenta and destroy fetal cells bearing the foreign antigen. Rhesus incompatibility is the commonest cause of haemolytic disease but it can be caused by ABO incompatibility when small molecule alpha and beta haemolysins are present, or by the presence of other antibodies such as anti-Duffy and anti-Kell. Pregnancy is the time when a woman is most likely to be exposed to the stimulating antigen by the escape of fetal cells into the maternal circulation. This occurs at times of placental separation, notably the third stage of labour. It may also occur however with abortion or ante-partum haemorrhage or due to surgical procedures such as amniocentesis or external version. Inappropriate blood transfusion should no longer be a cause of Rhesus sensitisation.

FISHER CLASSIFICATION OF RHESUS FACTOR

In each individual Rhesus genes are carried on two chromosomes, either of which may be handed on to the succeeding generation. There are six main Rhesus genes, three carried on each chromosome. Of the six, three are dominant C, D and E and three, their alleles, c, d, e are recessive. Each chromosome has a C locus, a D locus and an E locus which may be occupied by a dominant or recessive gene of the particular type.

The most important gene in Rhesus incompatibility is the dominant D gene. Because of this people possessing the D antigen are commonly described as rhesus positive. When it is absent from both chromosomes its place is occupied by the recessive allele and the individual is termed rhesus negative. Formerly more than 95% of cases of rhesus disease were due to anti-D antibodies. With the introduction of anti-D prophylaxis (see page 109), however, the incidence of the disease due to this antibody has fallen sharply and haemolytic disease due to Rhesus antibodies other than D, anti-c and anti-E notably, is relatively more important. The term genotype means the mixture of genes on two chromosomes. For example:

CDe/cDE – Homozygous Rhesus (D) positive.
CDe/cde – Heterozygous Rhesus (D) positive.
cde/cde – Rhesus negative.

83% of the UK population are rhesus positive, i.e. they possess at least one dominant D gene and of these 42% are homozygous and 58% heterozygous. This is of fundamental importance in pregnancy as all the offspring of a homozygous positive man will be rhesus positive, while there is a 50% chance of a rhesus negative child if the father is heterozygous positive and the mother Rhesus negative.

RHESUS INCOMPATIBILITY

The other factor which determines whether the process of immunisation is initiated in the mother or not, is the ABO blood group of the mother and fetus. The immunisation of the mother is brought about by the escape of fetal red cells into the maternal circulation. If the fetal cells are ABO compatible with those of the mother they will persist in her circulation and will stimulate antibody formation. If they are ABO incompatible they will be destroyed rapidly and no immunisation will occur.

The circumstances might be as follows.

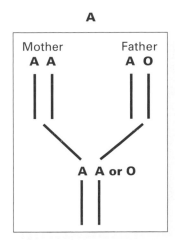
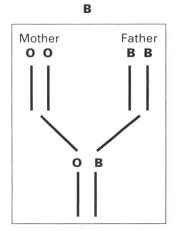

In family A the fetal blood is compatible with maternal group and fetal cells will continue to circulate in the maternal circulation. If the mother is Rhesus negative and the fetus is Rhesus positive then antibodies will form. The fetal cells in example B are incompatible with the maternal blood and will be rapidly destroyed on entering the maternal circulation. No antibodies are likely to form even if there is Rhesus incompatibility.

Before Rhesus immunisation is likely to occur the red cells of the fetus must have a blood group either the same as the mother or group O, and must possess a Rhesus gene not found in the mother.

ANTIBODY FORMATION AND DETECTION

When fetal cells enter and persist in the mother's circulation two antibodies are formed. The first, the Saline Antibody (IgM), generally appears seven days after stimulation. It agglutinates Rhesus positive cells suspended in saline. It is a large molecule and does not cross the placenta. Twenty-one days after stimulation the Albumin Antibody (IgG) appears in the maternal blood. It is a small molecule and crosses the placenta easily and attacks the Rhesus positive red cells of the baby. It generally agglutinates Rhesus positive cells provided they are suspended in plasma, serum or albumin. Frequently, however, it is difficult to read tests for the antibody formed in this way and its detection is made easier if the Rhesus positive cells are first treated with enzymes such as papain.

Kleihauer Test

The presence of fetal cells in the mother's circulation can be demonstrated by this test. It depends on the fact that fetal haemoglobin is more resistant than adult to acid elution. When a blood film is stained following elution the fetal cells will stand out against the adult 'ghost' cells. It is roughly quantitative by counting the number of fetal cells per 50 low power fields. Five cells per 50 fields = a bleed of 0.5 ml.

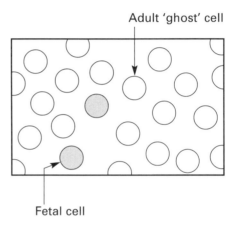

Adult 'ghost' cell

Fetal cell

Coombs' Test

This test depends on the fact that antibodies are globulins. If these globulins are injected into an animal antibodies to them will be formed. These antibodies can in turn be used to detect the presence of the original antibodies. The Coombs' reagent therefore is immune anti-globulin.

The **DIRECT** test is used to detect an affected fetus at birth. Cells from cord blood are suspended with the reagent and if the baby is affected (has maternal antibody attached) agglutination will occur.

The **INDIRECT** test (IAGT) is used to detect and measure antibody in the mother's serum. This is suspended with test cells. Antibody in the serum will coat the cells and agglutination will occur when the Coombs' reagent is added. By using dilutions of the mother's serum a measure of the amount of antibody (titre) is obtained.

EFFECTS ON FETUS AND NEONATE

The basis of the disease is haemolytic anaemia brought about by the action of maternal anti-Rhesus albumin antibody. Levels of unconjugated bilirubin rise and there is a compensating erythropoiesis.

In its most severe form the process produces Fetal Hydrops which is fatal either in utero or after birth unless it can be detected at an early stage in utero and treated by direct transfusion. Here the severity of the anaemia has resulted in cardiac failure with widespread oedema, ascites and pleural effusions. The diagnosis may be made in utero by ultrasound.

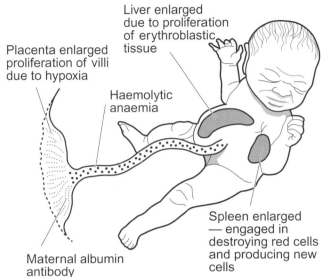

Liver enlarged due to proliferation of erythroblastic tissue

Placenta enlarged proliferation of villi due to hypoxia

Haemolytic anaemia

Spleen enlarged — engaged in destroying red cells and producing new cells

Maternal albumin antibody

Fetal Hydrops

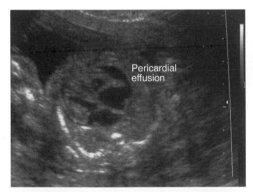

Pericardial effusion

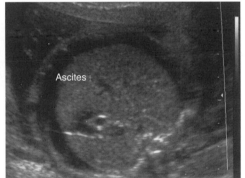

Ascites

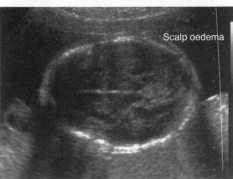

Scalp oedema

Ultrasound features of Fetal Hydrops

EFFECTS ON FETUS AND NEONATE

In less severe degrees of the condition the baby may be born alive and quickly becomes jaundiced. Treatment by exchange transfusion (see page 112) may be needed. In the least affected babies jaundice does not occur but the child becomes progressively anaemic and may require top-up transfusion.

	MILD HAEMOLYSIS	SEVERE HAEMOLYSIS
Child	Pale	Golden yellow jaundice appears within minutes of birth
Liver	Slightly enlarged	Greatly enlarged
Spleen	Slightly enlarged	Much enlarged
Blood	Mild anaemia	Rapidly increasing anaemia
	Hb 13–15 g per dl	
	Few reticulocytes	Numerous reticulocytes, erythroblasts, normoblasts, and early white cells
	Bilirubin scarcely increased	Indirect & direct bilirubin increased and rising
Urine	Negative test for bile	Positive test for bile

Kernicterus is a condition which may arise in any form of neonatal jaundice when the unconjugated bilirubin level rises above 340 microMoles/l. Rhesus incompatibility is the main cause. Bilirubin enters the fetal brain tissue causing necrosis of neurones especially in the basal ganglia. The infant becomes lethargic and refuses to suck. Convulsions, rolling of eyes and head retraction develop. Death may occur. Physical and mental handicap usually follow if the baby survives.

PREVENTION OF RHESUS HAEMOLYTIC DISEASE

The initiation of antibody formation starts in the first Rhesus incompatible pregnancy. Although small numbers of fetal red cells escape into the maternal circulation during pregnancy, the important immunising dose is usually received by the mother at the time of delivery when the placenta is compressed and separated. It is for this reason that Rhesus sensitisation is uncommon in first pregnancies.

If the fetus is Rh +ve these red cells will stimulate antibody formation. The aim is to 'hide' the D antigen so that the maternal immune mechanism does not recognise the cells as 'foreign' and antibodies will not then be formed. This is done by giving the mother anti-D which attaches itself to the D antigens of the fetal red cells making them unrecognisable by the immune mechanism and therefore incapable of stimulating antibody formation.

Anti D for administration is prepared from immunised rhesus negative individuals in the United States who have produced their own Anti D. In the UK manufactured anti D is obtained from The Scottish Fractionation Centre or the Bioproducts Laboratory. One manufacturer imports anti D from the United States.

Procedure. Tests are carried out as in flow diagram.

All rhesus negative women, without antibodies on re-testing, giving birth to rhesus positive babies, are given an injection of anti D immunoglobulin. This is done even if the Kleihauer test is negative. The standard dose is 500 i.u. by intra-muscular injection within 72 hours of delivery.

A rough estimate of the amount of fetal blood escaping into the mother's circulation is made by the Kleihauer test and the dose of anti D may be adjusted accordingly.

Where the pregnancy ends before 20 weeks the blood group of the fetus will not usually be known and 250 i.u. of anti D should be given.

Similarly, when invasive procedures such as amniocentesis or external version are carried out anti D is given. Other episodes of placental separation such as threatened miscarriage and antepartum haemorrhage should be covered by anti D administration, the dosage being determined by the stage of pregnancy and the estimated volume of the bleed.

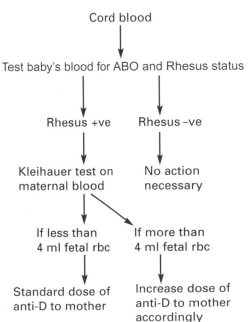

MANAGEMENT OF PREGNANCY

1. Rhesus negative without antibodies
   (a) First visit: Rhesus group and screening test for immune antibodies.
   (b) Repeat antibody check monthly from 24 to 36 weeks.
   (c) Give anti D immunoglobulin for complications as above.
   (d) Delivery: Mother's blood — antibody check and Kleihauer.
                   Cord blood — ABO and Rhesus group,
                                Haemoglobin,
                                Coombs' test,
                                Bilirubin.
   (e) Give anti D if blood negative for antibodies and baby Rhesus positive. If Kleihauer suggests bleed more than 4 ml, further anti D given.
2. Rhesus negative with antibodies
   a) First visit — antibody identified and measured by IAGT and, preferably, direct quantitation of antibody level.
   (b) Antibody test repeated monthly or until management decided on by other investigations e.g. amniocentesis.
   (c) Rhesus genotyping of partner — if heterozygous Rhesus positive the possibility of an unaffected child exists.
   (d) Amniocentesis — the bilirubin level in the liquor, measured by spectrophotometry, is a useful prognostic indicator as it reflects the excretion of bilirubin by the baby and thus

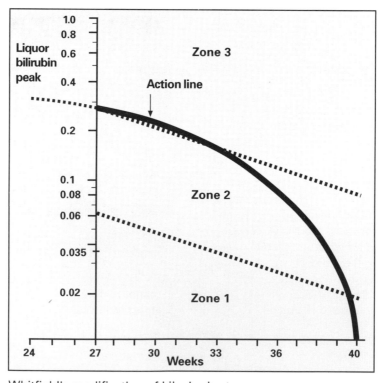

Whitfield's modification of Liley's chart

MANAGEMENT OF PREGNANCY

the degree of haemolysis. The result obtained is plotted on a prediction graph such as Whitfield's modification of Liley's chart and a second examination will usually be done 2–3 weeks later to establish a trend. By extrapolating the line through two results towards the 'Action Line' guidance on the timing of intervention is obtained.

Amniocentesis is the preferred method of assessment after 27 weeks but may be combined with ultrasound examination and fetal blood sampling when severe disease is suspected before this. Special investigations such as these are indicated in all patients with a history of a significantly affected baby or, in the absence of such a history, in patients with antibody levels of 2.5 i.u. per ml or more or with IAGT titre of 1:8.

The timing of the first amniocentesis is crucial. A rough guide is to perform it 10 weeks before the time of the earliest previous death or delivery of a severely affected baby. If there is no such history the first test should be performed at 28 to 30 weeks. The test will usually be repeated to establish the trend in 2 to 3 weeks but may be done sooner in severe cases.

(e) Ultrasound — can detect fetal ascites and oedema, indicating a severely affected fetus, at a very early stage in the pregnancy, e.g. less than 20 weeks. Such findings indicate the need for fetal blood sampling by cordocentesis.

(f) Cordocentesis (see page 88)

Blood may be obtained from the fetus in patients with a history of severe early rhesus disease and in those in whom ultrasound has demonstrated ascites. A haematocrit reading is at once available and treatment by direct intravascular transfusion can be given if indicated by the result.

Umbilical vein

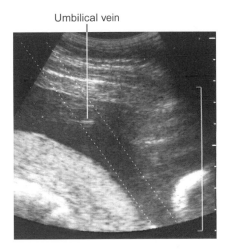

TREATMENT

1. Delivery

Delivery of the baby, prematurely if necessary, followed by assessment of its condition and exchange transfusion, as required, is the traditional treatment of rhesus sensitised patients. Those with very low levels of antibody (less than 2.5 i.u./ml) may be safely allowed to proceed to term when labour should be induced. The timing of intervention in other cases depends on the patient's history and the results of liquor or blood analysis. If treatment by fetal transfusion is given, the aim is usually to continue treatment to achieve a maturity of 36 weeks before delivery.

After birth the cord blood is examined:
   a. Coombs' test.
   b. Blood grouping and Rhesus typing.
   c. Haemoglobin estimation.
   d. Serum bilirubin.

A positive Coombs' test indicates an affected baby.

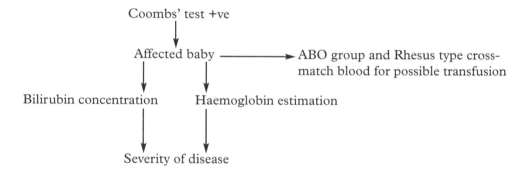

Mild degrees of anaemia (not below 12 g/dl) may not require treatment and mild degrees of jaundice may respond to phototherapy. More seriously affected babies will require an EXCHANGE TRANSFUSION. This means the withdrawal of blood through the umbilical vein and its replacement with healthy compatible blood. It thus corrects anaemia and reduces high levels of circulating bilirubin which would cause kernicterus, and washes out any free circulating antibodies. The decision to perform transfusion is not based simply on cord blood findings. The patient's history, the maturity of the baby and the rate of increase in the bilirubin level in the baby are all critical.

TREATMENT

2. Fetal Transfusion

Intraperitoneal fetal transfusion has been used for many years to treat severely affected babies at a gestation when delivery and exchange transfusion would not be possible. Packed cells, usually O negative, are injected into the fetal peritoneal cavity under ultrasound guidance and are readily absorbed into the circulation. The volume injected depends on the maturity of the pregnancy but as much as 120 ml can be absorbed in a few days. The procedure may be repeated as required at intervals of about 2 weeks.

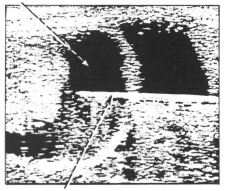

Fetal peritoneal cavity

Needle through abdominal wall

Direct intravascular transfusion, again directed by ultrasound, may be used at very early stages of pregnancy (less than 22 weeks). The availability of a direct measure of the degree of fetal anaemia allows careful determination of the volume of blood to be transfused. Specialised fetal medicine centres have achieved remarkable results in such cases, sometimes with 6 or more transfusions.

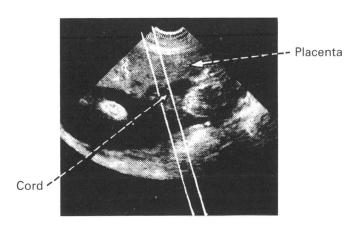

Placenta

Cord

NON RHESUS ISO-IMMUNISATION

Other red cell antigens expressed in the fetus and not the mother are also associated with haemolysis. As the toll of Rhesus disease is reduced by prophylaxis the importance of these blood systems is becoming proportionately greater. The more severe of these include the Kell, Duffy and MNS antigen systems.

HYPERTENSION IN PREGNANCY

Raised blood pressure in pregnancy is a common and potentially dangerous complication, associated with an increase in both maternal and fetal mortality. Blood pressure readings of 140/90 mmHg or more are generally considered abnormal. The reported overall incidence varies widely, but usually lies between 12 and 25% of all pregnancies.

The normal resting blood pressure is virtually never above 120/80, and since the plasma volume increase averages 1200 ml, there must be some vasodilatation to allow the peripheral pressure to remain low. If this vasodilatation is counteracted by arteriolar spasm, hypertension results and there is a reduction in the perfusion of all organs, including the uterus and thus the placental site.

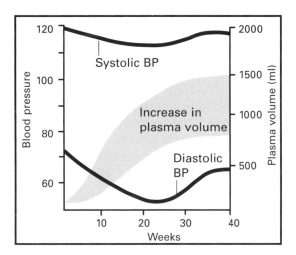

Hypertension is conventionally divided into:
a) **Pre-existing hypertension** where there is an elevated blood pressure before pregnancy or in the first 20 weeks. This may be due to essential hypertension, renal disease, connective tissue disorders and other rare causes.
b) **Pre-eclampsia.** This is a condition of unknown aetiology, occurring chiefly in primigravidae and presenting in the second half of pregnancy. Women may be considered as having pre-eclampsia if:
1) they have a blood pressure of 140/90 mmHg or greater in the second half of pregnancy and were normotensive before this and
2) they demonstrate a rise of 25 mmHg over the diastolic level in the non-pregnant state or in the first half of pregnancy.

HYPERTENSION IN PREGNANCY

Pregnancy induced hypertension may be considered as synonymous with pre-eclampsia. Some workers restrict the use of the term pre-eclampsia to women who have proteinuria as well as hypertension and yet others use the term **Proteinuric Pregnancy Induced Hypertension** for such cases.

Proteinuria is a serious complication of hypertension. It indicates impaired renal function and, by inference, impaired placental function with consequent threat to the baby. A small amount of protein in the urine may be normal in pregnancy but the level should be less than 300 mg per volume in a 24 hour collection.

Other causes of proteinuria should be noted:
Contamination.
Urinary tract infection.
Renal disease.
Connective tissue disorders.
Orthostatic proteinuria.
The term Pre-eclampsia has much to commend it as it serves to remind the clinician of one of the major complications of the condition, namely, **eclampsia.**

Oedema may be associated with pre-eclampsia but swelling of the feet and ankles is almost invariable in late pregnancy, and even generalised oedema involving the face and hands is sufficiently common to be considered normal if unassociated with raised blood pressure. It should not, however, be ignored. The presence of oedema may give early warning of developing pre-eclampsia and, when associated with a hypertensive pregnancy, may be a sign of deterioration or progression to eclampsia.

AETIOLOGY
Pre-eclampsia is a multisystem disorder and in severe cases results in disturbances of liver function and the clotting system. Although the aetiology remains unclear the trophoblast is causative since the condition may be seen before 20 weeks in conditions such as multiple pregnancy or hydatidiform mole, and it is cured by delivery.

The incidence is 5 to 7% of primigravid pregnancies where the disease is 'primary' i.e. occurring in a patient whose blood pressure was previously normal and disappearing after pregnancy. In women with chronic hypertension and especially those with renal disease, the incidence is much higher, the pre-eclampsia being superimposed on the existing hypertension.

While the cause of the condition remains unknown there is a clear pre-disposition in certain groups:
1. Primigravid patients or in the first pregnancy with a given partner.
2. Increased risk with age.
3. Family history of pre-eclampsia or hypertension.
4. Pre-existing hypertension, especially renal disease or connective tissue disorder.
5. Multiple pregnancy.
6. Diabetic pregnancy.
7. Hydatidiform mole.
8. Severe rhesus sensitisation.

HYPERTENSION IN PREGNANCY

PATHOPHYSIOLOGY

A great mass of data has been collected and many theories propounded over the years to try to explain this much-studied disease. It is accepted that the starting point is in the placental bed. In normal pregnancy the trophoblast invades the maternal spiral arteries and converts these vessels into low resistance arteries thereby increasing perfusion. In pre-eclampsia this process is defective and this so-called 'physiological change' does not occur.

Clinically there is evidence of widespread systemic disturbance.

a) Cardiovascular system. The maternal hypertension results from increased peripheral resistance due possibly to imbalance of vasoactive substances such as prostanoids and local disturbances in the control of the vessel tone by substances produced by the endothelium of the vessel wall.

In addition the normal expansion of the plasma volume (see Chapter 2) is reduced in pre-eclampsia and there may be a fall in plasma proteins due to renal dysfunction. Together this creates a state of hypovolaemia and tissue oedema.

b) Renal system. Impaired renal function has long been recognised in pre-eclampsia with evidence of both glomerular and tubular dysfunction. This is detected by the presence of protein in the urine and raised plasma urate levels:

> Proteinuria: > 300 mg per volume in a 24 hour collection
> Plasma urate: > 0.35 mmol/litre

Urea and creatinine levels may also rise. Levels of greater than 6 mmol/litre and 100 micro-moles per litre respectively are significant.

c) Clotting system. A falling platelet count and changes in many clotting factors have been reported in pre-eclampsia. In severe cases this may proceed to disseminated intravascular coagulation with micro-angiopathic haemolysis secondary to small vessel blockage, revealed by anaemia and the presence of fragmented red cells in the peripheral blood. Raised levels of fibrin degradation products are found.

d) Liver damage. Post-mortem examination of patients dying from eclampsia have long demonstrated evidence of liver damage with subcapsular haemorrhage and areas of necrosis seen microscopically in the peri-portal region of the liver lobules. Epigastric tenderness has always been described as a sign of impending eclampsia but in recent years awareness of the risk of liver damage has increased and evidence of it in the form of elevated enzymes in the mother's circulation should be sought.

The term HELLP syndrome has been coined to emphasise the dangerous combination of disseminated intravascular coagulation and liver damage in severe pre-eclampsia:

> **H**aemolysis — **E**levated **L**iver enzymes — **L**ow **P**latelets

HYPERTENSION IN PREGNANCY

e) Central nervous system – Eclampsia. Pre-eclampsia is largely a disease of signs rather than symptoms. Headache, visual disturbance and abdominal pain may indicate progression towards eclampsia. The first two of these reflect the effects of hypertension on the brain in terms of hypertensive encephalopathy and the last the effect on the liver of subcapsular haemorrhage.

The epileptiform fit, the defining aspect of eclampsia, also reflects hypertensive encephalopathy although there is no defining blood pressure at which a woman with pre-eclampsia will actually convulse.

In the United Kingdom in 1997–1999 there were 7.1 deaths from pre-eclampsia or eclampsia per million maternities.

Of the 15 deaths, two women died from rupture of the liver, one from adult respiratory distress syndrome and the remainder from intracranial haemorrhage. Some of these deaths are preventable by the availability of effective treatment to reduce blood pressure and prevent or control fits.

Units should encourage the development and use of specific packs or boxes containing first line drugs for management of this condition with other relevant equipment easily available.

It is not clear what causes the fit but it is not solely related to the level of the blood pressure. Death may occur from cerebral haemorrhage or cardiac failure. A recent United Kingdom survey of eclampsia recorded an incidence of 4.9 cases per 10 000 pregnancies, with a maternal mortality of 1.8% and a fetal loss of 7.8%.

f) Renin angiotensin system. In normal pregnancy there is a reduction in sensitivity to the vasopressor effects of angiotensin. This reduction does not occur in a high proportion of cases which subsequently develop pre-eclampsia.

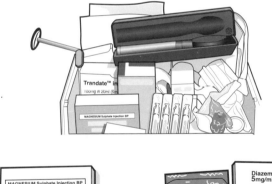

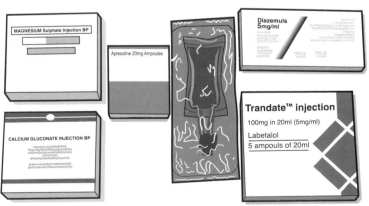

First line drugs

HYPERTENSION IN PREGNANCY

CLINICAL COMPLICATIONS OF HYPERTENSIVE PREGNANCY
1. Intra-uterine growth restriction — the risk is increased in cases with proteinuria.
2. Fetal hypoxia and intra-uterine death.
3. Abruption of the placenta.
4. HELLP syndrome.
5. Eclampsia.
6. Renal failure.
7. Cerebro-vascular accident.
8. Cardiac failure.

To these should be added the risks, to both mother and child, of operative and/or premature delivery.

MANAGEMENT OF HYPERTENSIVE PREGNANCY
1. Detection
There is no established, practical screening procedure other than good antenatal care. Regular supervision, especially of recognised high risk groups, may be shared between the general practitioner, midwife and obstetrician.

2. Observations
Below are listed the routine observations carried out on patients in whom hypertension has been confirmed. On them are based decisions about treatment. Nowadays many hypertensive patients are assessed on an out-patient basis in a Day Care Unit with only the more severe cases being admitted. Similarly the severity of the condition would determine frequency of these observations.

  a) Serial blood pressure recordings.
  b) Quantitation of proteinuria.
  c) Plasma urate levels.
  d) Platelet counts.
  e) Liver enzymes if b, c or d are abnormal.
  f) Assessment of fetal growth and well-being by kick charts, cardiotocography and ultrasound estimates of fetal weight and liquor volume (see Chapter 6).

HYPERTENSION IN PREGNANCY

3. Treatment

a) Admission to hospital — this is indicated if the diastolic blood pressure remains at 100 mmHg or more. The presence of proteinuria and evidence of fetal compromise are also indications for admission. Many patients with hypertension arising late in pregnancy require no other treatment before delivery. It must always be remembered, however, that the disease can run an unpredictable course and its severity may change very quickly.

b) Hypotensive agents — these may be used in three situations — chronic hypertension, severe pregnancy-induced hypertension and in the treatment of a hypertensive crisis or imminent eclampsia (see below). Many obstetricians are still cautious about such agents in spite of the risks of hypertension because of anxieties about the effects of the drugs on placental perfusion. This is particularly the case when medication is initiated in the mid trimester of pregnancy. Most would favour medication where the mother's diastolic blood pressure remains persistently above 100 mmHg.

   (1) Methyldopa is well established in the treatment of chronic hypertension and its safety in pregnancy is accepted. The usual dosage is 250 mg twice or three times daily.

   (2) Labetalol, a combined alpha and beta blocker, has become a popular drug in this situation. By blocking alpha-adrenoreceptors in peripheral arterioles it reduces peripheral resistance. At the same time the concurrent beta-blockade protects the heart from the reflex sympathetic drive normally induced by peripheral vaso-dilatation. The dosage by mouth is 100–400 mg twice daily. Atenolol may also be used though intra-uterine growth restriction has been reported with the use of beta blockers when employed before the third trimester.

   (3) Nifedipine is a calcium channel blocker and may be used as an alternative to labetalol. It is given orally in a dose of 10 mg three times daily and appears to be safe in late pregnancy.

c) Delivery is the ultimate treatment of hypertensive pregnancy and its timing depends on the observations of fetal and maternal well-being noted above. Prolongation of the pregnancy by drug therapy may reduce the risks of prematurity and improve the chances of vaginal delivery. Epidural block for both analgesia in labour and delivery by caesarean section is excellent providing the platelet count is satisfactory.

SEVERE PRE-ECLAMPSIA AND ECLAMPSIA

The dangers of severe pre-eclampsia and eclampsia have been decribed. If premonitory signs are observed then the woman should be entered into a specific protocol for this situation and all institutions should have such a protocol subject to regular revision.

a) Observations and investigations
Maternal
   i) Blood pressure should be measured every 15–20 minutes (initially using a mercury sphygmomanometer to exclude cases in which automated machines underestimate pressure)
  ii) Oxygen saturation should be monitored continuously
 iii) Urine output measured hourly
  iv) Urea and electrolytes, full blood count, liver function tests and coagulation screen at least every 24 hours and more often as clinically indicated.

Fetal
Ultrasound biophysical assessment
(Fetal maturity and estimate of fetal size if not known.)
Continuous cardiotocography

b) Treatment
   i) Magnesium sulphate reduces the risk of eclampsia by around half in women with pre-eclampsia before delivery or presenting within 24 hours of giving birth. Intravenous access should be established as part of the admission protocol, ideally using the cannula used for obtaining initial blood samples, and 4 g of magnesium sulphate given over 5–10 minutes. This should be followed by a maintenance infusion of 1 g per hour. This should be continued until 24 hours after the last fit or if the deep tendon reflexes are absent (check hourly) or the respiratory rate is 14 per minute or less. Repeat fits may be treated by using further boluses of magnesium sulphate or diazepam.

SEVERE PRE-ECLAMPSIA AND ECLAMPSIA

ii) Hypotensive therapy
Hydralazine, 5 mg over 15 minutes and repeated to a maximum cumulative dose of 20 mg is the approach of choice.
A Labetalol infusion also has a role as a second line agent.

iii) Fluid balance
Fluid overload can readily occur and pulmonary oedema rapidly develop.
Standard fluid regimes should be used and monitored. A CVP line may be required to assess fluid balance and aid management.

iv) Delivery
If the condition is one of severe pre-eclampsia then the timing of delivery will depend on the rate of deterioration of the mother's condition and the maturity of the pregnancy.
If an eclamptic fit has occurred then, if the baby is alive and viable, delivery should be expedited, often by caesarean section. If the cervix is favourable then induction of labour still has a role, particularly in parous women.

v) Depending on the coagulation status consideration should be given to prophylaxis of DVT and even during the assessment period compression stockings should be provided.

COAGULATION FAILURE IN PREGNANCY

Normal haemostasis depends on healthy vasculature, the aggregation of platelets in response to damage to the vascular endothelium and the presence of normal clotting factors in the blood to allow the generation of fibrin to form clot. This system is balanced by the presence of natural anticoagulants such as anti-thrombin III, protein C and protein S, and the fibrinolytic mechanism which removes fibrin and restores vascular patency.

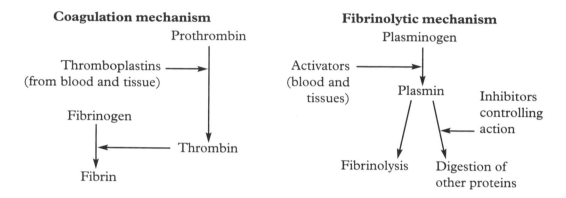

These two mechanisms are normally in a state of dynamic equilibrium. The coagulation mechanism is activated whenever vascular endothelium is breached. Fibrinolysis prevents vascular occlusion as soon as endothelial integrity is restored and removes the fibrin scaffold when no longer required in areas of repair.

In a normal pregnancy there is an increase in some coagulation factors, notably fibrinogen. Fibrin is laid down in the utero-placental vessels and fibrinolysis is suppressed. These changes presumably help to reduce the risk of haemorrhage at delivery.

A deficiency or absence of blood clotting can be brought about by the depletion of fibrinogen and other factors due to the formation of a large blood clot as in abruption of the placenta or multiple small intravascular thrombi (disseminated intravascular coagulation). Often both lesions are present due to the escape of tissue thromboplastins into the blood stream. Additionally excessive production of plasminogen activators can result in the lysis of any clot formed. These usually form two phases of the coagulation defects syndrome. Phase I, depletion of fibrinogen, is always present and, by the nature of the lesion causing it, is apt to initiate the phase of fibrinolysis.

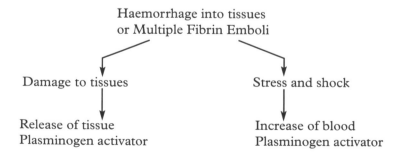

COAGULATION FAILURE IN PREGNANCY

Phase II is particularly liable to occur in pregnancy since activator is present in high concentration in the uterus and lungs.

The position may be summarised as follows:

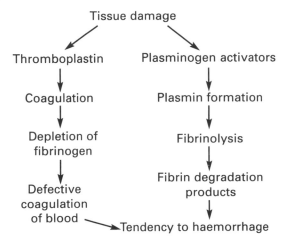

Aetiology
The coagulation failure syndrome is associated mainly with four conditions in pregnancy.

1. **Concealed Accidental Haemorrhage**

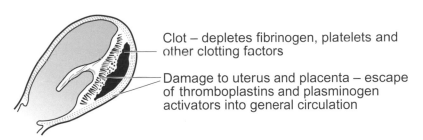

Clot – depletes fibrinogen, platelets and other clotting factors

Damage to uterus and placenta – escape of thromboplastins and plasminogen activators into general circulation

2. **Amniotic fluid embolism** This catastrophic event is often fatal but fortunately rare. The diagnosis may only be made with certainty at post-mortem when emboli of vernix and bundles of squamous cells are identified in pulmonary vessels. It is a complication of artificial rupture of the membranes, Caesarean section and occasionally external version. There is sudden collapse associated with tachycardia, tachypnoea, cyanosis and hypotension. Multiple small emboli lodge in the lungs and venous pulmonary arterial pressures are increased. Multiple small intravascular fibrin clots are formed as well as amniotic emboli. Fibrinolysins are probably released from the damaged lung.
3. **Retention of a dead fetus** A coagulation defect may occur in this condition but only if the dead fetus is retained for at least one month. Thromboplastins causing intravascular thrombi, and plasminogen activators are liberated from the degenerating placenta and fetus.
4. **Septic abortion** The mechanism is similar in this condition, various factors being liberated by the necrotic tissues. The condition is complicated by the presence of infection which may cause a kind of Schwartzmann reaction.

COAGULATION FAILURE IN PREGNANCY

Diagnosis and Treatment

The proper treatment of coagulation defects in pregnancy requires expert haematological guidance. The essential screening tests required are:

Platelets
Partial thromboplastin time
Prothrombin time
Thrombin time
Fibrinogen

Acute hypovolaemia, as in abruption of the placenta, can be treated initially by a gelatine infusion (Haemaccel or Gelofusine) pending the arrival of blood. Whole blood is now virtually unavailable in the United Kingdom and fresh frozen plasma and concentrates of red cells are given. Concentrates of platelets may also be required.

CHAPTER 8

SYSTEMIC DISEASES
IN PREGNANCY

CARDIAC DISEASE

GENERAL CONSIDERATIONS

The obstetric population is generally fit and healthy with a small proportion of women in this age group having pre-existing disease. When there is pre-existing disease the ideal approach would be for the patient to be assessed before pregnancy as described for pre-pregnancy care. Either at this stage, or when pregnancy has occurred, the approach of the obstetrician must be to involve a multidisciplinary team of colleagues. Thus management of conditions such as diabetes, epilepsy or heart disease must involve the expertise of the appropriate physicians.

In considering systemic diseases in pregnancy consideration must be given to two basic issues:

1. The effect of the pregnancy on the disease.
2. The effect of the disease (and its treatment) on the pregnancy.

CARDIAC DISEASE

Between 1997 and 1999 there was a total of 35 deaths as a result of heart disease in pregnancy in the UK. Because of the reduction in the numbers of deaths from other causes, heart disease now equals thromboembolism as one of the leading reported causes of maternal death. Of these deaths, 10 resulted from congenital causes and 25 from acquired disease.

One third of the causes of congenital heart disease contributing to death comprised women with primary pulmonary hypertension. Some of these cases are hereditary and at least one gene responsible for some cases has been identified.

Of the 25 cases of acquired cardiac disease the majority, seven, resulted from puerperal cardiomyopathy. This represents a significant change over the years in the underlying pathology of cardiac disease in pregnancy and its contribution to maternal death.

Further older motherhood and lifestyle habits have led to an increasing number of cases of ischaemic heart disease.

EFFECTS OF PREGNANCY ON HEART DISEASE

The physiological changes in the cardiovascular system have been described in Chapter 2. In summary it can be said that there is an early and sharp rise in cardiac output in the first trimester and a further slower rise to a maximum of 40% above normal in mid-pregnancy. During labour, cardiac output rises even higher during contractions but falls again between contractions. There is a significant rise after delivery when dramatic changes take place in the uterine blood flow due to reduction in flow to the placental bed. This acts almost like a sudden autologous blood transfusion and, in cases of heart disease, may result in considerable myocardial compromise.

The effect of pregnancy on heart disease in general then, is to increase the risk of cardiovascular compromise, most noticeably in labour and the third stage in particular. Cardiac failure may occur gradually, however, throughout pregnancy as the heart fails to meet the demands on the circulation.

Left heart failure, presenting as pulmonary oedema, may present early in pregnancy in those with moderate or severe disease. More commonly acute failure is precipitated when situations such as marked tachycardia of 110 per minute reduce the interval for ventricular filling with resulting pulmonary vascular congestion.

Common aggravating factors are:

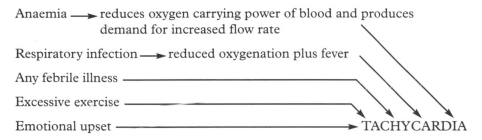

Anaemia ⟶ reduces oxygen carrying power of blood and produces demand for increased flow rate

Respiratory infection ⟶ reduced oxygenation plus fever

Any febrile illness ⟶

Excessive exercise ⟶

Emotional upset ⟶ TACHYCARDIA

In mitral valve disease the third stage and puerperium are particularly dangerous due to the increasing circulatory volume.

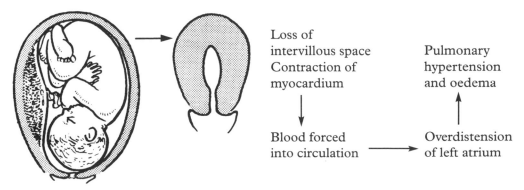

Loss of intervillous space
Contraction of myocardium

↓

Blood forced into circulation ⟶ Overdistension of left atrium

↑

Pulmonary hypertension and oedema

Infective endocarditis is a significant risk indicating the need for antibiotic prophylaxis during labour. Other infections during pregnancy may cause endocarditis and women with cardiac disease who are febrile should be treated with appropriate antibiotics and carefully observed.

EFFECT OF HEART DISEASE ON PREGNANCY

Severe heart disease is associated with preterm labour and with intra-uterine growth restriction. Cyanosis and poor functional capacity are indicators of significant maternal and fetal risk.

PRE-PREGNANCY AND EARLY PREGNANCY ASSESSMENT

a) Pre-pregnancy counselling is important for women with known heart disease. It allows a detailed assessment of their cardiac status and the likely effect of pregnancy on it. Women with certain conditions such as Eisenmenger's syndrome should be told that pregnancy is absolutely contraindicated.

b) A heart murmur may be detected for the first time at the booking antenatal visit. Haemic systolic murmurs are common in pregnancy and the significance of such a finding can be difficult to determine. Careful enquiry should be made for any history which might suggest organic heart disease. Assessment by a cardiologist should be requested.

c) Patients with known heart lesions should be supervised throughout the pregnancy jointly by obstetrician and cardiologist.

TERMINATION AND SURGICAL TREATMENT

Termination of pregnancy is not usually indicated on grounds of cardiac disease alone. Exceptions to this are lesions such as Eisenmenger's syndrome (mortality 30–50%). Fallot's tetralogy also carries a small but appreciable mortality (1%) in corrected cases.

After 12 weeks gestation the risks of termination are as great as continuing the pregnancy.

The decline in the incidence of rheumatic heart disease means that mitral valve disease, and consequently valvotomy, are very rare. Minor lesions such as uncomplicated septal defects and patent ductus arteriosus rarely justify surgical treatment during pregnancy.

ANTENATAL CARE

This is shared between the obstetrician and the cardiologist. The principles are simple: plenty of rest and avoidance of the aggravating factors mentioned earlier.

1. The majority of cardiac patients may be managed as out patients or attend a day care assessment unit. Admission for rest and treatment must be available at any time. Any deterioration in the cardiac state is an indication for admission and expert cardiological opinion.

2. Any infections should be treated vigorously. Smoking should be strongly discouraged and any chest infection managed by admission, antibiotic treatment and physiotherapy.

3. Anaemia should be avoided and, when found, treated appropriately.

4. Good dental care is essential. All dental surgery should be covered with antibiotics to avoid the risk of bacterial endocarditis.

5. Patients with prosthetic cardiac valves or in atrial fibrillation may be receiving anticoagulants. Warfarin is the most appropriate anticoagulant but carries the risk of fetal damage. Conversion to intravenous heparin may be considered for the first trimester although fetal effects of warfarin are not restricted to the first trimester.

HEART DISEASE — LABOUR AND DELIVERY

Most cardiac patients may be allowed to labour. If, however, obstetric factors make the outcome of labour more speculative than normal, planned caesarean section may be the safest choice.

The aim should be to make the labour as easy and non-stressful as possible. Prolonged labour is physically and emotionally draining and increases the risk of infection.

1. Position
The patient should labour in a propped-up, comfortable position. She may maintain this position for delivery, even when this has to be assisted. The lithotomy position should be avoided because of the sudden increase in venous return to the right side of the heart when the legs are raised above the level of the atria.

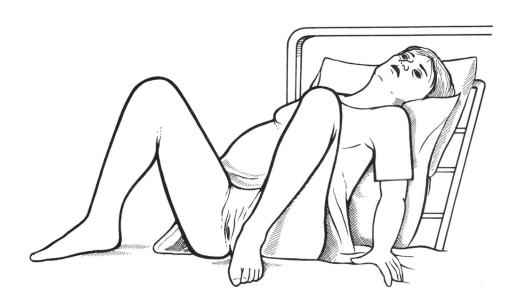

2. Analgesia
Good analgesia is essential in order to avoid the tachycardia associated with labour pain.

Epidural anaesthesia is the method of choice provided hypotension is avoided. This also facilitates operative delivery should this become necessary. Morphine or diamorphine given intramuscularly have much to commend them if an epidural service is not available.

3. Antibiotics
It is now standard practice to give antibiotic prophylaxis to protect against the dangers of bacterial endocarditis in women with structural cardiac lesions. Intra-muscular administration of Ampicillin and Gentamicin is recommended.

HEART DISEASE — LABOUR AND DELIVERY

4. Second Stage

If the second stage proceeds easily and quickly then normal delivery is allowed. Episiotomy should be resorted to if there is delay due to perineal rigidity. The patient should not be required to make substantial expulsive efforts and assisted delivery, by forceps or vacuum extractor, should be used readily. The latter has the advantage of ease of use when the patient is upright.

5. Third Stage

There should be no hurry at this point. Time should be allowed for circulatory adjustment as blood returns from the uterine circulation as the uterus contracts. The risks of atonic post partum haemorrhage must be balanced against the risk of tachycardia and hypotension associated with the use of oxytocin.

In women with severe heart disease a maximum of 5 units of oxytocin should be given over some minutes. In the UK women with such severe disease delivery will often be by caesarean section with a multidisciplinary team in attendance. Delivery by section permits direct uterine compression following delivery if an atonic situation persists following circulatory redistribution of blood.

ACUTE PULMONARY OEDEMA

The patient quickly becomes dyspnoeic and may have frothy sputum or haemoptysis. She should be propped up and if possible, the legs allowed to hang over the edge of the bed. Oxygen should be given by face mask.

Morphine (5–15 mg) may be given intra-muscularly and frusemide (20–40 mg) given intravenously. Venous return can be reduced by applying inflatable cuffs to the limbs. These measures will reduce the need for more invasive techniques. A cardiology opinion should be obtained about further management.

PUERPERIUM

Early ambulation with appropriate rest are advised. Vigilance should be maintained for signs of infection. Pyrexia merits blood cultures.

Counselling about the risks of future pregnancies should be provided.

PERIPARTUM CARDIOMYOPATHY

This condition occurs in the last month of pregnancy or first five months after delivery. The cause is unknown but may be autoimmune or post viral in origin. Its management is largely of cardiac failure and anticoagulants may be required to prevent thrombi forming in the dilated cardiac chambers.

RESPIRATORY DISEASES

ASTHMA

The incidence of asthma in the obstetric population is increasing. The effect of pregnancy on asthma is variable. In most cases the condition is unaffected and the pregnancy proceeds uneventfully.

The patient's usual medication can be maintained. Inhaled sympathomimetics such as Salbutamol remain the mainstay of treatment. Inhaled steroids may be continued if required.

Systemic steroids should be given without hesitation if indicated for acute severe asthma since the dangers of hypoxia to mother and fetus greatly outweigh any disadvantage.

CYSTIC FIBROSIS

Young women with cystic fibrosis (CF) are increasingly entering the reproductive age group due to advances in treatment. Mild or moderate CF is not a contraindication to pregnancy but ideally these women should be seen preconceptionally and respiratory function optimised.

In the presence of pulmonary hypertension risks are increased both for the woman and her fetus.

Treatment is multidisciplinary with attention to adequate nutrition, appropriate antibiotic use and, when required, vigorous physiotherapy.

TUBERCULOSIS

See under infectious disease (p. 155).

VENOUS THROMBO-EMBOLISM

Deaths from thrombo-embolic disease constitute 17% of all maternal mortality in the UK. Thrombo-embolism is said to be five times commoner in pregnancy and puerperium than in non-pregnant women of similar age.

The pathologist Virchow described a triad of causes of venous thrombosis:

1. Changes in the composition of blood.
2. Changes in the rate of blood flow.
3. Lesions of the vascular intima.

In general, **changes in the composition of the blood** play a minor role in venous thrombosis in pregnancy except in situations such as dehydration, as in hyperemesis gravidarum, and in pre-eclampsia, in which the intravascular fluid volume is reduced.

Increasingly the hereditary thrombophilias, such as Protein S and Protein C deficiency and Anti-thrombin III deficiency are being recognised as contributors to ante-natal venous thrombosis.

Changes in Rate of Flow

The rate of flow in the leg veins is much reduced in the later weeks of pregnancy, partly from pressure on the pelvic veins by the gravid uterus, and also from the reduced activity of the woman advanced in pregnancy. Bed-rest in pregnancy for any reason will increase this risk. Early mobilisation after delivery is now invariable.

Changes in Vascular Intima

These can result from hypertensive disease, surgery and local or blood borne infection which can follow any delivery, spontaneous or operative. The risk of thrombo-embolism after caesarean section is 5 times higher than after vaginal delivery.

Sites of thrombus formation:

1. Calf veins (often extending to the popliteal vein).
2. Common femoral vein.
3. Iliofemoral (perhaps extending to the vena cava).
4. Saphenous vein at or above the knee.
5. Superficial thrombosis in varices.

Emboli may come from any of these sites except the last. Unfortunately, in many cases of pulmonary embolism there are no preceding signs of venous thrombosis. Diagnosis of venous thrombosis is difficult and many cases suspected on clinical examination prove normal on investigation.

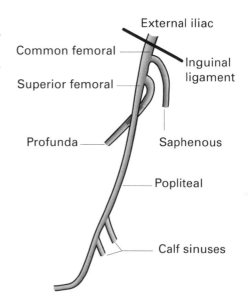

VENOUS THROMBO-EMBOLISM

SUPERFICIAL THROMBO-PHLEBITIS

This is easily diagnosed. There is a reddened, tender superficial vein with a surrounding area of inflammation and oedema. It may be accompanied by a mild pyrexia. As long as the condition remains superficial there is no risk of thrombo-embolism. Conservative management with support stockings should be given. In postnatal cases non-steroidal anti-inflammatory agents can be given with good effect.

DEEP VEIN THROMBOSIS

1. Clinical Features

There may be no complaint, but examination of the legs either as a routine or in search of the cause of a mild pyrexia may reveal signs.

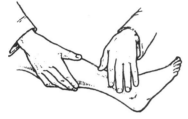

Palpation of the calf demonstrates tenderness and oedema

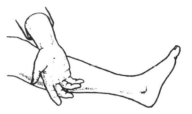

The affected leg may feel warmer to the back of the hand

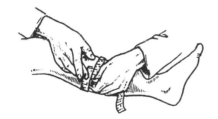

Careful measurement may reveal some swelling compared with the other leg

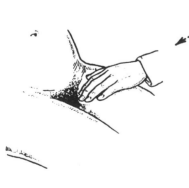

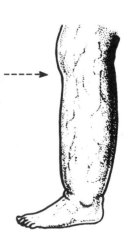

The femoral vein must be palpated in the groin. It may be palpable in the condition known as *Phlegmasia Alba Dolens* (painful white inflammation). This is an old name for an extreme degree of thrombosis which completely blocks the femoral vein, causing solid oedema which does not pit on pressure. The superficial veins give a marbled appearance, but arterial supply is not affected. The condition is very painful and gives rise to what is now called the post-phlebitic syndrome.

133

VENOUS THROMBO-EMBOLISM

2. Complications of thrombosis

a) Pulmonary embolism — this can be mild or severe, isolated or recurrent and in more than 50% of cases is not preceded by clinical signs of thrombosis.

b) Post-phlebitic syndrome — a result of the damage sustained by the vein, in particular, the loss of functioning valves. It includes swelling, varicose veins, eczema, ulceration and is much more severe if the acute condition is not energetically treated.

3. Diagnosis

This is not always easy as the clinical signs are unreliable. Because of the dangers of the condition, the risks of treatment and the implications for the future it is important to establish the diagnosis accurately.

a) Venography

Venography is the most established technique for diagnosis. Unfortunately it relies on the use of X-rays following the injection of a radio-opaque dye. When used in pregnancy the fetus must be shielded from irradiation.

b) Duplex ultrasound

Compression ultrasonography of the deep veins. Repeat testing may be required to identify thrombi extending into the proximal deep veins since it is these which are thought to be clinically significant. The test is easily repeatable and non-invasive.

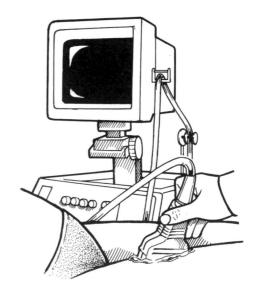

Duplex ultrasound as used for compression studies

VENOUS THROMBO-EMBOLISM

4. Treatment

The dangers of deep vein thrombosis are sufficiently great that treatment with intra-venous heparin should be commenced until the diagnosis is refuted by further investigation. The aim of treatment is to prevent extension of the thrombus and reduce the risk of embolism. In the acute phase treatment is begun with intravenous heparin 24 000 to 40 000 units/day. Maintenance treatment with either subcutaneous heparin or warfarin is required for the remainder of the pregnancy.

As warfarin crosses the placenta, heparin is preferred as it carries no risk to the fetus. If warfarin is used it should be replaced with heparin for the last three weeks of pregnancy to reduce the risk of fetal intra-cranial haemorrhage.

Osteoporosis and thrombocytopenia are complications of prolonged heparin therapy and careful monitoring of heparin levels is required. The former is not common with low molecular weight heparins but platelet levels must be checked regularly in all women receiving heparin.

Anticoagulation can be discontinued during labour and, after delivery, warfarin can be commenced for a period of at least 6 weeks.

5. Prophylaxis

Preventing stasis. Patients with varicose veins should wear full length elasticated stockings. Bed rest should be discouraged both before and after delivery. All puerperal patients should be seen by the physiotherapist. A short post natal stay, if mother and baby are well, should be encouraged.

PULMONARY EMBOLISM

Diagnosis

Neither a chest X-ray nor ECG are immediately diagnostic of pulmonary embolism. Blood gases in which the partial pressure of both oxygen and carbon dioxide are low, strongly suggest an embolism.

In the non-acute situation a ventilation/perfusion scan may be helpful. In severe cases in which surgery may be required, pulmonary angiography is indicated. The role of spiral computed tomography in the evaluation of pulmonary embolism is still being evaluated. These cases should be managed with the aid of physicians with an interest in chest disease.

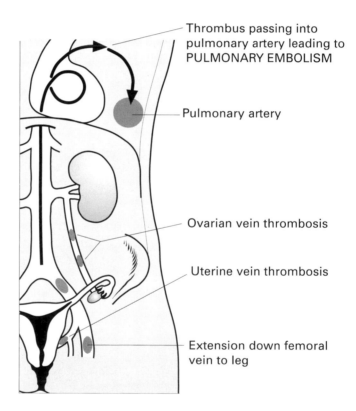

Thrombus passing into pulmonary artery leading to PULMONARY EMBOLISM

Pulmonary artery

Ovarian vein thrombosis

Uterine vein thrombosis

Extension down femoral vein to leg

Treatment

Continuous intravenous heparin, as described earlier, is employed. Admission to an intensive care unit may be advised.

ANAEMIA

Pregnancy makes considerable nutritional demands on the mother. As a consequence anaemia is very common, particularly when consecutive pregnancies are not well spaced. The presence of anaemia increases morbidity in pregnancy, the risk of infection and, should it occur, the hazards of post-partum haemorrhage. The main nutritional factors involved are iron, folic acid and B group vitamins.

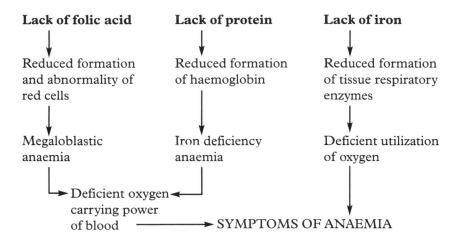

There are two main anaemias seen in pregnancy: iron deficiency causes a hypochromic, microcytic anaemia and folic acid deficiency is associated with megaloblastic anaemia. In obstetric practice most cases involve a combined anaemia although the haematological features may be more typical for one than the other. Automated assays for serum iron, ferritin, folic acid and vitamin B12 levels have made investigation of anaemia in pregnancy more rapid and allow correction of haematinic deficiency early in pregnancy.

Haematinic deficiency may result from:

1. Diminished intake.
2. Abnormal absorption.
3. Reduced storage.
4. Abnormal utilisation.
5. Abnormal demand.

The aetiology of anaemia must be considered in relation to these principles.

The average UK diet just meets the daily requirement for iron in women who are regularly menstruating. Heavy periods and the demands of pregnancy readily lead to anaemia. The increased demands for iron amount to 1000 mg.

ANAEMIA

Factors operating to cause anaemia in pregnancy

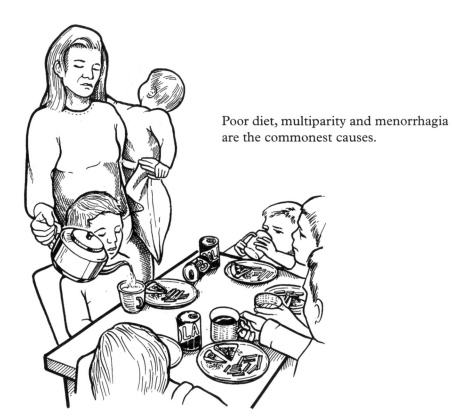

Poor diet, multiparity and menorrhagia are the commonest causes.

Symptoms

Since lethargy and tiredness are common in pregnancy, many women will consider these as normal and make no complaint suggestive of anaemia.

Peripheral vasodilatation makes pallor less common and clinical diagnosis difficult.

Regular measurement of haemoglobin reduces the risk of a woman entering labour in an anaemic state.

IRON DEFICIENCY

Blood changes in pregnancy

These have already been discussed and the effect of haemodilution on haemoglobin levels is important. Nevertheless it is desirable that women at term have a haemoglobin level of 110 g/l or greater.

Diagnosis

Blood films will show hypochromic microcytosis. Automated blood counting will give low values for mean red cell volume and mean red cell haemoglobin. The serum iron and ferritin will be reduced.

Treatment

Oral iron is the treatment of choice. In many UK centres prophylaxis against anaemia in pregnancy is given in the form of preparations of 100 mg elemental iron with 400 micrograms of folic acid daily.

In these circumstances, anaemia is usually associated with failure to take the preparation. This may be simply poor compliance, or poor absorption, because of nausea and vomiting.

Failure to respond to treatment requires further evaluation.

When oral iron is not suitable, for whatever reason, then intramuscular iron sorbitol may be given by intramuscular injection.

Total dose intravenous infusions of iron, once popular for poorly compliant multiparae, are no longer advocated because of the high incidence of anaphylaxis.

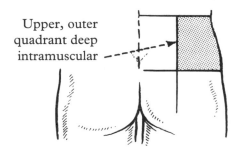

Upper, outer quadrant deep intramuscular

Severe anaemia near to estimated time of delivery

Up to the 35th week parenteral iron may be given. After this the uncertainty of the time of delivery and the possibility of preterm labour may require transfusion to be given in severely anaemic and symptomatic women. Packed red cells should be given slowly and may be given in stages. The oxygen carrying capacity of transfused red cells is low for the first 24 hours following transfusion and it is important to remember that the red cells are being given to prevent complications of blood loss at the time of delivery.

In less severe cases blood should be available during labour and transfused at or after delivery depending on the clinical condition.

FOLIC ACID DEFICIENCY

Folic acid is necessary for nucleic acid formation and inadequate levels leads to a reduction in cell proliferation. The main effects are seen in tissues which rapidly proliferate such as the bone marrow.

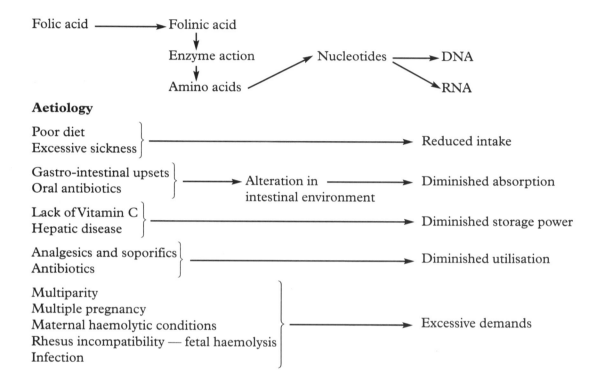

Aetiology

Poor diet
Excessive sickness } ⟶ Reduced intake

Gastro-intestinal upsets
Oral antibiotics } ⟶ Alteration in intestinal environment ⟶ Diminished absorption

Lack of Vitamin C
Hepatic disease } ⟶ Diminished storage power

Analgesics and soporifics
Antibiotics } ⟶ Diminished utilisation

Multiparity
Multiple pregnancy
Maternal haemolytic conditions
Rhesus incompatibility — fetal haemolysis
Infection } ⟶ Excessive demands

Clinical Findings

These depend on the severity of the deficiency. There may be no symptoms and only moderately low haemoglobin. Folic acid deficiency and iron deficiency often co-exist and iron treatment given alone will only increase haemoglobin levels slightly.

FOLIC ACID DEFICIENCY

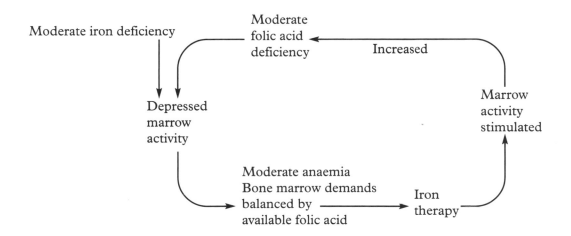

Severe folic acid deficiency is now less common than formerly. The use of folic acid prophylaxis for prevention of neural tube defects reduces the risk of anaemia in pregnancy. Unfortunately those most likely to take prophylaxis are not the population at greatest risk of dietary deficiency.

Consequently folic acid is now often prescribed in a combined preparation with iron and given throughout pregnancy.

When severe cases do present, the features may co-exist with other signs of nutritional deficiency such as glossitis.

Laboratory Diagnosis
Automated testing will reveal macrocytosis and these cells may be hypochromic. A blood film will occasionally show megaloblasts. Hypersegmentation of the neutrophils may be seen.

Treatment
Established deficiency should be treated with oral folic acid 5 mg three times daily throughout pregnancy.

Vitamin B12 deficiency is exceedingly rare in pregnancy as pernicious anaemia causes infertility.

HAEMOGLOBINOPATHIES AND IDIOPATHIC THROMBOCYTOPENIA

HAEMOGLOBINOPATHIES

The haemoglobinopathies are a group of genetic disorders of globin synthesis.

Heterozygotes for haemoglobinopathies may be mildly affected but homozygotes may be severely anaemic.

The two common haemoglobinopathies in the UK are becoming commoner because of immigration. Sickle cell disease is seen in the African and Afro-Caribbean communities and Thalassaemia in those from the Mediterranean and Far East. In these populations haemoglobin electrophoresis may be offered at the booking visit.

In homozygous sickle cell disease there is chronic anaemia and increased risk of haemolytic crises.

Alpha thalassaemia is less common and, in the homozygous form, lethal in utero.

Homozygous beta thalassaemia causes death in childhood but the heterozygous form causes chronic anaemia and may only be diagnosed in pregnancy. Folic acid should be given but iron is not required.

Women who are heterozygotes for a haemoglobinopathy should be offered screening of their partner to determine the chance of an affected fetus. Chorion villus sampling or amniocentesis can be used to establish the diagnosis in the fetus.

IDIOPATHIC THROMBOCYTOPENIA

Idiopathic, or immune thrombocytopenic purpura (ITP) is commoner in women and in those below 30 years. It is not rare in the obstetric population. The presence of antiplatelet IgG causes a reduction in both maternal and fetal platelets.

Treatment, if required, is by glucocorticoids. The risk to the fetus is difficult to assess but neonatal handicap from intra-uterine intra-cranial haemorrhage has been reported. Many obstetricians advocate elective Caesarean section for these women to reduce this risk.

Intravenous gammaglobulin may be given to the mother some days before delivery as this transiently increases platelet counts.

DIABETES

Pregnancy is a diabetogenic state

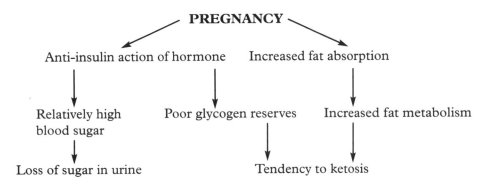

These effects will aggravate established clinical diabetes and may reveal impaired glucose tolerance.

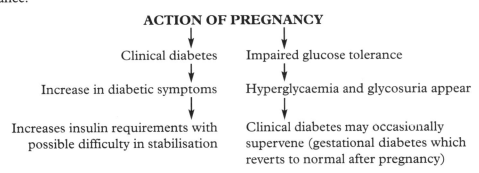

The World Health Organisation reviews diagnostic criteria for the diagnosis of diabetes and impaired glucose tolerance using a 75 g glucose tolerance test.

	Venous Plasma Glucose (mmol/l)	
	Fasting	2 h Post-glucose
Impaired Glucose Tolerance	<7.0	7.8–11.1
Diabetes	>7.0	>11.1

Criteria are subject to revision: see http://www.who.int/home-page/

DIABETES

The implications of maternal diabetes are such that some authorities recommend checking random blood sugar levels at booking and 28 weeks. This may identify those requiring a full glucose tolerance test (GTT). Others recommend GTTs on high risk groups.

A widely accepted list of indications is:

1. Two or more episodes of glycosuria on routine testing.
2. Diabetes in a first degree relative.
3. Maternal weight of greater than 85 kg.
4. Previous baby of 4.5 kg or more.
5. Previous unexplained perinatal death.
6. Previous congenital abnormality.
7. Polyhydramnios.

Effect of Pregnancy on Diabetes
1. Control is more difficult with the rise in insulin requirements.
2. Diabetic nephropathy appears to be largely unaffected by pregnancy. Untreated retinopathy significantly worsens. Treatment by laser photocoagulation is safe in pregnancy. Pre-existing treated retinopathy is not usually a significant problem.

Effect of Diabetes on Pregnancy
1. Increased miscarriage rate.
2. Increased perinatal loss. There is a higher incidence of abnormality in the offspring of diabetics and this reflects the quality of glycaemic control around conception and during organogenesis. The increased risk of intra-uterine death from metabolic upset in the last few weeks of pregnancy has long dictated delivery at 36–37 weeks though good control may allow continuation beyond this.
3. Macrosomia. Infants of diabetic mothers tend to be macrosomic and are at risk of dystocia.
4. Fetal lung maturation may be delayed.
5. Increased risk of pregnancy complications:
   Pre-eclampsia.
   Polyhydramnios.
   Infections, notably urinary tract infection and candidal vaginitis.

All of the adverse effects of diabetes may be reduced by good diabetic control from conception onwards.

MANAGEMENT OF PREGNANCY
1. Pre-pregnancy
General practitioners and physicians should take every opportunity to advise diabetic women about the importance of good control even before conception. Glycosylated haemoglobins, HbA1c, in particular, reflect control over the previous ten weeks. High levels of HbA1c are associated with an increased rate of fetal abnormality.

DIABETES

2. Pregnancy

Supervision should be shared between obstetrician and diabetic physician. If control is not adequate then admission for stabilisation should be arranged. Blood sugar profiles, in which levels are checked before each meal and at 21.30 hours, should be obtained. Blood sugar levels of less than 8 mmol/l should be maintained with a mixture of short and medium acting insulins. The frequency of administration may be increased.

Home blood level monitoring is now widely available. Urine testing for glucose is of no value in pregnancy.

Regular assessment of fetal growth and wellbeing, screening for retinopathy and HbA1c levels should be performed. The frequency of monitoring increases with gestation.

Admission to hospital in the last 4 weeks is indicated if frequent day care assessment is not possible.

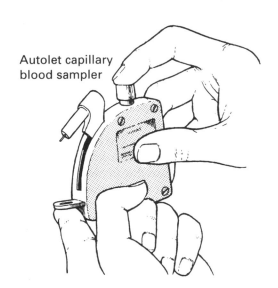

Autolet capillary blood sampler

LABOUR AND DELIVERY

Delivery at 38–40 weeks is possible if sugar control is good and there are no other complications. Tests for fetal lung maturity are only indicated if gestational age is uncertain.

The intention is to achieve vaginal delivery. On the day of planned induction the morning dose of insulin is omitted. A dextrose infusion is set up with 5 units of insulin per 500 ml. Alternatively insulin can be given by controlled infusion pump. Blood sugar and potassium levels should be measured 2 hourly.

Artificial rupture of the membranes is performed and syntocinon commenced if uterine activity does not become established.

Caesarean section should be performed for standard obstetric indications.

Epidural anaesthesia is ideal, both for labour and if section is required.

Following delivery, insulin requirements reduce quickly and the pre-pregnancy dose may be begun the day after delivery if the patient is eating.

BABY

Macrosomia is common, though reduced with good control. Fetal islet cell hyperplasia is common and the neonate must be observed for signs of hypoglycaemia. Blood sugar levels should be checked regularly in the neonate.

URINARY TRACT INFECTION

Pregnancy predisposes to urinary tract infection through increased urinary stasis.

Progesterone reduces tone in the ureters and these become dilated. With the mechanical effect of uterine pressure on the ureters at the pelvic brim, the risk of stasis and infection are increased.

The risk of cystitis proceeding to pyelonephritis is greater and the commonest pathogens are *E. coli*, Proteus species, bacteroides and the enterococci.

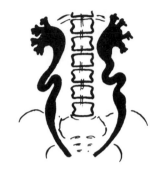

Pyelogram in pregnancy

Bacterial Counts in Urine

A mid stream specimen of urine (MSU) always contains some contaminating organisms but levels of 100 000 per ml, or greater, indicate infection.

A variety of proprietary culture systems are available and allow bacterial count to be obtained on the basis of the number of colonies counted on a slide.

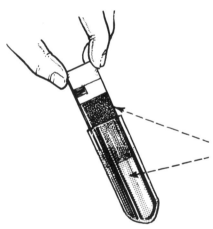

Techniques of counting

Various methods are used to provide a simple screening test. The 'Uricult' system uses a slide coated with agar which is dipped into the fresh urine, cultured overnight and read the next day.

Asymptomatic Bacteriuria

About 6–7% of asymptomatic women attending a booking antenatal clinic have infected urine. These women have increased risk of developing clinical pyelonephritis in pregnancy. Screening all women at booking allows identification of this high risk group. Around 10% of women with asymptomatic bacteriuria will have a renal tract abnormality on intravenous pyelography.

URINARY TRACT INFECTION

Clinical Features
These are variable and often vague.

1. Dysuria.
2. Fever and tachycardia.
3. Loin pain. This is diagnostic and tenderness may be elicited over one or both kidneys.
4. Abdominal pain, often in the lower abdomen and probably reflecting ureteric inflammation.
5. Nausea and vomiting. This can be sufficiently severe to cause dehydration.

Laboratory Investigations
A mid stream specimen of urine must be collected. Vaginal swabs may be obtained at the same time.

Differential Diagnosis
Premature labour. Placental abruption.
Appendicitis.
Cholecystitis (rare).

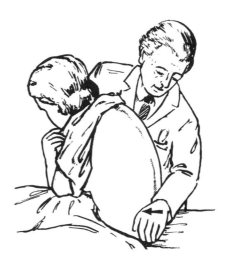

To elicit loin tenderness, first palpate the spine gently to accustom the patient to the touch, then tap gently with the thenar eminence over the loin. If positive, the patient gives an unmistakeable wince.

Treatment
The patient should be admitted to hospital and, if dehydrated, intravenous fluids commenced. A high fluid intake should be encouraged, if possible. A broad spectrum antibiotic, such as cephradine, may be given while awaiting culture results. Analgesia should be prescribed as appropriate and treatment continued for 7 days. The urine should be re-checked to confirm that it is negative on culture.

Patients developing pyelonephritis should provide mid stream specimens for culture at every subsequent attendance.

Repeated infection requires renal tract investigation three months after delivery.

CHRONIC RENAL DISEASE/EPILEPSY

CHRONIC RENAL DISEASE

Chronic pyelonephritis and chronic glomerulonephritis both increase perinatal mortality and morbidity. Hypertension, if not already present, usually develops and intra-uterine growth restriction is common.

In severe renal disease infertility often results. Should pregnancy occur then termination may be indicated on medical grounds.

Renal transplantation may restore fertility in women with severe disease and they should be counselled about contraception. Successful pregnancy is possible but pre-eclampsia is common and careful supervision by both the obstetrician and renal physician is required.

EPILEPSY

Women with epilepsy should be strongly advised to seek pre-pregnancy counselling.

In women who have been fit-free for 2–3 years it may be possible to discontinue treatment since all anticonvulsants are teratogenic.

Women with idiopathic epilepsy have increased rates of fetal abnormality even when not receiving treatment. Anticonvulsants increase this risk further so that the incidence of abnormality is 4–6% and this group of women should be offered detailed ultrasound examination of the fetus.

Phenytoin, carbamazepine and sodium valproate are all associated with severe fetal abnormalities.

These drugs also alter fetal vitamin K metabolism and increase the risk of haemorrhagic disease of the new-born. Vitamin K should be given to women taking these agents from around 35 weeks gestation.

Pregnancy does not have any constant effect on the clinical course of epilepsy but there is an increased incidence (2.5%) of epilepsy in offspring.

JAUNDICE

Jaundice is uncommon in pregnancy.

Aetiology
a) Pregnancy jaundice
1. Acute fatty liver.
2. Cholestatic jaundice.
3. Complicating pre-eclampsia (such as HELLP syndrome — Haemolysis, Elevated Liver enzymes, Low Platelets).
b) Intercurrent jaundice
1. Viral hepatitis.
2. Obstructive jaundice.
c) Iatrogenic jaundice
1. Hepatotoxic drugs.
2. Drugs interfering with bilirubin conjugation.
3. Drugs causing haemolysis.

The most common causes of jaundice are
1. Viral hepatitis (41%).
2. Cholestatic jaundice (21%).
3. Obstructive jaundice (less than 6%).

VIRAL HEPATITIS
See section on infectious diseases, p. 155.

CHOLESTATIC JAUNDICE OF PREGNANCY
Intrahepatic cholestasis is characterised by pruritus and mild jaundice, usually in late pregnancy. There is a significant variation in prevalence world-wide.

Serum bile acids are elevated. The effects on pregnancy are greater than once thought; preterm labour and intra-uterine death are recognised complications.

There is a high recurrence rate and, if previously associated with poor outcome, is an indication for close fetal surveillance.

JAUNDICE

ACUTE FATTY LIVER OF PREGNANCY
This is a rare but usually fatal disease in which the liver cells are filled by lipid vacuoles.

The presentation is with severe nausea and vomiting, abdominal pain, jaundice and haematemesis. Coagulopathy may develop. Treatment is by delivery and management of complications such as renal failure, by standard methods.

The differential diagnosis includes severe pre-eclampsia but the jaundice is more usually of the haemolytic type.

GALL-STONES
Jaundice due to gall-stones is rare in pregnancy. Treatment is as for the non-pregnant.

BIOCHEMISTRY OF JAUNDICE IN PREGNANCY

	Serum Bilirubin	Serum Transaminases	Alkaline Phosphatase
Viral Hepatitis	Increased	Very high	Slightly increased
Cholestatic Jaundice	Increased conjugated Bilirubin	Normal Occasionally high	Increased
Acute Fatty Liver	Increased	Moderate increase	Moderate increase
Gall-stones	Increased conjugated Bilirubin	Normal	Increased

OTHERS
Jaundice may occur in pregnancy for other reasons such as drug-induced cases, either by causing haemolysis or cholestasis. Hereditary jaundice such as Dubin Johnson syndrome and Rotor syndrome may be identified for the first time in pregnancy.

THYROID DISEASE

Infertility is a common consequence of thyroid dysfunction and overt disease is uncommon.

HYPERTHYROIDISM

Diagnosis of hyperthyroidism developing during pregnancy is difficult as many of the features, e.g. tachycardia, goitre and peripheral vasodilatation, are common in normal pregnancy. A severe anxiety state may also be the presenting feature. This may be disproportionate to the clinical picture and suggest a psychological problem. Thyroid function should be checked in such women.

Diagnosis depends on biochemical investigation of free thyroxine, free T3 and TSH levels.

Treatment

Carbimazole and propylthiouracil are the mainstays of treatment although, rarely, surgery may be required. These drugs can result in fetal goitre.

Propylthiouracil is theoretically preferable due to reduced placental transfer.

Antithyroid antibodies can also cross the placenta and cause fetal goitre and exophthalmos. The former may, rarely, cause an abnormal presenting part in labour, i.e. brow presentation. The baby should be examined carefully after birth. The baby's thyroid function should be checked.

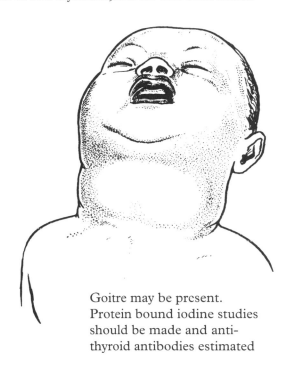

Goitre may be present. Protein bound iodine studies should be made and anti-thyroid antibodies estimated

HYPOTHYROIDISM

The obstetrician is more likely to meet a woman currently being treated rather than a new presentation in pregnancy.

Thyroxine will be required and dosage may need to be increased as pregnancy advances. In a proportion of women, thyroid growth in pregnancy is sufficient to meet needs and treatment may be stopped.

INFECTIONS

1. SEXUALLY TRANSMITTED DISEASES

a) Syphilis

Infection of the fetus with syphilis causes miscarriage, stillbirth or delivery of a baby with the stigmata of congenital syphilis.

All women should be screened pre-natally for syphilis. The tests used include VDRL (Venereal Disease Reference Laboratory) test and Rapid Plasma Reagin (RPR) which are non-specific together with the TPHA (Treponema Pallidum Haemagglutinating Antibody) test and the FTA-ABS (Fluorescent Treponemal Antibody Absorption) test. The last is the most sensitive and becomes positive early in primary syphilis and remains so. The presence of IgM in this test indicates recent infection.

The VDRL test is non-specific and the majority of abnormal results are biological false positives. The Lupus Inhibitor syndrome, one of the anti-cardiolipin syndromes and a cause of recurrent miscarriage and IUGR, may be associated with a false positive result.

Clinical Signs

These are rarely seen in the UK. The primary chancre is usually seen on the labia and there may be condylomata lata around the vulva and anus. There is usually inguinal lymphadenopathy.

Treatment

Procaine penicillin may be given daily for two weeks. When there is poor compliance then benzathine penicillin may be given weekly for three weeks. First doses should be given under supervision as the Jarisch Herxheimer reaction may occur.

Contact tracing is essential and the child should be followed up after delivery.

In subsequent pregnancies many authorities would repeat the treatment.

b) Gonorrhoea

Symptoms

These may be slight or unnoticed in the female. Postnatal salpingitis may occur with considerable tubal damage.

Babies become infected during delivery and may develop gonococcal ophthalmia. This should be treated.

Diagnosis

Swabs should be cultured from the cervix, urethra and rectum. Chlamydial swabs should be taken concurrently.

Treatment

Third generation cephalosporins, penicillin or erythromycin may be given subject to local antibiotic sensitivities

The baby's eyes should be swabbed and treatment commenced.

Contact tracing should also be provided. The aid of genito-urinary medicine physicians is invaluable.

INFECTIONS

c) HIV Infection

World wide 34 million people have acquired Human Immunodeficiency Virus type 1 and each year two million are women who become pregnant. Of the 1.3 million children currently infected the majority will die before their teenage years. Thus the priorities in the care of pregnant women with HIV are:

1. Maintenance of good general health and treatment of intercurrent infection including sexually transmitted diseases.
2. Antibiotic prophylaxis for women with low CD4 counts.
3. Prevention of vertical transmission. This can be achieved by three principal approaches:

a) Antiretroviral treatment. Treatment antenatally, either in long course or short course protocols reduces transmission. Zidovudine and nevirapine both reduce vertical transmission when given antenatally and post partum to the baby. Short course treatment is especially important in developing countries with limited resources.

b) Delivery by caesarean section. In the European setting, delivery by caesarean section reduces infant infection to 1.8% from the 10.5% rate seen in vaginally delivered babies.

c) Avoidance of breastfeeding. Transmission through breast milk is associated with a doubling of infection rates. In developing countries this may be impossible.

If a woman chooses to deliver vaginally and fetal monitoring is required then non-invasive suction electrodes permit cardiotocography.

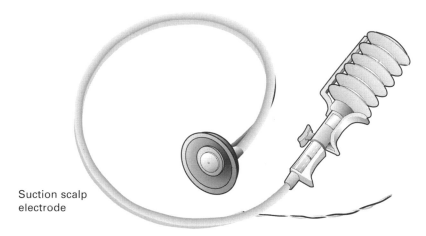

Suction scalp
electrode

2. FETOTOXIC INFECTIONS

a) Toxoplasmosis

There are around 50 cases of severe congenital toxoplasmosis annually in the UK. These cases result from maternal ingestion of this parasite, usually through undercooked meats and unpasteurised dairy products. Miscarriage, intrauterine death, growth restriction, hydrocephalus, neurological disability and retinitis may all result. Diagnosis is by observing seroconversion in the mother. Termination of the pregnancy may be offered. If the pregnancy is to continue, spiramycin daily may reduce the degree of disability. In cases where fetal infection is confirmed by ultrasound scan or by identifying the parasite in amniotic fluid more aggressive treatment with sulphadiazine and pyrimethamine can be used.

INFECTIONS

b) Rubella

The dangers of rubella infection are now well recognised. Cardiovascular abnormalities, cataract and deafness are the main lesions resulting from infection in early pregnancy. The risk of damage is greatest in the first trimester though infection later can cause mental and physical handicap. The introduction of Measles, Mumps, Rubella (MMR) vaccination in early childhood will reduce the need for this although current uptake rates are worryingly low.

85% of the population are immune but non-immune women who give a history of possible exposure should have serial testing to identify seroconversion. Where infection is confirmed, termination is commonly offered.

c) Cytomegalovirus

This is a common infection which is usually sub-clinical. Miscarriage, stillbirth, growth restriction, microcephaly and cerebral palsy may result. Intra-uterine infection is usually transplacental but can result during birth. Two thirds of infected women do not transmit the virus to the fetus and the majority of infected neonates do not develop features of the disease. Molecular analysis of amniotic fluid may identify fetal infection after 21 weeks.

Unfortunately there are no techniques which determine if the fetus of an infected mother is likely to be damaged making counselling difficult.

d) Herpes Simplex

This is a common infection in the female genital tract. Primary infection causes small ulcerating lesions around the vulva and perineum which are intensely painful and may cause urinary retention. Vaginal delivery in the presence of active herpetic lesions carries significant risk of neonatal infection. The consequences can be devastating and caesarean section is advocated in the presence of active lesions. It may be possible to allow vaginal delivery in women treated for the last four weeks of pregnancy using aciclovir but data are preliminary.

e) Parvovirus

Parvovirus B 19 is now recognised as causing aplastic crises in utero. Hydrops fetalis may result and frequent ultrasound assessment is indicated. Treatment of the fetus by intrauterine transfusion may be life saving.

f) Varicella (Chickenpox)

Maternal chickenpox is not common but may be more severe in adult life and fatal pneumonia is a well recognised risk.

The commonest problem with regard to varicella in pregnancy is when there is a history of recent exposure and uncertainty regarding the woman's immunity. Significant exposure of a non-immune woman means face to face contact with a case for five or more minutes or contact indoors for more than fifteen minutes. Antibody levels can quickly be checked and immunity confirmed. Any non-immune women should receive varicella zoster immune globulin.

INFECTIONS

Nevertheless some cases of infection occur in pregnancy and in the first trimester carries a 0.4% chance of fetal varicella syndrome and between 13 and 20 weeks a 2% chance of the condition. Aciclovir may be used during pregnancy and may reduce the incidence of fetal varicella syndrome which causes eye defects and limb hypoplasias as well as neurological impairment.

OTHER INFECTIONS

a) Group B Streptococcus (GBS)

GBS is a common vaginal organism and may be isolated from the vagina in around 15–20% of the population. GBS is implicated in preterm labour and in urinary tract infection. The significance to the fetus is that 1–2% of neonates of infected women will themselves become infected. In the early onset form of the disease this causes pneumonia, septicaemia and meningitis. This carries a 30–50% mortality.

Identification of GBS in low vaginal swabs at any time in a woman's life indicates the need for treatment during labour, and supervision of the neonate with antibiotics being given until bacteriological swabs from the baby are negative.

b) Viral Hepatitis

Hepatitis B and C may present in pregnancy but more commonly the clinician will be presented with a woman with a history of previous disease. The infant of a woman of high infectivity for Hepatitis B should receive a full course of immunisation to prevent later cirrhosis or hepatic cancer. There is no vaccine for the C virus and the long term outcome remains uncertain.

c) Malaria

Malaria may account world wide for 10% of all maternal deaths, usually resulting from anaemia. In chronic situations miscarriage, preterm birth and IUGR occur.

The acute maternal disease may result in cerebral malaria, hypoglycaemia, pulmonary oedema and coma.

Treatment options are determined by local sensitivities since chloroquine resistance is now common. Travellers to malarial areas should be advised about avoiding exposure and seek the latest advice about effective prophylaxis in the region they are visiting. Immigrants to Europe who revisit their home countries are a particular risk group since the interval from their last exposure may lead to reduced immunity.

d) Tuberculosis (TB)

This is uncommon but due to immigration and co-infection with HIV may become more frequently seen. TB causes miscarriage, preterm labour and growth problems in the newborn. Fetal infection is extremely rare but newborns of infected mothers should receive chemoprophylaxis.

Isoniazid and rifampicin remain the mainstay of treatment but drug resistance means that management should be coordinated with a specialist in infectious diseases.

MANAGEMENT OF THERAPEUTIC DRUG EXPOSURE IN PREGNANCY

When considering systemic medical disorder in pregnancy the potential for teratogenesis should be carefully considered.

When women have, or may have been, exposed to drugs in pregnancy it is important to determine if this may have an adverse effect on fetal development. Key points in the management plan are:

1. Has exposure actually occurred during pregnancy? When an adequate history, examination and ultrasound examination have been obtained a number of women will be identified who have not been exposed.
2. Are the drugs actually teratogenic?
3. Was exposure during or beyond the stage of organogenesis?
4. Is prenatal diagnosis possible?

These may be summarised thus:

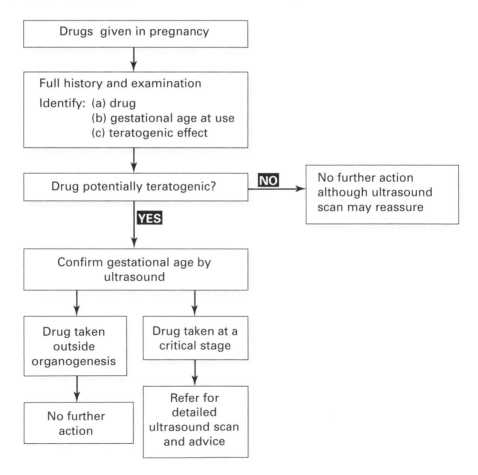

ACUTE ABDOMINAL CONDITIONS

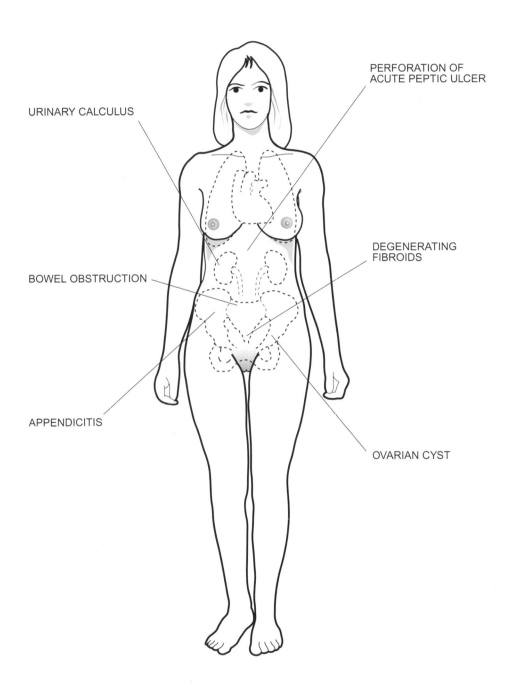

PERFORATION OF
ACUTE PEPTIC ULCER

URINARY CALCULUS

DEGENERATING
FIBROIDS

BOWEL OBSTRUCTION

APPENDICITIS

OVARIAN CYST

ACUTE ABDOMINAL CONDITIONS

BOWEL OBSTRUCTION

Usually caused by adhesion bands altering in position with the rising uterus, but volvulus is sometimes found. Colic, distension, vomiting, diminished or absent bowel sounds are signs that laparotomy is required.

APPENDICITIS

The point of maximum tenderness is higher in pregnancy, and the high steroid levels will reduce the usual response to inflammation. There is usually sickness and, if doubt persists after a period of observation, laparatomy should be carried out. If pus is present, wound drainage should be continued for at least a week. Acute pyelonephritis may present much the same clinical picture, but loin tenderness and urine findings help in diagnosis.

URINARY CALCULUS

This causes acute pain radiating to the groin and haematuria is present. Treatment is conservative unless hydronephrosis develops and ureteric drainage is required.

DEGENERATING FIBROIDS

Necrobiosis causes pain, vomiting, tenderness and pyrexia, and diagnosis is difficult. The condition should settle with rest and sedation, and operation is only likely to be indicated when there is torsion of the pedicle of a fibroid.

PERFORATION OF ACUTE PEPTIC ULCER

This is very rare in pregnancy because of the high steroid level. The clinical appearances in the early months are unmistakably of perforation, but are less clear in the 3rd trimester. There is little rigidity, but shock is marked and air may be shown by X-ray, under the diaphragm.

OVARIAN CYST

Torsion of the pedicle causes acute pain, tenderness, vomiting and often pyrexia. Under anaesthesia a mass separate from the uterus may be distinguished, and laparotomy must be performed.

Laparotomy for these conditions may induce miscarriage or labour, although removal of an ovarian cyst is usually safe enough in this circumstance.

Caesarean section is not advisable in the presence of intra-abdominal infection. In late pregnancy however delivery by section may be indicated if laparotomy is needed since requiring a recently post operative patient to sustain a labour may be inappropriate.

CHAPTER 9

VAGINAL BLEEDING IN PREGNANCY

SUMMARY OF CAUSES

ECTOPIC PREGNANCY

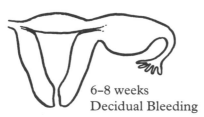

6–8 weeks
Decidual Bleeding

MISCARRIAGE
Usually before
16 weeks

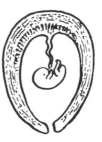

HYDATIDIFORM MOLE
Usually before 16 weeks

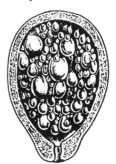

ANTE-PARTUM HAEMORRHAGE
After 24 weeks

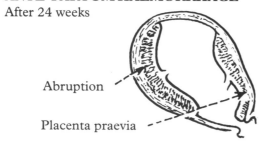

Abruption

Placenta praevia

Placental abnormalities

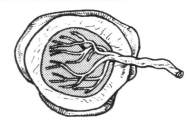

INTRA-PARTUM HAEMORRHAGE

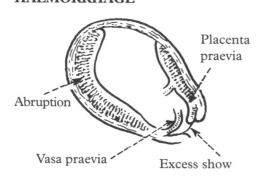

Abruption

Vasa praevia

Placenta praevia

Excess show

INCIDENTAL CAUSES

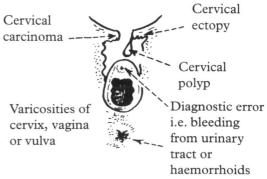

Cervical carcinoma

Cervical ectopy

Cervical polyp

Varicosities of cervix, vagina or vulva

Diagnostic error i.e. bleeding from urinary tract or haemorrhoids

May present at any stage of pregnancy

ECTOPIC PREGNANCY

Ectopic pregnancy is one in which the products of conception develop outside the uterine cavity. By far the commonest site is the fallopian tube.

The fallopian tube is about 10 cm long. The diameter of the lumen varies from 1 mm in the interstitial portion to about 5 mm at the fimbriated end.

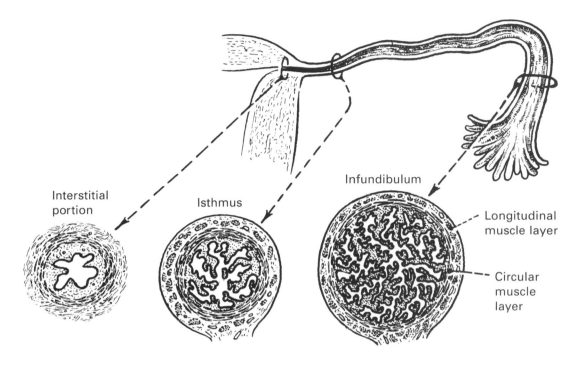

The musculature is of two layers, an inner circular and an outer longitudinal, and peristaltic movements are particularly strong during and after ovulation. The mucosa is arranged in plications or folds which become much more complete and plentiful as the infundibulum is approached.

The mucosa consists of a single layer of ciliated and secretory cells, resting on a thin basement membrane. There is little or no submucosa and no decidual reaction, so muscle is easily invaded by trophoblast.

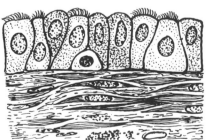

TUBAL PREGNANCY — AETIOLOGY

Ectopic implantation may be fortuitous or the result of a tubal abnormality which obstructs or delays the passage of the fertilised ovum.

1. Preceding tubal or pelvic inflammation with residual endothelial damage or distortion by adhesions.

2. Previous tubal surgery e.g. attempted sterilisation, reversal of sterilisation or salpingostomy.

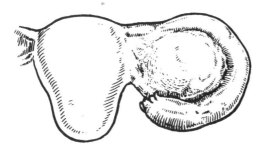

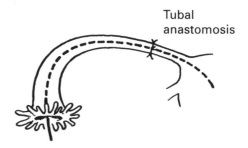

Tubal anastomosis

3. Intra-uterine contraceptive device (IUCD).

Women who conceive with an IUCD in situ have an increased risk of ectopic pregnancy. This may be due to infection or an effect on tubal motility.

4. Congenital abnormality of the tube such as hypoplasia, elongation or diverticulum.

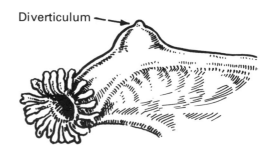

Diverticulum

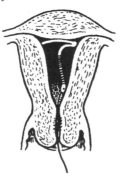

5. Migration of ovum across the pelvic cavity to the fallopian tube on the side opposite to the follicle from which ovulation occurred.

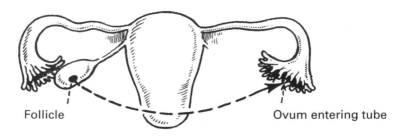

Follicle   Ovum entering tube

TUBAL PREGNANCY — IMPLANTATION

Because there is no decidual membrane in tubal mucosa, and no submucosa, the ovum rapidly burrows through the mucosa and embeds in the muscular wall of the tube, opening up maternal blood vessels and causing necrosis of muscle and connective tissue cells.

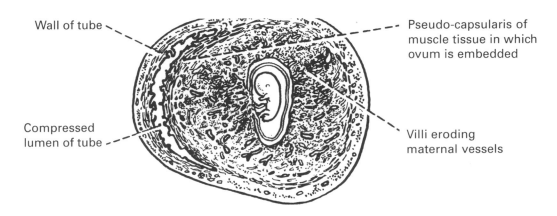

Wall of tube

Pseudo-capsularis of muscle tissue in which ovum is embedded

Compressed lumen of tube

Villi eroding maternal vessels

The ampulla is the commonest site of implantation, followed by the isthmus.

Interstitial implantation is rare but very dangerous because it ends in rupture of the uterine muscle with severe haemorrhage.

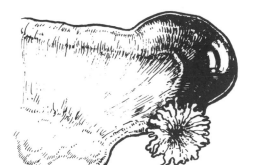

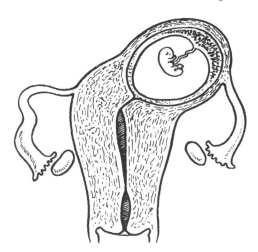

TUBAL PREGNANCY — OUTCOME

The muscle wall of the tube has not the capacity of uterine muscle for hypertrophy and distension and tubal pregnancy nearly always ends in rupture and the death of the ovum.

RUPTURE INTO LUMEN OF TUBE (TUBAL ABORTION)

This is usual in ampullary pregnancy at about 8 weeks. The conceptus is extruded, complete or incomplete, towards the fimbriated end of the tube, probably by the pressure of accumulated blood.

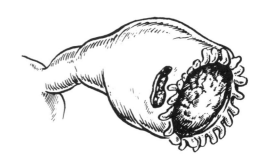

There is a trickle of bleeding into the peritoneal cavity, and this may collect as a clot in the pouch of Douglas. It is then called a pelvic haematocele.

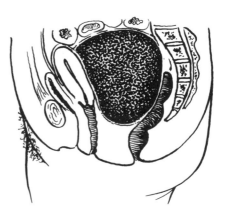

TUBAL PREGNANCY — OUTCOME

RUPTURE INTO THE PERITONEAL CAVITY

This occurs mainly from the narrow isthmus before 8 weeks, or later from the interstitial portion of the tube. Haemorrhage is likely to be severe.

Sometimes rupture is extraperitoneal between the leaves of the broad ligament — broad ligament haematoma. Haemorrhage in this site is more likely to be controlled.

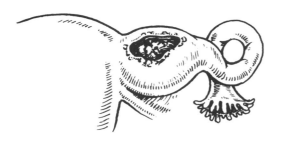

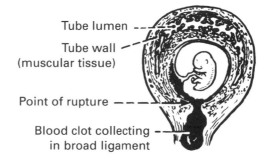

Tube lumen

Tube wall
(muscular tissue)

Point of rupture

Blood clot collecting
in broad ligament

TUBAL PREGNANCY — EFFECT ON UTERUS

The uterus enlarges in the first three months almost as if the implantation were normal and may reach the size of a gravid uterus of the same maturity. This is a source of confusion in diagnosis.

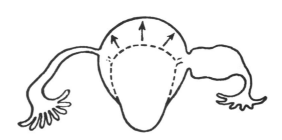

The uterine decidua grows abundantly and when the embryo dies bleeding occurs as the decidua degenerates. Rarely it is expelled entire as a decidual cast.

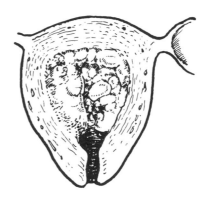

TUBAL PREGNANCY — SYMPTOMS AND SIGNS

Tubal pregnancy can present in many ways and misdiagnosis is common.

PAIN in the lower abdomen is always present and may be either constant or cramp-like.

It may be referred to the shoulder if blood tracks to the diaphragm and stimulates the phrenic nerve, and it may be so severe as to cause fainting. The pain is caused by distension of the gravid tube, by its efforts to contract and expel the ovum, and by irritation of the peritoneum by leakage of blood.

VAGINAL BLEEDING occurs usually after the death of the ovum and is an effect of oestrogen withdrawal. It is dark brown and scanty and its irregularity may lead the patient to confuse it with the menstrual flow and thus, inadvertently, give a misleading history. In about 25% of cases tubal pregnancy presents without any vaginal bleeding.

INTERNAL BLOOD LOSS can be severe and rapid and the usual signs of collapse and shock will appear.

Acute internal bleeding is the most dramatic and dangerous consequence of tubal pregnancy, but it is less common than the condition presenting by a slow trickle of blood into the pelvic cavity.

PELVIC EXAMINATION in the conscious patient will demonstrate extreme tenderness over the gravid tube or in the pouch of Douglas if a haematocele has collected. If the pregnancy is sufficiently advanced and rupture has not occurred, a cystic (and very tender) mass may be felt in the fornix; but often tenderness is the only sign elicited.

PERITONEAL IRRITATION may produce muscle guarding, frequency of micturition, and later a degree of fever, all leading towards a misdiagnosis of appendicitis.

SIGNS and SYMPTOMS of EARLY PREGNANCY may be present and help to distinguish the condition from other causes of lower abdominal pain. The menstrual history may be confusing, as noted above, and when implantation occurs in the isthmus, tubal rupture may occur before the patient has missed a period.

ABDOMINAL EXAMINATION will demonstrate tenderness in one or other fossa. If there has been much intraperitoneal bleeding there will be general tenderness and resistance to palpation over the whole abdomen.

TUBAL PREGNANCY — DIFFERENTIAL DIAGNOSIS

1. Salpingitis.
2. Miscarriage.
3. Appendicitis.
4. Torsion of pedicle of ovarian cyst.
5. Rupture of corpus luteum or follicular cyst.
6. Perforation of peptic ulcer.

1. SALPINGITIS

Swelling and pain are bilateral, fever is higher and a pregnancy test is usually negative. There may be a purulent discharge from the cervix.

2. MISCARRIAGE (threatened or incomplete)

Bleeding is the dominant clinical feature and usually precedes pain. The bleeding is red rather than brown and the pain is crampy or colicky. The uterus is larger and softer and the cervix patulous or dilated. Products of conception may be recognised on vaginal examination.

3. APPENDICITIS

The area of tenderness is higher and may be localised in the right iliac fossa. There may be a swelling if an appendix abscess was formed but is not so deep in the pelvis as a tubal swelling. Fever is greater and the patient may appear toxic. A pregnancy test will usually be negative although pregnancy and appendicitis can, of course, co-exist.

4. TORSION OF PEDICLE OF OVARIAN CYST

The mass so formed can usually be felt separate from the uterus, while a tubal pregnancy usually feels attached. Tenderness may be marked, and intraperitoneal bleeding may produce fever. Signs and symptoms of pregnancy are absent but there is a history of repeated sudden attacks of pain which pass off.

5. RUPTURE OF CORPUS LUTEUM

It is virtually impossible to distinguish this, by examination, from a tubal pregnancy, but such a severe reaction is rare.

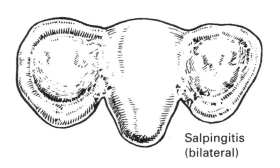

Salpingitis (bilateral)

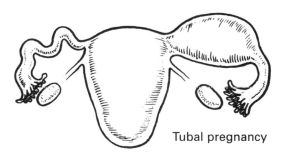

Tubal pregnancy

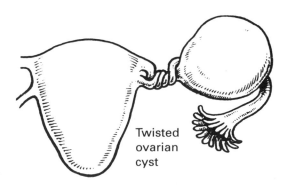

Twisted ovarian cyst

167

TUBAL PREGNANCY — AIDS TO DIAGNOSIS

1. Always take a **careful history.** Inquire in detail about supposed LMP, its timing and appearance.

2. Always **think** of tubal pregnancy; a woman with lower abdominal pain in whom there is a possibility of pregnancy should be regarded as having an ectopic until proved otherwise.

3. **Pregnancy test.** Highly-sensitive modern pregnancy tests have made the early diagnosis of ectopic pregnancy much easier. A positive test will nearly always be found by the time of clinical presentation.

4. **Ultrasound.** The main value of ultrasound is to exclude an intra-uterine pregnancy. If this is done in the presence of a positive pregnancy test, ectopic pregnancy is likely. Increasingly, however, high resolution ultrasound machines and transvaginal scanning may actually demonstrate the pregnancy outwith the uterus.

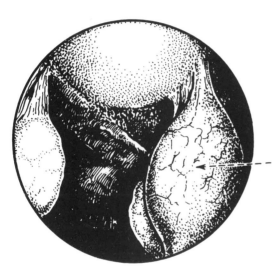

5. **Laparoscopy.** This remains the main means of diagnosis in suspected ectopic pregnancy although the increased use of transvaginal ultrasound and better pregnancy testing may make it unnecessary. The laparoscope is particularly useful for identifying an unruptured tubal pregnancy which is producing equivocal symptoms, and for excluding salpingitis and bleeding from small ovarian cysts. Laparoscopy may also enable operative treatment using minimally invasive methods.

6. **Culdocentesis.** This means passing a needle through the posterior fornix into the pouch of Douglas. This may be helpful if laparoscopy is not available. Intraperitoneal blood does not readily clot and if such blood is obtained it is an indication for laparotomy.

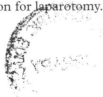

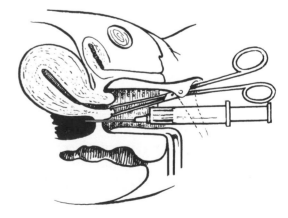

TUBAL PREGNANCY — TREATMENT

1. If haemorrhage and shock are present, restore the blood volume by the transfusion of red cells or a volume expander and proceed with operation. The patient's condition will improve as soon as the bleeding is controlled.

2. Laparotomy will usually be required where there is extensive intra-peritoneal bleeding. Blood and clot should be removed and a severely damaged tube excised (salpingectomy). This may, however, be effected by means of a laparoscope without recourse to open surgery.

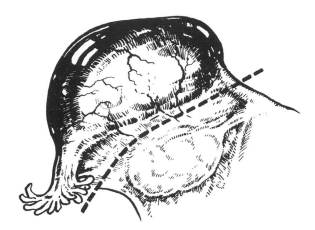

The earlier diagnosis of tubal pregnancy has allowed a more conservative approach to management permitting greater prospects of less intervention such as laparoscopic salpingectomy or greater chance of future intrauterine pregnancy by using methotrexate, a chemotherapeutic agent which destroys the abnormally sited trophoblast. This is usually given intramuscularly and its use results in resorption of the conceptus. If methotrexate is used then careful follow up, to identify declining levels of HCG, is essential to determine that treatment has been effective and that surgical removal of the ectopic pregnancy is not indicated.

ABDOMINAL PREGNANCY

Abdominal pregnancy is very rare in the United Kingdom. The embryo may be expelled from the tube, having implanted there initially, and re-implants elsewhere on the peritoneal surface or within the broad ligament. Primary implantation on the peritoneum may occur. In either case the trophoblast develops its connection with the nearest blood supply, with the subsequent risk of severe haemorrhage when placental separation occurs.

Clinical Features

1. There is a history of 'threatened miscarriage' with irregular bleeding.
2. Continued abdominal discomfort is felt and fetal movements are painful.
3. Fetal abnormality is common and fetal mortality is high.

Diagnosis is difficult.

1. Palpation is unreliable even when fetal limbs are easily felt.
2. Ultrasound may show the fetus outwith the uterus and an abnormal fetal attitude due to lack of liquor.

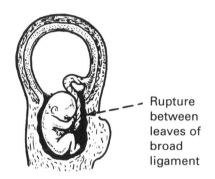

Rupture between leaves of broad ligament

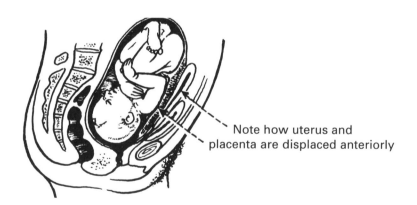

Note how uterus and placenta are displaced anteriorly

Treatment

Once diagnosed or strongly suspected, it is better to perform laparotomy in the interests of the mother. The fetus is removed, the cord tied and the abdomen closed. No attempt is made to detach the placenta unless it is clear that bleeding can be controlled.

If the condition is diagnosed around the time of fetal viability then delivery may be deferred to improve the prognosis for the fetus. This approach requires careful supervision and laparotomy may be required at any time.

MISCARRIAGE

Miscarriage is the expulsion, dead, of the products of conception before 24 weeks' gestation.

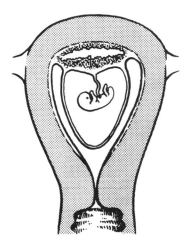

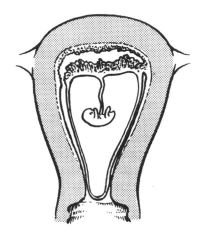

1. Haemorrhage occurs in the decidua basalis leading to local necrosis and inflammation.

2. The ovum, partly or wholly detached, acts as a foreign body and initiates uterine contractions. The cervix begins to dilate.

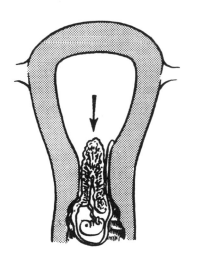

3. Expulsion complete. The decidua is shed during the next few days in the lochial flow.

Up to 12 weeks, before the placenta is independently developed, miscarriage may be complete as shown, but from the 12th to 24th week the gestation sac is likely to rupture leading to expulsion of the fetus, while the placenta is retained.

MISCARRIAGE

Miscarriage becomes inevitable because of the amount of blood loss or dilatation of the cervix. Then it becomes either:

COMPLETE

Uterine contractions are felt, the cervix dilates and blood loss continues. The fetus and placenta are expelled complete, the uterus contracts and bleeding stops. No further treatment is needed.

or   INCOMPLETE

In spite of uterine contractions and cervical dilatation, only the fetus and some membranes are expelled. The placenta remains partly attached and bleeding continues. This miscarriage must be completed by surgical methods.

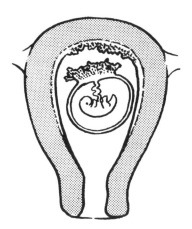
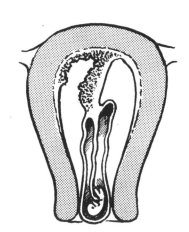

Classification is based on a mixture of clinical and pathological concepts, and is sufficiently flexible to suit a condition in which diagnosis is often only presumptive. Sepsis can complicate any type of abortion and, in countries with restrictive laws on abortion, must often be due to criminal interference.

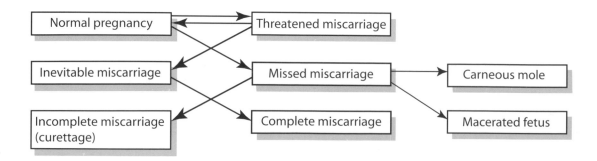

Normal pregnancy — Threatened miscarriage

Inevitable miscarriage — Missed miscarriage → Carneous mole

Incomplete miscarriage (curettage) — Complete miscarriage — Macerated fetus

MISCARRIAGE — AETIOLOGY

In many cases the cause is unknown.

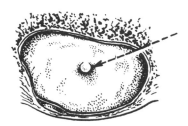

1. Abnormal development of the ovum
Of those fetuses recovered from miscarriage about half are said to be abnormal either chromosomally or structurally.

2. Maternal condition
Pyrexial illness, infection, severe rhesus iso-immunisation and any chronic maternal disease have all been associated with an increased risk of pregnancy loss. A deficiency of progesterone or human chorionic gonadotrophin have both been postulated and used as a rationale for treatment though without any significant evidence of benefit.

3. Uterine causes
Mechanical causes are rare but recognised:

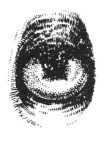

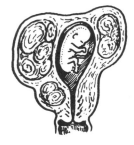

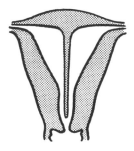

Cervical Incompetence
Lacerations or functional incompetence may make it impossible for the uterus to contain a gestation normally. Miscarriage occurs in midtrimester.

Fibroids
Although the majority of women with fibroids do not experience mechanical cause of pregnancy loss a uterus distorted by fibroids may be unable to accommodate the growing fetus.

Congenital abnormality of the uterus may interfere with the development of the growing fetus.

MISCARRIAGE — CLINICAL FEATURES

1. Haemorrhage is usually the first sign and may be very heavy if placental separation is incomplete.
2. Pain is usually intermittent, 'like a small labour'. It ceases when the miscarriage is complete.

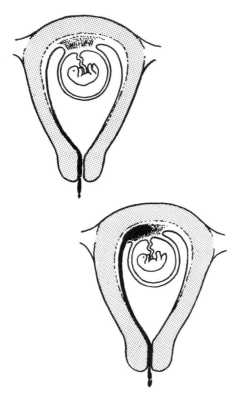

Threatened miscarriage

Miscarriage is said to threaten when any bleeding, usually painless, occurs before the 24th week. It may be impossible to distinguish it from partial shedding of the decidua at the time of a missed period which can occur up to 12 weeks.

Bed rest has been traditionally advised as treatment but there is no evidence that it affects the outcome. An ultrasound scan should be carried out and if the fetus is alive, the mother can be reassured.

Inevitable miscarriage

Here the bleeding may still be slight but uterine contractions have started to dilate the cervix. This can be detected on vaginal examination. Ultrasound may diagnose an inevitable miscarriage at an earlier stage by demonstrating fetal death. Treatment is by evacuation of the uterus.

Incomplete miscarriage

The patient will have had substantial bleeding and painful contractions. Tissue and blood clot may be found in the vagina. Bleeding may be controlled by an intramuscular injection of ergometrine 0.5 mg. This is often combined with an analgesic such as pethidine or morphine. This will usually control the bleeding until surgical evacuation can be performed. Hypovolaemia may necessitate blood transfusions.

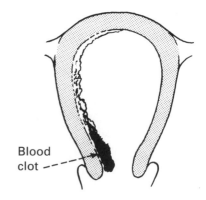

Blood clot - - -

MISCARRIAGE — DIFFERENTIAL DIAGNOSIS

The diagnosis is not usually difficult but tubal pregnancy, hydatidiform mole (see page 178) and some menstrual disorders (e.g. oligomenorrhoea) may need to be considered.

MISCARRIAGE — TREATMENT

SURGICAL TREATMENT OF INCOMPLETE MISCARRIAGE

1. It must be done in theatre with the patient anaesthetised.

2. The patient may bleed:

   (a) before admission to hospital
   (b) while in hospital
   (c) during the operation

   Blood loss may be large and facilities for blood transfusion must be at hand.

3. The operator must, at all times, remember the ease with which a gravid uterus can be perforated by a metal instrument.

'Digital Curettage' is tried first.

The surgeon presses on the fundus with the external hand and clears out as much of the cavity as he can reach with the internal finger.

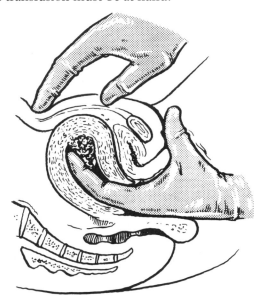

Removal of placental tissue with ovum forceps.

The open blades are rotated to grasp tissue and then gently withdrawn. Before using any instrument inside the uterus an oxytocic, Syntocinon 10 units or Ergometrine 0.25 mg, should be given intravenously to cause contraction and hardening of the uterine wall.

Evacuation is completed by careful exploration of the cavity with a sharp curette.

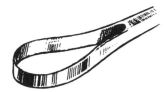

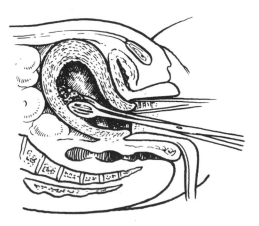

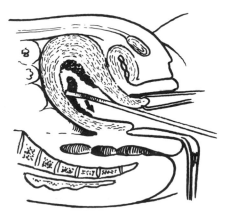

MISSED MISCARRIAGE

This term is used to describe the retention of a fetus, after its death, for a period of several weeks.

Death of the fetus occurs unnoticed or is marked by some vaginal bleeding which is regarded as a threat to miscarry. Symptoms of pregnancy regress, however, and the uterus shrinks as liquor is absorbed. The pregnancy test will become negative and ultrasound confirms the diagnosis.

If retained long enough the gestation may end up as a

CARNEOUS MOLE

A carneous mole is a lobulated mass of laminated blood clot. The projections into the shrunken cavity are caused by repeated haemorrhages in the chorio-decidual space. In very early pregnancies (up to 12 weeks) complete absorption of the dead ovum may occur.

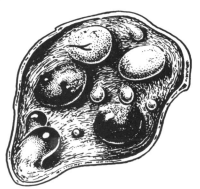

or MACERATED FETUS

The skull bones collapse and override and the spine is flexed and there is little or no amniotic fluid on ultrasound examination. The internal organs degenerate and the abdomen is filled with bloodstained fluid. The skin peels very easily.

Pathological changes in the fetus such as mummification (fetus papyraceous) and calcification (lithopaedion) are exceedingly rare.

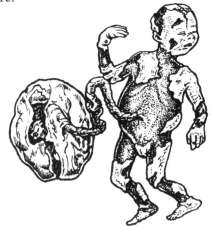

Treatment

If left alone most missed miscarriages will be expelled spontaneously, but during the waiting period there is a slight risk of coagulation defect and this should be investigated before embarking on evacuation of the uterus in cases of fetal death of more than four weeks.

Surgical. If the uterus is not larger than the size of an eight to ten week pregnancy it may be emptied by curettage. This operation requires experience and as bleeding is free until the uterus is emptied, transfusion facilities must be available.

Medical. Mifepristone, a progesterone receptor blocker may be used to 'prime' the uterus for miscarriage and be followed by the use of gemeprost or misoprostol and medical management of this condition is highly effective in producing complete miscarriage.

SEPTIC MISCARRIAGE

Infection may complicate miscarriage once the cervix starts to dilate or instruments are introduced into the uterine cavity.

Causes

1. Delay in evacuation of the uterus. Either the patient delays seeking advice, or the surgical evacuation has been incomplete. Infection occurs from vaginal organisms after 48 hours.

2. Trauma, either perforation or cervical tear. Healing is delayed and infection is more likely to be a peritonitis or cellulitis. Criminal abortions are, of course, particularly liable to sepsis.

Infecting Organisms

These are usually the vaginal or bowel commensals.

1. Group B haemolytic streptococcus.
2. Anaerobic streptococcus.
3. Coliform bacillus.
4. *Clostridium welchii.*
5. *Bacteroides necrophorus.*

Any of these organisms but particularly the last two may be the cause of septic shock.

Treatment

This should be active to minimise the risk of septic shock. Cervical and high vaginal swabs and blood cultures are taken and a broad spectrum antibiotic such as a cephalosporin together with an agent effective against anaerobes prescribed. Curettage should be carried out as soon as possible; there is nothing to be gained by leaving infected material in utero. The septic uterus is particularly vulnerable to trauma.

HYDATIDIFORM MOLE/CHORIOCARCINOMA

Hydatidiform change in the placenta is a form
of trophoblastic neoplasia which may change
to a frankly malignant proliferation of
trophoblast cells, known as choriocarcinoma.

Histology
To the naked eye the mole looks like a bunch
of whitish grapes, often interspersed with
blood clot. Microscopically, the villi show three
changes:

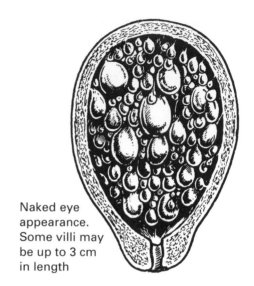

1. Trophoblastic proliferation of both the
   cytotrophoblast (Langhan's cells) and the
   syncytiotrophoblast.
2. Hydropic changes in the stroma, with
   'cistern' formation.
3. Absence of fetal vessels.

Naked eye
appearance.
Some villi may
be up to 3 cm
in length

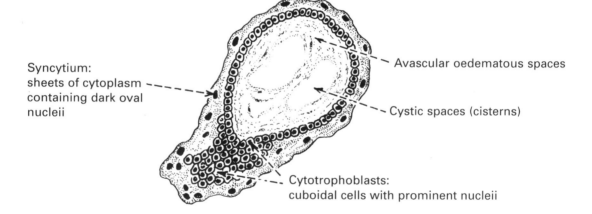

Syncytium:
sheets of cytoplasm
containing dark oval
nucleii

Avascular oedematous spaces

Cystic spaces (cisterns)

Cytotrophoblasts:
cuboidal cells with prominent nucleii

In a normal villus, the trophoblastic layers
are single-celled with no proliferation, the
stroma contains numerous cells, and there
are fetal vessels.

Normal villus

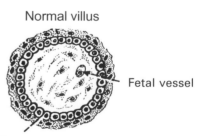

Fetal vessel

Chorionic epithelium

HYDATIDIFORM MOLE

Hydatidiform moles are now classed as complete or partial. The distinction is made on histological and karyotype evidence and is of considerable clinical significance.

Complete Mole

This shows total hydatidiform change with no evidence of fetal circulation. Proliferation of the trophoblast cells is marked.

The karyotype is in most cases 46XX, derived entirely from the paternal contribution. Fertilisation is by haploid (23X) sperm which duplicates its chromosomes without cell division. Why there should be failure of the ovum contribution is not yet known. Complete moles are more likely to develop malignant change.

Partial Mole

This mole is associated with a fetus even if the only evidence is traces of a microscopic fetal circulation. Hydatidiform change is variable, and trophoblast proliferation, although present, is of moderate degree. The karyotype is abnormal and the commonest finding is triploid (69XXX or XXY), the result of fertilisation by more than one sperm. Partial moles are less likely to develop malignant change.

HYDATIDIFORM MOLE — AETIOLOGY

This is not known but factors include age, environment and probably genetic constitution. Mole is commoner in Asians than in Caucasians, and the European incidence is about 1:2000 compared with an extreme of 1:250 in the Philippines.

Maternal age

Hydatidiform mole occurs most commonly in women under 20 and over 45, the women in whom congenital abnormalities are most likely to be found. In Asian countries where there is a high birth rate, women tend to continue child-bearing until late in their reproductive life.

High parity and malnutrition

Although there is no evidence of any specific dietary deficiency as a cause, these factors are associated in every society with congenital abnormality. Asian countries have high birth rates and high perinatal and infant mortality rates. They also have to deal with the problems caused by malnutrition.

CLINICAL FEATURES

This uncommon condition tends to be unsuspected, but should always be considered in cases of threatened miscarriage and hyperemesis gravidarum.

Symptoms

1. Bleeding

This is almost the rule. A minor degree of intravascular coagulation appears to accompany molar pregnancy, platelets are reduced, and FDPs increased.

2. Hyperemesis

This is probably due to the increase in HCG secretion, although this has never been established definitely as the cause of hyperemesis in normal pregnancy.

3. Pallor and dyspnoea

4. Anxiety and tremor

HCG, which is a glycoprotein similar to TSH, has weak thyroid stimulating properties.

Signs

1. Uterine enlargement

Most patients present at about 14 weeks, and in a majority of cases the uterus is larger than expected. The presence of theca-lutein cysts in the ovary, which occurs in about 10% of cases, may add to this impression.

2. Absent FH

Very rarely a mole and fetus will coexist.

3. Absent fetal parts

The uterus has a doughy feel.

4. Signs of pre-eclampsia

Hypertension and proteinuria before 20 weeks suggest the possibility of a mole.

5. Unexplained degree of anaemia.

6. Passage of vesicles per vaginam (which make the diagnosis).

7. Signs of hyperthyroidism.

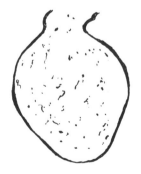

HYDROPIC MISCARRIAGE

This occurs in the first trimester. In the products of conception there is usually a mixture of normal chorionic villi and hydropic villi, but in the latter the chorionic epithelium is atrophic. This may be confused with partial mole but the trophoblast is atrophic and the condition is non-neoplastic.

HYDATIDIFORM MOLE — DIAGNOSIS

ULTRASONOGRAPHY

Ultrasound has become the main method of diagnosing hydatidiform mole. It is extremely accurate provided that the mole is sufficiently developed, as the echoes produced from the mass of vesicles produce a characteristic 'snowstorm' appearance. The scan must be carried out by an experienced operator as the appearances of vesicle tissue can be mimicked by a septic miscarriage or a fibroid.

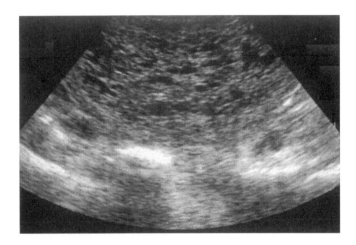

HUMAN CHORIONIC GONADOTROPHIN

Since most of the trophoblast cells secrete HCG, its assay is a measure of the amount of tumour tissue. Grossly elevated levels of HCG are found with hydatidiform moles. HCG is a glycoprotein of two polypeptide chains, alpha and beta. Beta is unique to HCG, and very accurate radio-immunoassays can now be made of beta HCG. For ordinary diagnostic and follow-up purposes however the standard HCG assay is satisfactory.

There are wide variations of the levels in normal pregnancy which reach a peak at about 14 weeks and thereafter fall.

HYDATIDIFORM MOLE — DIAGNOSIS

Once hydatidiform mole is diagnosed, the uterus should be evacuated. Risks before evacuation:
1. Haemorrhage.
2. Trophoblastic invasion and perforation of myometrium.
3. Dissemination of possibly malignant cells.

Risks during evacuation:
1. Haemorrhage.
2. Perforation by instruments.
3. Dissemination of possibly malignant cells.

There seems no doubt that active methods of evacuation such as hysterectomy, hysterotomy and the use of oxytocics are associated with a threefold increase in the need for subsequent chemotherapy to deal with varying degrees of malignancy. However the immediate safety of the patient may call for some of these measures, and the following plan of management is suggested.

1. After miscarriage, the uterus should be completely emptied by suction.
2. If miscarriage does not occur, an attempt should be made to empty the uterus by suction. This is usually quite simple up to about 14 weeks size.
If bleeding becomes severe, oxytocics must be given, and on rare occasions an emergency hysterectomy or hysterotomy may be unavoidable.
3. If the uterus is of such a size as to deter the obstetrician from attempting suction curettage, abortion should be induced using prostaglandin together with oxytocin if necessary. Subsequent surgical evacuation of the uterus may also be required.
4. In the case of the older woman whose family is complete, hysterectomy may be justified, especially as dissemination of trophoblast cells can be almost completely prevented by early clamping of the uterine vessels.

HYDATIDIFORM MOLE — FOLLOW UP

Hydatidiform mole, although it can cause serious immediate complications, is particularly important because in about 10% of cases it will persist and undergo malignant change in varying degrees. This outcome is much more common after complete rather than partial moles, but all patients must be followed up for prolonged periods by radioimmune assays of serum or urinary HCG. In the United Kingdom this is organised around three centres with whom all cases of mole are registered and which organise follow up by serial HCG measurements. These are done with diminishing frequency for up to 2 years. Failure of HCG levels to fall quickly after evacuation of the mole means the persistence of trophoblastic tissue and treatment with chemotherapy will be required.

Indications for chemotherapy

1. The high HCG levels associated with mole persist for two months after evacuation.
2. Any detectable HCG in the serum after 6 months.
3. Persistent uterine bleeding, even if no trophoblastic material is obtained by curettage. This is an indication of myometrial invasion.
4. Evidence of trophoblastic metastases usually to the brain or lungs.

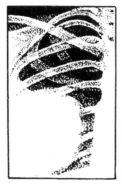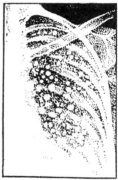

X-ray of the lung field may show one large shadow (cannon-ball metastasis) or numerous trophoblastic emboli (snowstorm).

INVASIVE MOLE AND CHORIOCARCINOMA

The classification of the various degrees of malignant change in hydatidiform mole is not universally agreed. A simple system of nomenclature would be:

1. Hydatidiform mole.
2. Intermediate degrees of neoplastic change (Invasive mole, Destructive mole, Villous choriocarcinoma).
3. Choriocarcinoma.

Both invasive mole and choriocarcinoma are rare conditions. The symptoms and signs are similar to those associated with hydatidiform mole but metastatic lesions occur; the more malignant the growth the earlier its appearance. Haemoptysis and cerebral haemorrhage are the normal results but local metastases to the vagina are also common.

INVASIVE MOLE (Destructive mole, Villous choriocarcinoma)

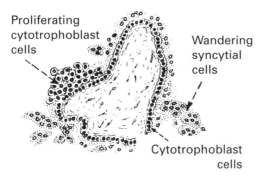

The trophoblast retains its villous structure but it invades the myometrium and may produce metastases.

CHORIOCARCINOMA (Chorionepithelioma, Avillous choriocarcinoma)

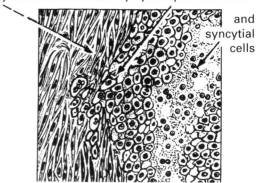

Villous formation is absent. Trophoblast cells invade the myometrium and blood vessels resulting in gross haemorrhage and metastases.

It must be emphasised that the histological patterns vary widely. The more malignant growths show the greater cellular irregularity and mitotic activity. Choriocarcinoma is usually found early in pregnancy arising in association with a mole but can follow miscarriage or even normal pregnancy.

INVASIVE MOLE AND CHORIOCARCINOMA — CHEMOTHERAPY

Immediate chemotherapy is indicated if either of the conditions described above, invasive mole or choriocarcinoma, is diagnosed. Chemotherapy is also indicated where there is any evidence of persistence of trophoblastic tissue, as shown by the continuing presence of HCG in the urine or serum. Chemotherapy is intended to cure and this may be said to have occurred when HCG becomes undetectable and remains so over a prolonged period of follow-up.

The following prognostic factors should be taken into account in determining the type of chemotherapy employed:

ADVERSE
1. Histological evidence of choriocarcinoma.
2. Large tumour masses or widespread secondaries.
3. Delay in detection of persisting tumour cells.
4. Very high HCG levels.
5. Previous unsuccessful chemotherapy.

FAVOURABLE
1. Evidence of invasive mole only.
2. No evidence of recurrence or spread: small tumour mass.
3. Early diagnosis of persistence.
4. Relatively low and falling HCG levels. (HCG excretion is roughly indicative of the amount of tumour.)

METHOTREXATE, combined with folinic acid, is the treatment of choice in low-risk cases. Dosage is limited by side-effects on the bone marrow and alimentary tract. Treatment is monitored by assay of HCG and blood cell counts. Methotrexate is excreted unchanged in the urine and renal function must be adequate. Combination therapy again is employed in high-risk situations. Methotrexate may be combined with agents such as actinomycin, etoposide, cyclophosphamide and vincristine. Other agents may be employed in non-responding cases.

Trophoblastic disease chemotherapy is a highly specialised service confined in the United Kingdom to a single unit to which all cases may be referred.

ANTE-PARTUM HAEMORRHAGE

Ante-partum haemorrhage is bleeding from the genital tract after the 24th week of pregnancy and before the birth of the baby. This is a practical definition as it includes the incidental causes of bleeding illustrated in summary at the beginning of this chapter. These are dealt with elsewhere. An alternative definition, no longer favoured, is bleeding from the placental site. This encompasses the two conditions of Placenta Praevia (inevitable haemorrhage) and Placental Abruption (accidental haemorrhage). A substantial number of cases of ante-partum haemorrhage remain unexplained even when the placenta is examined after delivery for signs of premature separation.

PLACENTA PRAEVIA (INEVITABLE HAEMORRHAGE)

A low implantation of the placenta in the uterus, causing it to lie alongside or in front of the presenting part.

The cause is unknown. The incidence rises with maternal age and parity and the condition is commoner in women who have previously been delivered by caesarean section. Twin pregnancy, with its large placental bed, is prone to low implantation of at least part of the placenta. Placenta praevia is divided into four types or degrees, of which the first two are commonest.

Type 1

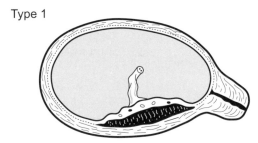

The lower margin of the placenta dips into the lower segment. ('Low implantation'.)

Type 2

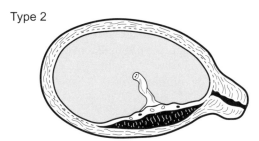

The placenta reaches the internal os when closed but does not cover it. ('Marginal'.)

Type 3

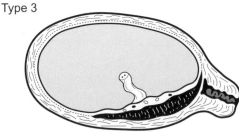

The placenta covers the internal os when closed, but not when fully dilated. ('Partial' or 'Incomplete'.)

Type 4

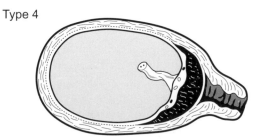

The placenta covers the os even when the cervix is fully dilated. ('Central' or 'Complete'.)

Allocation to a particular type is usually made by palpation prior to delivery, or by observation at caesarean section; so there is a subjective bias. In addition the degree of dilatation of the cervix at the time of assessment may alter a classification; what was type 1 at 2 cm dilatation may become type 2 at 4 or 5 cm.

PLACENTA PRAEVIA (INEVITABLE HAEMORRHAGE)

Signs and Symptoms
The formation of the lower segment by stretching leads to separation of the placenta and escape of blood from the maternal sinuses. This commonly occurs around the 32nd week but may begin as early as the late mid-trimester of pregnancy.

The loss may be slight or considerable and tends to be recurrent. The bleeding is painless because blood is not normally retained within the uterine cavity.

Diagnosis
The presence of the placenta in the lower segment pushes the presenting part upwards and may encourage malpresentation or an oblique or transverse lie. The abdomen is soft and non tender. The patient's general condition should reflect the amount of visible blood loss. Confirmation of the diagnosis is obtained by localisation of the placenta by ultrasound. This is very accurate but in minor degrees of placenta praevia (especially on the posterior wall) it may be impossible to be sure if the placenta encroaches on the lower segment.

Management
If the pregnancy is immature (less than 37 weeks) the aim is to treat conservatively. The patient must remain in hospital and cross-matched blood should be available. Conservative management will be abandoned if the bleeding becomes severe or persistent. Placenta praevia is a treacherous condition and bleeding is unpredictable.

If preterm delivery seems likely then steroids may be given to accelerate fetal lung maturation.

Examination in Theatre and Delivery
If the pregnancy continues to 37–38 weeks, the degree of placenta praevia can be confirmed by vaginal examination in theatre. This is carried out under anaesthesia and the theatre is set and staffed for caesarean section. The vaginal fornices are carefully palpated for evidence of the placenta and, if not encountered, a finger is then passed through the cervix to explore the lower segment. If the obstetrician is convinced of the diagnosis and the degree of placenta praevia he may omit this examination for fear of provoking haemorrhage. The treatment of placenta praevia today is invariably caesarean section except in type 1 when the membranes may be ruptured and, if no bleeding occurs, spontaneous delivery may be awaited.

As a rule the lower segment operation is done even with an anterior placenta when the operator passes his hand around or below the placenta to extract the baby. If the examination has provoked torrential haemorrhage classical section may have a slight advantage in speed. Because of the poor retractile quality of the lower segment there is sometimes difficulty in obtaining control of bleeding after delivery of the baby and placenta. Hysterectomy may be ultimately necessary.

If dangerous haemorrhage occurs and facilities for caesarean section are not available, attempts might be made to control the bleeding by pressure of the presenting part on the placenta. Where the head is presenting, Willett's forceps may be applied to the fetal scalp and traction maintained. With a breech presentation it may be possible to bring down a leg if at least two fingers can be passed through the cervix.

These are desperate measures which will almost certainly result in fetal death. They are only applicable when the mother herself is at risk from uncontrollable haemorrhage.

PLACENTAL ABRUPTION (ACCIDENTAL HAEMORRHAGE)

This means the separation of a normally situated placenta. It usually leads to bleeding per vaginam ('revealed') but often blood remains in the uterus as a retro-placental clot and sometimes there is no external bleeding ('concealed'). Where there is both external bleeding and evidence of retro-placental clot the haemorrhage is described as 'mixed'.

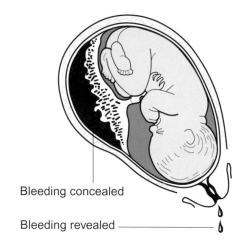

Bleeding concealed

Bleeding revealed

Aetiology

The aetiology of abruption is unknown but several factors have been postulated as linked causes:

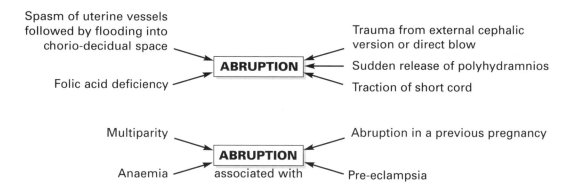

Spasm of uterine vessels followed by flooding into chorio-decidual space

Folic acid deficiency

ABRUPTION

Trauma from external cephalic version or direct blow

Sudden release of polyhydramnios

Traction of short cord

Multiparity

Anaemia

ABRUPTION associated with

Abruption in a previous pregnancy

Pre-eclampsia

Certain patients seem susceptible to abruption but again the reason is unknown.

The incidence of abruption has fallen greatly with the reduction in the number of multiparous patients and better health of the pregnant population.

Signs and Symptoms

1. The patient complains of abdominal pain which may be severe and constant. Pain is greatest when there is a substantial 'concealed' bleed and may be minimal or absent where bleeding is entirely 'revealed'.
2. Vaginal bleeding, where present, usually makes the diagnosis straightforward.
3. The uterus may be tense and tender due to the retention of clot and the extravasation of blood into the uterine wall. The term, 'Couvelaire uterus' is used to describe this condition. In severe cases blood may spread into the broad ligament or peritoneal cavity. It is difficult to detect the fetal heart by ordinary stethoscope or to feel uterine contractions.
4. There may be evidence of hypovolaemia depending on the extent of haemorrhage.
5. In severe cases the fetus is dead.

PLACENTAL ABRUPTION (ACCIDENTAL HAEMORRHAGE)

Differential Diagnosis

Mild and early cases of abruption are difficult to distinguish from normal labour with excessive 'show'. The diagnosis of an established mixed haemorrhage is not usually difficult but concealed abruption may need to be distinguished from:

(a) Acute polyhydramnios
(b) Degeneration of fibroid
(c) Peritonism from perforation of a peptic ulcer, appendicitis or other cause.

Complications of Abruption

1. Coagulation failure

In severe cases of mixed and concealed abruption coagulation failure may supervene due to the consumption of clotting factors and/or the development of fibrinolysis (see Chapter 7).

All patients with ante-partum haemorrhage should have a clotting screen carried out on admission to hospital. An undetected coagulation defect may lead to catastrophic bleeding and shock. It is essential to correct the defect before delivery occurs. Transfusion with whole blood is the best treatment. Fresh-frozen plasma and concentrates of platelets may also be indicated. Expert haematological guidance is desirable.

2. Renal failure

Severe hypovolaemic shock may cause ultimate renal failure with first haemoglobinuria, then oliguria or anuria. This may be due to either tubular damage or cortical necrosis. Urinary output should be monitored carefully in all cases of severe abruption.

The complications and dangers of this condition may be summarised as follows:

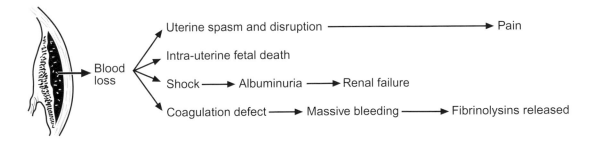

It is recognised that the risk of either coagulation failure or renal failure occurring will be reduced by rapid and liberal transfusion to restore the circulating blood volume together with speedy emptying of the uterus. Similarly the baby's chances of survival will be increased by improved perfusion of the placental site.

PLACENTAL ABRUPTION (ACCIDENTAL HAEMORRHAGE)

Management
1. Minor or uncertain cases

Minor retro-placental bleeding sometimes occurs producing a tender area in the uterus. There is a complaint of pain but little systemic upset. Similarly slight external bleeding will cause little disturbance. In both of these situations treatment is by bed-rest, sedation if required and observation. The haemoglobin should be estimated and a clotting screen carried out. Confirmation of placental separation may be obtained by a positive Kleihauer test, indicating fetomaternal bleeding. (See Chapter 7.)

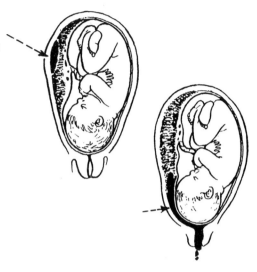

Placenta praevia is excluded by ultrasound scan. Symptoms usually settle quickly and the patient is mobilised and the pregnancy may safely be allowed to continue. Fetal growth should be closely observed and at delivery the placenta should be examined for evidence of old blood clot or the presence of a crater.

2. Established Abruption

(a) Rapid assessment of maternal and fetal state.
(b) Blood taken for haemoglobin, cross-match and clotting screen.
(c) Analgesia to treat shock and pain.
(d) Blood transfusion to correct hypovolaemia. The rate and volume of transfusion are best monitored by a central venous pressure (CVP) line in severe cases as blood loss is always likely to be underestimated.
(e) Expedite delivery.

3. Delivery

If the baby is dead an attempt should be made to achieve vaginal delivery. Vaginal examination and amniotomy are performed and labour is usually rapid. It is quite common to find on vaginal examination that the cervix is already considerably dilated. The presence of uterine contractions may not have been detected due to the hardness of the uterus caused by the abruption. If the fetal heart is detected on admission by ultrasound, caesarean section is increasingly favoured to deliver the baby. As already noted the baby's condition will be improved by rapid restoration of the circulating blood volume. There may be poor retraction of the uterus following the delivery of the placenta due to high levels of circulating fibrin degradation products, and thus an atonic post partum haemorrhage may add to the dangers the mother already faces. Intravenous oxytocics should therefore be given and ergometrine, with its tonic action on the uterus, is the drug of choice. Following delivery careful supervision of urinary output is essential and the presence of anaemia should be sought.

A CLINICAL APPROACH TO ANTE-PARTUM HAEMORRHAGE

Many cases of relatively minor ante-partum haemorrhage do not fit clearly into the descriptions of placenta praevia and placental abruption already given. The diagnosis is not obvious and both mother and baby appear well. Conservative or 'expectant' management is appropriate and the following approach is suggested:

1. **Hospital admission** Prescribe anti-embolism stockings.

2. **General assessment** of the mother and baby including haemoglobin estimation, coagulation screen and Kleihauer test.

3. **Localise the placenta** by ultrasound and perform biophysical assessment of the fetus.

4. **An early speculum examination** to exclude local causes or confirm that the bleeding is from the uterine cavity (i.e. the placental site). A digital examination should NEVER be done.

5. Mobilise when fresh bleeding has stopped.

6. **Give anti-D immunoglobulin to Rhesus negative mothers** without antibodies.

7. The patient may go home when the bleeding has stopped and **placenta praevia has been excluded.**

8. Continue ante-natal supervision to exclude **growth restriction.**

9. **Examination in theatre at 38 weeks,** finally to exclude placenta praevia, may be advisable if ultrasound is not confirmatory, as may be the case with a posterior praevia.

10. **Careful examination of the placenta** and membranes after delivery to try to identify the cause of the bleeding.

CHAPTER 10

MULTIPLE PREGNANCY AND OTHER ANTENATAL COMPLICATIONS

MULTIPLE PREGNANCY

Multiple pregnancy is the term used to describe pregnancy with more than one fetus. The vast majority of such pregnancies are cases of twins. The rate of twinning in different populations is determined by racial predisposition to double ovulation and hence nonidentical twinning.

Thus, among the Caucasian population, twins are found in 1 in 80 pregnancies. The ratio of binovular (dizygotic) twins, to monovular (monozygotic) twins, is around 3 to 1. In contrast, in West Africans, who have the highest rates in the world (1 in 44 pregnancies is a case of twins) the ratio of dizygotic to monozygotic twinning may be between 4–6 to 1. The lowest rates of twinning are seen in Asia.

The incidence of twin pregnancy has risen slightly over the last 10 years. In contrast, the rate of triplets and higher order multiple pregnancy (quadruplets, sextuplets etc.) has increased dramatically. Theoretically by 'Heilin's rule' the incidence of triplets should be 1 in 80^2 (6400) and that of quadruplets 1 in 80^3 (512 000). From 1982 to 1993 the incidence of multiple pregnancies rose dramatically due to the widespread introduction of assisted conception programmes encompassing ovulation induction and in vitro fertilisation.

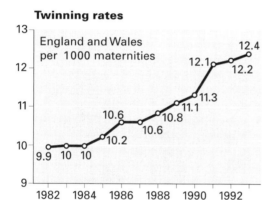

Twinning rates

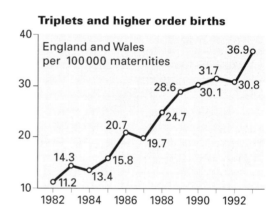

Triplets and higher order births

AETIOLOGY

Monozygotic twinning appears to be a chance event and is poorly understood although the rate of monozygotic twinning is uniform throughout all populations. Dizygotic twinning is commoner in the female relations of women who are, or have had, dizygotic twins. There does not appear to be any male factor, familial or otherwise, which increases the rate of twin pregnancy.

Twins are commoner in women of high parity and in those who are older at the time of conception. Dizygotic twinning is also commoner in women who are tall and in the obese. The importance of multiple pregnancy lies in the observation that almost all complications are commoner than in singleton pregnancies. The high incidence of prematurity and fetal abnormality in particular result in a sixfold increase in perinatal mortality.

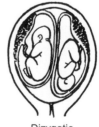

Dizygotic twins

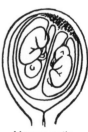

Monozygotic twins

MULTIPLE PREGNANCY

DIAGNOSIS IN EARLY PREGNANCY

The diagnosis of multiple pregnancy may be suspected on history and clinical examination: a history of infertility treatment or severe hyperemesis in early pregnancy are suggestive. Suspicion may be further raised if the uterus if found to be large for dates.

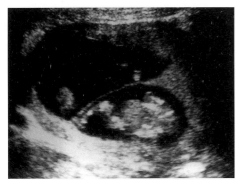

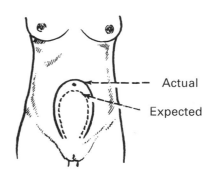

Twin gestation sacs at 8 weeks

Other causes of apparently abnormal uterine enlargement in early pregnancy are:

(a) **Mistaken Dates** — bleeding after conception being considered as a period.

(b) **Polyhydramnios** — rare in early pregnancy.

(c) **Fibroids** — These tend to flatten and soften in pregnancy but may be irregular.

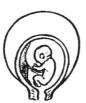

(d) **Abdominal Cyst** — It is usually possible to differentiate two masses.

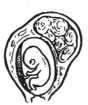

(e) **Hydatidiform Mole** — Usually accompanied by staining. Urinary HCG excretion will be much elevated.

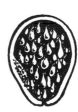

(f) **Retention of Urine** — 'Catheter will cure'. It may be associated with retroversion and incarceration of the uterus.

Ultrasound examination in early pregnancy will differentiate these conditions and is the only method of diagnosing multiple pregnancy reliably.

MULTIPLE PREGNANCY

DIAGNOSIS IN LATE PREGNANCY

The uterus is more globular and larger than normal for the dates. Polyhydramnios may be present. It is commoner in monozygotic than in dizygotic twins.

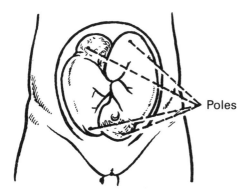

Poles

If there is no evidence of polyhydramnios, an apparent 'excess' of fetal parts may be noted. It may be difficult to define the lie of the fetuses but three fetal poles (head or breech) must be identified to be sure of the diagnosis.

Clinical suspicion of twin pregnancy must always be confirmed by ultrasound, if this has not already been performed.

MULTIPLE PREGNANCY

COMPLICATIONS

The major complications are illustrated below but it must be remembered that the so-called minor complications of pregnancy such as heartburn, varicose veins, haemorrhoids and other pressure effects may all add to the mother's burden.

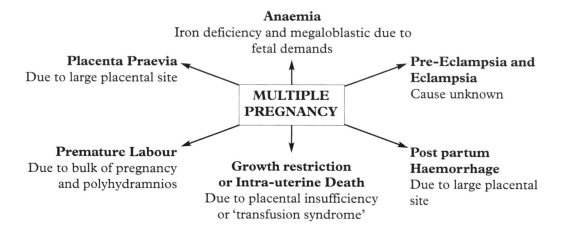

Anaemia
Iron deficiency and megaloblastic due to fetal demands

Placenta Praevia
Due to large placental site

MULTIPLE PREGNANCY

Pre-Eclampsia and Eclampsia
Cause unknown

Premature Labour
Due to bulk of pregnancy and polyhydramnios

Growth restriction or Intra-uterine Death
Due to placental insufficiency or 'transfusion syndrome'

Post partum Haemorrhage
Due to large placental site

MANAGEMENT OF MULTIPLE PREGNANCY
Before 20 weeks
Antenatal care is conducted in the usual fashion with particular attention to identifying the complications mentioned above. A good diet is advised and iron and folic acid supplementation should be prescribed.

Ultrasound enables an early diagnosis to be made but should not be shared too early with the patient as a significant number of apparently multiple pregnancies when scanned at 8 weeks are singleton pregnancies at 12 weeks as a result of fetal death.

Threatened miscarriage is more likely to proceed to inevitable miscarriage in multiple pregnancy.

Fetal abnormality is commoner in multiple pregnancies; AFP screening is of use in some respects since the normal range is twice that of a singleton pregnancy and elevated values are associated with the same abnormalities. Biochemical screening for Down's syndrome is not currently possible in multiple pregnancy.

Detailed fetal assessment is usually offered around 18 to 20 weeks.

Identification of abnormality in one of a set of twins presents a number of difficulties. The parents are presented with one of three choices: the first, is to await events. The second is to opt for termination of the pregnancy and sacrifice of the healthy fetus. The third option is selective feticide in which the heart of the abnormal fetus is injected with potassium chloride to cause asytole. Clearly the management of such problems is very difficult and requires considerable expertise.

MULTIPLE PREGNANCY

MANAGEMENT OF MULTIPLE PREGNANCY *(continued)*
After 20 weeks

Routine hospital admission does not improve perinatal outcome although it may be indicated for either geographical reasons, if the patient lives some distance from hospital care, or social reasons, when admission for rest may be valuable.

Complications, such as preterm labour and pre-eclampsia, should be managed as for singleton pregnancies but consideration given to the problems associated with multiple pregnancy. Placentography should be performed to exclude placenta praevia.

When fetal compromise is suspected fetal monitoring may be more technically demanding but current cardiotocography equipment allows tracing of both babies simultaneously.

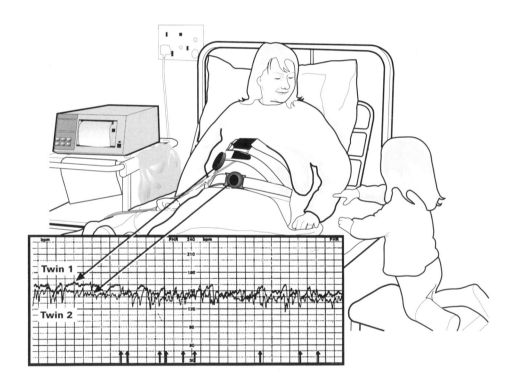

MULTIPLE PREGNANCY

Regular assessment of fetal growth is indicated to identify IUGR. This is commoner in multiple pregnancy. When this occurs in one of twins, delivery may be required in that baby's interest. If both babies are mature this decision is straightforward. When preterm delivery is indicated then the larger, appropriately grown, baby is put at risk of the complications of prematurity in the interest of its sibling. This is a problem unique to multiple pregnancy and can present ethical, emotional and practical difficulties. The degree of difficulty is influenced by gestational age; a growth discrepancy at 34 weeks gestation means that the risk to the larger fetus of early delivery, though not negligible, is relatively small in a well equipped obstetric unit. In contrast, such a problem in twins at 26 weeks gestation may result in loss of both babies from extreme prematurity.

Another cause of growth discrepancy between twins is Twin to Twin Transfusion Syndrome. This condition, in which there are vascular anastomoses between the placentae of monochorionic twins, results when one baby acts as a blood donor to its twin. The result is an anaemic, growth restricted fetus and a polycythaemic, macrosomic twin which may develop hydrops. The ideal management when this occurs in early pregnancy is unclear. When the onset is later in pregnancy, delivery is indicated in the interests of both babies.

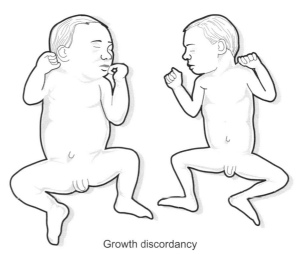

Growth discordancy

MULTIPLE PREGNANCY

ZYGOSITY AND ITS DIAGNOSIS

In singleton pregnancies the membranes surrounding the fetus are chorion and amnion. In dizygotic twinning each fetus will each have both membranes, i.e. the placentae will be *dichorionic and diamniotic.*

In monozygotic twinning, if separation of the fetal poles occurs early enough, the placentae will be diamniotic and dichorionic. Later separation will result in each fetus being within its own amniotic sac but may share a chorion, a diamniotic, monochorionic placenta. When very late separation occurs both babies may share amnion and chorion.

Such monoamniotic pregnancies have a very high perinatal mortality.

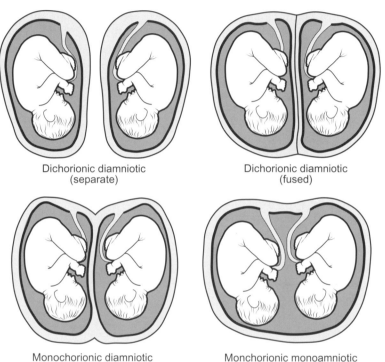

Dichorionic diamniotic
(separate)

Dichorionic diamniotic
(fused)

Monochorionic diamniotic

Monchorionic monoamniotic

The most extreme type of late separation of the fetal poles causes conjoined (so-called Siamese) twins.

The finding on ultrasound examination of a pyramidal area of placental tissue at the site of insertion of the separating membranes between twins, the so-called Lambda sign, suggests a dichorionic placentation. Because of the comment above this is not synonymous with dizygosity.

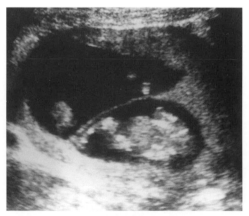

Lambda sign

MULTIPLE PREGNANCY

LABOUR AND DELIVERY

Malpresentations are common in twin pregnancy but in 75% of cases twin 1 presents by the vertex.

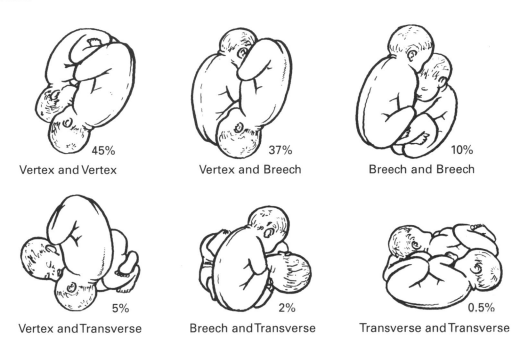

45%	37%	10%
Vertex and Vertex	Vertex and Breech	Breech and Breech
5%	2%	0.5%
Vertex and Transverse	Breech and Transverse	Transverse and Transverse

The lie of the second baby is unimportant until the first is born.

Labour is usually straightforward though the higher incidence of malpresentation increases the risk of cord prolapse. Vaginal examination should be carried out when the membranes rupture.

Both fetal hearts should be monitored, the first by a scalp electrode and the second externally, ideally using ultrasound cardiotocography. Epidural analgesia is ideal, if available, as it permits any necessary intervention, especially with the second twin, during delivery. This should take place in an operating theatre with appropriate facilities and staff available. In addition to the obstetrician and midwives, an anaesthetist and paediatrician should be present. After the delivery of the first baby the cord is double clamped in case there are monozygotic twins and a risk of the second baby bleeding from the cord of the first due to placental vascular anastomoses.

MULTIPLE PREGNANCY

When the first baby is delivered, the lie of the second is checked and if necessary corrected by external version to a vertex or a breech; if that is not possible then internal podalic version and breech extraction is performed (see Ch. 12).

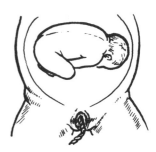

If the second baby has a satisfactory presentation and there is no evidence of fetal distress then, although the interval between delivery of first and second babies should not be prolonged, descent of the presenting part may be awaited. An oxytocin infusion may be commenced as uterine activity may reduce after delivery of twin 1. When the head or breech has descended into the pelvis the membranes may be ruptured and delivery proceeds.

If there is evidence of fetal distress then the second baby may be delivered more promptly by rupturing the second set of membranes and applying forceps or the ventouse, or, if required, internal podalic version and breech extraction may be performed.

Active management of the third stage only begins at delivery of the anterior shoulder of the second baby.

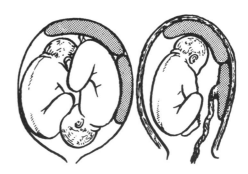

Placental site shrinking

Rarely the first placenta is born before the second baby. Bleeding is not usually severe. The uterus is actively contracting and the reduction in size of the placental site and the pressure of the fetus on it helps to control the blood loss.

Vigilance is required during the third stage to prevent atonic post-partum haemorrhage.

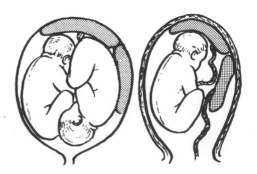

Placenta separating

MULTIPLE PREGNANCY

OTHER COMPLICATIONS
Locked Twins
Locked twins is a very rare condition in which parts of one interlock with the other causing an impasse. It most commonly occurs with the first as breech and the second as a vertex. The head of the second slips down with the shoulders of the first and prevents the engagement of the head of the first in the pelvis.

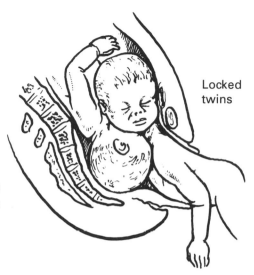

Locked twins

Early recognition is essential as the condition has a high fetal mortality. The treatment is to push the lower head out of the pelvis to free the head of the first fetus and allow delivery. If displacement is not possible the first baby will die. A destructive procedure may be performed to allow delivery of the trunk and then the second twin. Such expertise is uncommon in the UK and the psychological sequelae to a destructive procedure (decapitation of twin 1) are significant in this population. Consequently, upon diagnosis caesarean section may be undertaken.

If performed promptly this may also salvage twin 1.

Conjoined twins are due to imperfect separation of monozygotic twins. Vaginal delivery is possible particularly when delivery is preterm. Nevertheless most authorities would advocate elective caesarean section in a major paediatric/maternity unit.

Triplets and quadruplets have similar problems and difficulties. Premature labour is much commoner. The perinatal mortality rate is higher. Vaginal delivery is possible in triplet pregnancy although caesarean section remains the method of choice. Delivery by caesarean section is invariably the method of choice in quadruplet pregnancy.

Risk of Preterm Delivery

No of Fetuses	Median Gestation (Days)	Perinatal Mortality per thousand
1	280	11
2	245	60
3	231	150
4	203	

Fetus Papyraceous
Sometimes a twin does not develop but becomes amorphous or shrivelled and flattened. This is called fetus papyraceous or compressus. It may be readily apparent or may be found wrapped in the membranes of the placenta.

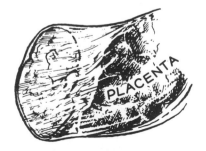

PLACENTA

PRETERM LABOUR

Preterm labour is defined as the onset of labour before 37 completed weeks of pregnancy.

INCIDENCE
5–10% of births but a major cause of peri-natal loss.

CAUSES
Certain conditions are associated with an increased risk of premature labour:

(a) Social factors:
    Low socio-economic groups.
    Low maternal age.
    Low maternal weight.
    Smoking.
(b) Overdistension of the uterus:
    Multiple pregnancy
    Polyhydramnios.
(c) Uterine anomaly:
    Congenital.
    Cervical incompetence.
(d) Fetal anomaly
(e) Infection:
    Maternal pyrexial illness.
    Amnionitis (premature rupture of the membranes)
(f) Antepartum haemorrhage
(g) Trauma:
    Injury.
    Surgery during pregnancy.

Many cases are unexplained and the mechanisms involved in stimulating uterine action are not clear.

PREVENTION
Improvements in the nutrition and general health of the population and a reduction in smoking should be beneficial.

Cervical suture is employed where there is evidence of incompetence of the cervix.

PRETERM LABOUR

TREATMENT
The decision to attempt to stop pre-term labour will depend on the period of gestation, the estimated fetal weight and the neonatal paediatric facilities available.

Improvements in paediatric care have reduced the need for efforts to postpone delivery.

Key points in the management of preterm labour
1. Need for tocolysis
2. Need for time to administer corticosteroids to accelerate fetal lung maturity
3. Need for time to transfer to Tertiary centre)

Beta-sympathomimetic Drugs
Betamimetics such as Salbutamol and Ritodrine inhibit sympathetic control of myometrium and delay delivery for between 24 and 48 hours but do not alter perinatal mortality rates. They are of value in delaying delivery until transfer to a facility with adequate paediatric support has taken place, and in allowing the administration of corticosteroids to accelerate fetal lung maturity.

They have several side-effects including maternal tachycardia, hyperglycaemia and hypokalaemia. A pulse rate of between 130–140 is acceptable, but overdosage may cause serious cardiac arrhythmias. There have been persistent reports of postpartum pulmonary oedema following the use of betamimetics in association with corticosteroids. Considerable caution should be exercised if these agents are used in combination.

Cardiac disease and diabetes are contraindications to the use of betamimetics.

Calcium Antagonists
This group of drugs also inhibit uterine muscle, but have not so far been found to offer any advantage over the betasympathomimetic drugs.

Prostaglandin Inhibitors
Drugs such as Indomethacin inhibit the production of prostaglandin synthetase and undoubtedly reduce uterine activity. Indomethacin appears to be a better tocolytic than betamimetics but there are risks of premature closure of the fetal ductus arteriosus and a reduction in fetal renal blood flow leading to renal failure if not adequately monitored. There have also been reports of increased rates of necrotising enterocolitis in the neonate if delivered within 48 hours of the last dose. Nevertheless, Indomethacin does appear to be an effective treatment for preterm labour and is being used increasingly. It may be given rectally as a 100 mg suppository twice daily for 48 hours.

In practice, the use of drugs to inhibit uterine activity has on the whole been disappointing. It is possible that more specific Cyclo-oxygenase 2 inhibitors may be more effective but these have still to be evaluated adequately.

PRETERM LABOUR

Assessment of effectiveness is difficult because of the uncertainty surrounding symptoms of labour. If the drug is given early enough to be followed by a cessation of activity, it is always possible that the patient was in 'false labour'. Further, when the cervix is 3 cm dilated and the existence of labour is not in doubt, it is likely to be irreversible anyway.

A more promising approach has been the introduction of oxytocin receptor blockers such as Atosiban but the development of this class of agents is at an early stage.

Corticosteroids

There is now clear evidence that corticosteroids given before 34 weeks gestation accelerate fetal lung maturity and decrease the incidence of respiratory distress syndrome and neonatal death. Betamethasone may be given, 24 mg in two divided doses, 12 hours apart.

PRETERM PREMATURE RUPTURE OF MEMBRANES

This means rupture of the membranes, in the absence of any uterine activity, prior to 37 completed weeks. The term 'Premature Rupture of the Membranes' is currently a potential source of confusion. Increasingly this term is being used to indicate rupture of the membranes in the absence of labour regardless of the gestational age and in North America may be used to describe this occurring, for example, at 42 weeks gestation.

CAUSES

Often the cause is not clear but bacterial vaginosis has been implicated. It may be that certain bacteria produce enzymes which exert a lytic effect on the fetal membranes. Other causes include cervical incompetence, fetal abnormality and polyhydramnios.

DANGERS

Intra-uterine infection (which may cause fetal death) and preterm labour.

MANAGEMENT

1. Admit to hospital.
2. Administer corticosteroids to accelerate lung maturation (in the absence of established infection).
3. Administer Erythromycin which reduces the number of births within 48 hours and number of babies infected.
4. 4-hourly temperature chart.
5. Detailed ultrasound scan to detect fetal abnormality.
6. Examine liquor for evidence of lung maturity (phosphatidyl glycerol). The specimen is obtained via sterile speculum and digital examination should be avoided.
7. Delivery is advised if lung maturity confirmed or clinical evidence of infection appears.

POSTMATURITY

This term applies to unduly prolonged pregnancy — commonly considered to be 294 days from the first day of the last menstrual period.

Postmaturity remains a common indication for induction of labour, mainly because of fears about fetal anoxia. The placenta shows signs of 'ageing' structurally and functionally after term. The perinatal mortality rate begins to rise in pregnancies running beyond 42 weeks. The risk of prolonged pregnancy will vary with other factors e.g. increased maternal age and hypertension.

A selective approach to intervention is, therefore, desirable and this is aided by modern methods of assessment:
1. Routine early ultrasound gives an accurate assessment of maturity.
2. A 'post dates' assessment of the fetus can be carried out at, e.g. term + 10 days.
   (a) Ultrasound will estimate fetal weight, fetal attitude (increased flexion with diminished liquor) and liquor volume (largest vertical pool).
   (b) Cardiotocography (repeated as considered appropriate) will give direct information about fetal well-being.
3. Even in the absence of concern about fetal well-being, the pregnant woman's views should be considered. Late pregnancy may be a time of great discomfort and induction of labour should be considered in her interest from ten days after the expected date of delivery.

PROLAPSE AND PRESENTATION OF THE CORD

Prolapse occurs after rupture of the membranes when the presenting part is ill-fitting or abnormal. It is associated with multiparity and prematurity, disproportion and malpresentation, fetal abnormality and polyhydramnios.

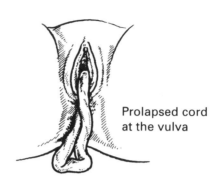

Prolapsed cord at the vulva

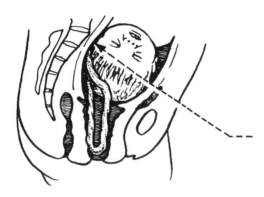

Once the cord is out of the uterus, and especially when out of the vagina, the fetal blood supply is obstructed, either because of the drop in temperature, and spasm of the vessels, or compression between the pelvic brim and the presenting part. If delivery is not effected promptly, fetal death is likely.

The presence of prolapse may not be recognised until cord appears at the vulva, or cord may be palpated on vaginal examination done to assess progress of the labour or because of the sudden onset of acute fetal distress. It is essential to make a vaginal examination as soon as the membranes rupture in all patients who display an ill-fitting or non-engaged presenting part.

Presentation of the cord means that the cord is palpable at the cervix through intact membranes. Occult presentation means that the cord is lying alongside the presenting part but will not be palpable on vaginal examination. It is a particularly dangerous condition and may be a cause of unexpected fetal distress.

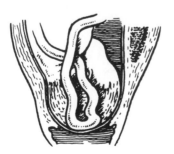

Presentation of the cord

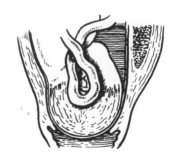

Occult presentation of the cord

PROLAPSE AND PRESENTATION OF THE CORD

TREATMENT

1. Determine the presence or absence of cord pulsation and fetal heart sounds. If the fetus is dead the labour may be left to proceed normally (if no other complication is present).

2. If the fetus is still alive, caesarean section must be carried out as soon as possible unless vaginal delivery by forceps or breech extraction is likely to be straightforward.

3. While arrangements are being made for operation, the cord should be pushed back into the vagina and kept up with a gauze pack or by hand. An attempt is made to prevent compression of the cord between the presenting part and the pelvis by getting the mother to adopt a suitable position. The foot of the bed should be raised.

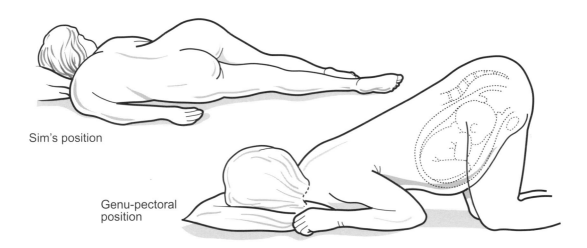

Sim's position

Genu-pectoral position

4. Handling of the cord should be minimised as far as possible.

5. Prolapse of the cord, although potentially fatal for the child, carries little risk for the mother unless proper precautions are neglected for the sake of saving time. However great the need for haste, the mother must be properly prepared for operation and appropriate blood products available.

6. Presentation of the cord when discovered by vaginal examination is an indication for section but, as the membranes are intact, there is no immediate danger for the fetus, and more time is available.

POLYHYDRAMNIOS

Normally the amniotic fluid volume is around 500–1500 ml and if it is excessive it is called polyhydramnios. Two litres will be detectable clinically as excessive.

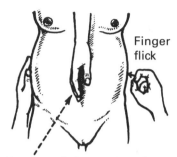

Finger flick

Hand on abdomen to cut transmission of impulse round abdominal wall

SIGNS

1. The uterus is bigger than expected.
2. Identification of the fetus and fetal parts is difficult.
3. The fetal heart is difficult to hear.
4. Ballottement of the fetus is easy.
5. A fluid thrill is detected.
6. Abdominal girth at the umbilicus is more than 100 cm before term. The abdominal girth varies a little — an ebb and flow.

CAUSES

Excess liquor amnii is associated with fetal abnormality — especially anencephaly, spina bifida, oesophageal atresia, hydrops fetalis and monozygotic twins. Haemangioma of the placenta is found on rare occasions with polyhydramnios.

Maternal conditions associated with polyhydramnios are diabetes and the more severe forms of heart disease and pre-eclampsia.

The development of polyhydramnios is usually gradual and in the last trimester. The symptoms are due to the bulk and weight of the uterus.

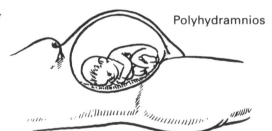

Polyhydramnios

1. Discomfort and dyspnoea.
2. Indigestion.
3. Oedema, increase of varicose veins and haemorrhoids.
4. There may be abdominal pain.

If polyhydramnios develops between 24 and 30 weeks it is often more acute. Acute abdominal pain and a feeling of 'bursting' are often the presenting symptoms. Frequently there is vomiting. The abdominal skin is glazed, sometimes oedematous and often with fresh striae. The uterus is tense and tender and may be mistaken for concealed accidental haemorrhage, but there is no shock.

Polyhydramnios, whether acute or chronic, may lead to late miscarriage or preterm labour.

POLYHYDRAMNIOS

MANAGEMENT

A detailed ultrasound scan of the fetus should be carried out in an attempt to find a cause for the condition. If the fetus appears anatomically normal then the aim is to prolong the pregnancy until maturity.

A glucose tolerance test should be performed to exclude gestational diabetes.

Indomethacin has been used successfully in the 50% of cases in which no cause is found. Careful fetal evaluation is needed to identify any fetal renal compromise. The role of other Cyclo-oxygenase selective inhibitors (COX-2) such as Rofecoxib is still to be evaluated. Rarely in monochorionic twin pregnancy complicated by twin transfusion syndrome, polyhydramnios develops in the sac of the recipient twin and repeated amniocentesis becomes necessary to relieve distressing symptoms and to prolong the pregnancy.

DIFFERENTIAL DIAGNOSIS

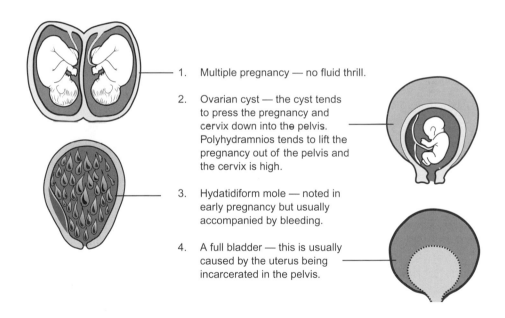

1. Multiple pregnancy — no fluid thrill.

2. Ovarian cyst — the cyst tends to press the pregnancy and cervix down into the pelvis. Polyhydramnios tends to lift the pregnancy out of the pelvis and the cervix is high.

3. Hydatidiform mole — noted in early pregnancy but usually accompanied by bleeding.

4. A full bladder — this is usually caused by the uterus being incarcerated in the pelvis.

Ultrasound will differentiate all these conditions if there is still doubt after clinical examination.

OLIGOHYDRAMNIOS

Oligohydramnios describes the finding, on clinical or ultrasound examination, of reduced liquor volume. It may be found as the result of fetal renal agenesis when there may be virtually no fluid, or in cases of IUGR.

Oligohydramnios also results from rupture of the membranes and in early pregnancy — around 18–24 weeks — results in pulmonary hypoplasia.

UNSTABLE LIE

This term is used when the longitudinal axis of the fetus is repeatedly changing in relation to the uterus. Variable lie is an alternative title. Transverse, oblique or longitudinal lies may be found but no lie persists. The patient is usually multiparous.

CAUSES
1. Lax abdominal and uterine muscles.
2. Polyhydramnios.
3. Distortion of lower uterine pole e.g. placenta or pelvic tumour.
4. Abnormal fetus.

Congenital malformation of the uterus tends to give a stable malpresentation.

Unstable lie is not a problem till the last four or five weeks of pregnancy. The foreseen danger is that labour will commence or that the membranes will rupture while there is a malpresentation leading to obstructed labour and/or cord prolapse. For this reason it is common practice to suggest hospital admission at about 38 weeks to patients with unstable lie. As the pregnancy proceeds the likelihood of the onset of labour or rupture of the membranes increases.

The liquor amnii is at a maximum about 35 weeks (approximately one litre) and less at term (0.5 litres or so). With fetal growth it appears even less relatively and this may stabilise the lie and presentation.

MANAGEMENT
1. Conservative — as the liquor decreases and the fetal size increases towards term the instability lessens and may lead to normal labour.
2. External version to longitudinal lie is usually easy but reversion to an abnormal lie is common. Version may be undertaken as part of the more active management at term; the patient is taken to theatre with full preparation made for caesarean section. When the lie is longitudinal oxytocin may be administered and controlled amniotomy performed. Liquor is allowed to drain, if possible at a slow rate. The main danger is of cord prolapse, in which case section can be immediately undertaken. Some workers remove the liquor transabdominally by amniocentesis in theatre in order to reduce this risk. Placental abruption may follow if the reduction in liquor volume is rapid.
3. Elective caesarean section may be performed.
4. An abnormal fetus incompatible with life such as an anencephaly would justify termination of pregnancy, but not the risk of a caesarean section.

Abnormal conditions such as tumours would be treated on their merits.

All cases which have had an unstable lie should be examined carefully in early labour to check that all is still satisfactory.

SPECIAL CASES

1. THE OLDER MOTHER

The uncomplimentary and rather emotive term 'elderly primigravida' should no longer be used but it had been commonly applied to a woman who becomes pregnant for the first time at the age of over 35 years. With healthy women often choosing to defer childbirth, older women are seen increasingly and, reasonably, object to this term.

It is of course an arbitrary term and the patients of this age who are young in mind and body, and have conceived without difficulty will usually do very well. Pregnancy in some women in this group, however, has occurred after a long period of infertility and there is an awareness in the minds of her attendants that the prospect of her conceiving again may be relatively low. The overall perinatal mortality in this group is raised as is the incidence of operative delivery.

The following antenatal complications are increased in frequency and may merit special investigation.

(a) Miscarriage.
(b) Down's syndrome.
(c) Hypertensive disorders.
(d) Intra-uterine growth restriction.
(e) Premature labour.
(f) Gynaecological disorders e.g. fibroids.
(g) Deep Vein Thrombosis and Pulmonary Embolism

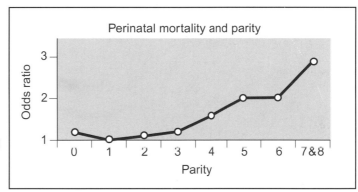

2. THE GRAND MULTIPARA

This term is rarely used in these days of limitation of family size, but it is worth remembering that rising parity is associated with a rising peri-natal mortality rate. The increase in fetal loss in fourth and subsequent pregnancies is striking (see graph above).

The mother of high parity is subject to the problems of increasing age and its effects, the harassment of a young family and the exhaustion this can cause, especially if there is little respite between pregnancies. The result may be self-neglect and poor attendance for antenatal care. Inevitably these factors are most harmful in lower socio-economic groups.

The incidence of the following complications is increased:
Anaemia.
Unstable lie due to muscular laxity.
Placental abruption.
Uterine rupture.
Post partum haemorrhage.

213

UTERINE DISPLACEMENTS AND ANOMALIES

RETROVERTED GRAVID UTERUS

This condition is probably a result of conception occurring in an already retroverted uterus. The commonest outcome is spontaneous correction between the 9th and 12th weeks, but sometimes the uterus becomes incarcerated in the pelvis as it grows, especially in the presence of some obstruction to correction, such as adhesions or pelvic contraction.

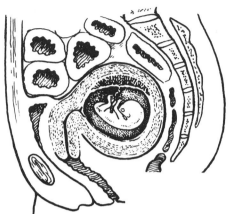

Incarcerated RGU

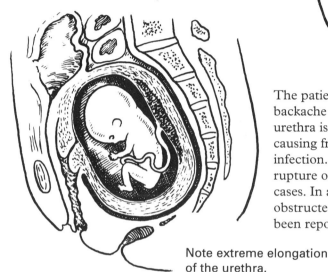

Note extreme elongation of the urethra.

The patient complains of pelvic pain and backache and defecation is painful. The urethra is compressed and elongated causing frequency, retention overflow and infection. Sometimes acute retention and rupture of the bladder occurs in neglected cases. In addition the vesical blood supply is obstructed and gangrene of the bladder has been reported.

Diagnosis

Urinary frequency and incontinence in early pregnancy always call for pelvic examination. In retroversion the cervix is high behind the symphysis and difficult to reach, the bladder is pushed up, and the soft uterus is felt in the pouch of Douglas.

Differential Diagnosis

Urinary retention and pouch of Douglas swelling may also be due to:

Haematocele from tubal pregnancy. Tenderness is extreme.

Fibroids are as a rule harder and more irregular.

An ovarian cyst may push the uterus up and forwards.

An ultrasound scan will help to differentiate these lesions.

Treatment

1. No action need be taken if the patient is asymptomatic but she should be warned of the dangers of urinary retention.
2. If urinary or other symptoms are present, the patient should be admitted and rested in bed for 48 hours with an indwelling catheter. This may allow the uterus to rise out of its abnormal position but catheterisation may sometimes need to be continued until the uterus has risen into the abdomen.

UTERINE DISPLACEMENTS AND ANOMALIES

FORWARD DISPLACEMENTS OF THE UTERUS ('PENDULOUS ABDOMEN')

If the pelvis is contracted and prevents descent, or if the abdominal muscles are weak (a consequence of repeated pregnancies) the uterus will project forward. A compensatory lordosis develops and the woman suffers great discomfort from backache and the stretching of the abdominal muscles. The condition causes delay in engagement of the presenting part apart from any disproportion, and may contribute to uterine rupture. A supporting corset may help during the pregnancy.

PROLAPSE OF THE UTERUS

This may co-exist with pregnancy and will be aggravated in the early months by the softening and stretching of the tissues. The cervix projects well beyond the vulva and becomes oedematous and ulcerated. A ring pessary will maintain the uterus in the correct position until it is too big to descend through the pelvis (usually about the 20th week).

TORSION OF THE UTERUS

Some dextro-rotation is normal in pregnancy, probably because the pelvic colon takes up some of the space available in the left pelvis. Occasionally this rotation reaches 90 degrees and if seen at caesarean section care must be taken not to incise the left broad ligament and arteries. Torsion so severe as to interfere with the blood supply is unknown except as a complication of pregnancy in one horn of a double uterus when it is usually mistaken for concealed accidental haemorrhage.

CONGENITAL ABNORMALITIES

These are the result of imperfect fusion of the two Mullerian ducts. The uterus, cervix and vagina, separately or together, can be single, double or intermediate; classification is difficult and nomenclature confused. The anomalies described here are representative.

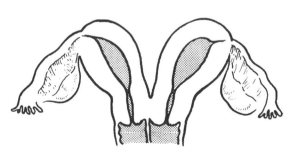

Double uterus, cervix and vagina
(Didelphys — 'double womb')

Uterus Didelphys

When both horns are well developed the pregnancy proceeds normally. Diagnosis is difficult but a double vagina and cervix may be observed, although easily missed at routine pelvic examination.

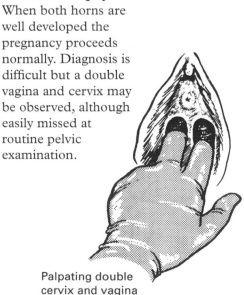

Palpating double cervix and vagina

Torsion of one horn can occur more easily than in the normal uterus and may occur during version, causing fetal death and symptoms of accidental haemorrhage. The nongravid horn develops its own decidua and hypertrophies, and has been known to occupy the pelvis and obstruct labour.

215

UTERINE DISPLACEMENTS AND ANOMALIES

CONGENITAL ABNORMALITIES *(continued)*
Uterus Bicornis Unicollis

It is impossible to diagnose this condition except at laparotomy or perhaps during removal of a retained placenta which is more common with these abnormalities. This uterus encourages breech presentation — the head occupies one horn, the feet the other.

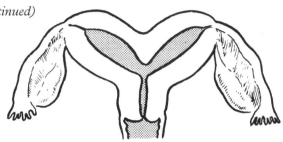

Uterus bicornis, unicollis, single vagina

Uterus Septus, Uterus SubSeptus, Uterus Arcuatus ('Cordiform Uterus')

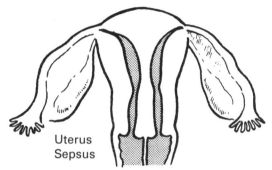

Uterus Sepsus

Uterus SubSepsus

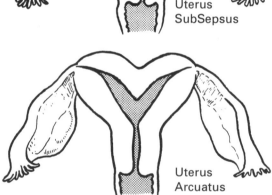

Uterus Arcuatus

This group can only be diagnosed when the uterus is opened at caesarean section, although the arcuate uterus is often suspected on abdominal palpation through a thin abdominal wall. As a group they predispose to miscarriage, and to some complications of later pregnancy such as abnormal or unstable lie, and retained placenta.

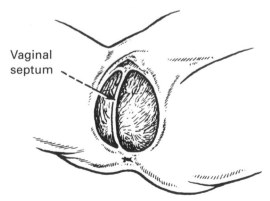

Vaginal septum

Vaginal Septa

These can occur on their own in otherwise normal genital tracts and are often incomplete. Sometimes the second stage may be delayed because of a septum preventing the advance of the head. The best treatment is to await this situation, and then when the septum is stretched, inject a little local anaesthetic, ligate, and divide with scissors.

TUMOURS COMPLICATING PREGNANCY

The important ones are carcinoma of the cervix, fibroids and ovarian cysts.

FIBROIDS

Pregnancy in the presence of fibroids is rather rare. They contribute to infertility and are usually found in older women.

Diagnosis

Fibroids are harder than any other pelvic mass likely to be met with and more likely to be multiple, but diagnosis is often presumptive. Twins, tubal pregnancy, ovarian cysts, salpingitis, cornual or angular pregnancies must all be considered. But fibroids are usually symptomless and can be left alone.

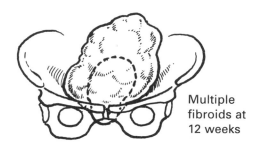

Multiple fibroids at 12 weeks

Degeneration. Fibroids are subject to 'red degeneration' (infarction) during pregnancy, when they become tender and painful and cause fever. Sedation only is required until the condition subsides in a few days but sometimes laparotomy may have to be performed to exclude appendicitis. Degeneration may also complicate the puerperium.

Pressure Symptoms. If the fibroids are very big or are impacted in the pelvis, dysuria, abdominal distension, varicose veins and even dyspnoea may be complained of. Treatment should always be conservative unless an obstruction develops. Myomectomy in pregnancy is a very haemorrhagic operation, and likely to be followed by miscarriage or even require hysterectomy.

Management of Labour. If the fibroid obstructs descent and engagement, caesarean section should be carried out, but if not, the labour should proceed normally. If there is doubt about obstruction the labour should be continued for a period to see if dilatation of the cervix causes the fibroid to be moved aside. If delivery is by section, myomectomy should not be done at the same time. Fibroids regress considerably in the months following pregnancy and the uterine incision may be placed anywhere, through the fundus if necessary, to avoid interfering with the fibroids which will bleed excessively.

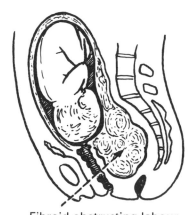

Fibroid obstructing labour

217

TUMOURS COMPLICATING PREGNANCY

OVARIAN CYSTS

Ovarian cysts are uncommon in pregnancy but are important clinically due to the complications associated with them.

Corpus luteum cysts may become quite large in early pregnancy. Unless they undergo haemorrhage, torsion or rupture they may be managed conservatively as they usually regress and removal may cause miscarriage. If cysts persist beyond 14 weeks gestation they are usually removed to prevent mechanical complications and the possibility of malignancy.

The commonest type, after corpus luteum cysts, is the simple cyst (70%) or the dermoid (25%). Ovarian cancer occurs in around 1 in 18 000 pregnancies.

Diagnosis

Palpation is much easier in early pregnancy before the uterus occupies most of the pelvis. An ovarian cyst is more mobile than a hydro- or pyosalpinx, and less tender than a tubal pregnancy.

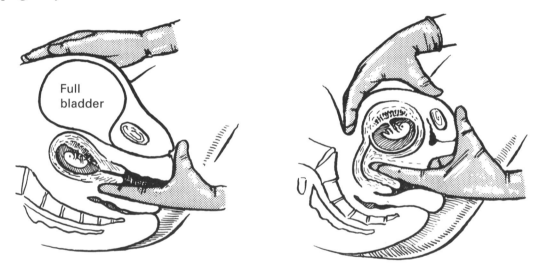

1. A full bladder especially when dislodged from the pelvis by the gravid uterus, is often mistaken for a cyst.
2. A normal gravid uterus from the 2nd to the 4th month has a very soft isthmic region and it is easy to mistake the cervix for the uterus and the corpus for a cyst.

Diagnosis of pelvic masses is accomplished by ultrasonography.

TUMOURS COMPLICATING PREGNANCY

Complications in the Cyst

1. Torsion is the commonest and may lead to rupture. The symptoms are acute, with sudden onset of abdominal pain, vomiting and pyrexia. These subside, to occur again a few days later. Pelvic examination will reveal a tender cystic mass and the distinction from tubal pregnancy may be impossible. Cyst torsion is likelier in the puerperium when the involuting uterus no longer limits movement of the cyst.
2. Pressure symptoms may arise if the cyst becomes incarcerated in the pelvis or is of very large size. These will include dysuria, pain, abdominal distension and varicose veins.
3. Infection. This is most likely in the puerperium as a result of trauma sustained during delivery.

Complications in the Pregnancy

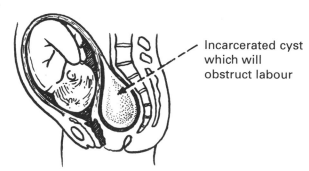

Incarcerated cyst which will obstruct labour

1. There is an increased tendency to miscarriage if the cyst is large.
2. A cyst in the pelvis will obstruct labour, causing malpresentation or non-engagement of the head.

Treatment

Laparotomy in early pregnancy is not usually a problem as little handling of the uterus is required to gain access to the cyst. If a cyst is discovered at or near term and is well clear of the pelvis, labour can be induced and the cyst removed a few days later. If the cyst is likely to obstruct labour, caesarean section and removal of the cyst should be performed.

The most difficult decisions arise in mid-pregnancy when laparotomy to remove the cyst might involve considerable uterine handling. The obstetrician must decide whether removal of the cyst can safely be postponed until the fetus is viable.

CARCINOMA OF THE CERVIX

Treatment

Proper treatment of the condition requires the termination of the pregnancy. The implications of delaying treatment for the sake of the fetus should be fully discussed with the mother. If the baby is viable, delivery should be by classical caesarean section following which normal treatment can be given. In early pregnancy hysterotomy may be carried out or external irradiation applied which will cause fetal death. Treatment in this case would be completed by the subsequent insertion of Caesium.

The positive cervical smear in pregnancy

The management of the positive cervical smear in pregnancy has been greatly simplified by the use of colposcopy. A colposcopic examination may provide adequate reassurance or allow a punch biopsy to be taken safely to make a definitive diagnosis.

RECURRENT MISCARRIAGE

Recurrent, or *habitual* miscarriage describes the occurrence of three consecutive spontaneous miscarriages. The causes of sporadic miscarriage may also be found in these cases though no specific aetiology is found in the majority of cases. In around 1–3% balanced chromosomal translocation will be found. Luteal phase defects, commonly causes of infertility, may also be associated with repeated early loss. Some workers have advocated treatment with progesterone for such cases. The antiphospholipid syndromes are associated with recurrent loss and the presence of Lupus Inhibitor in particular is a marker for poor outcome. Treatment with aspirin and heparin peri-conceptionally has been advocated.

Thyroid disorders are also associated with pregnancy loss though treatment may not improve pregnancy outcome if the disease is autoimmune in nature.

Congenital abnormalities of the uterus may be associated with some cases but the incidence of these conditions in the general population is small.

The role of alloimmune disease in recurrent miscarriage is currently the focus of some attention. Histocompatability between parents may, ironically, increase the risk of miscarriage since the maintenance of the pregnancy depends on the maternal immune system recognising the fetus as immunologically different. In women who do not develop antibodies to the paternally derived fetal antigens, miscarriage is commoner. Immunisation of women with their partners' white blood cells has been advocated as a treatment for recurrent loss but is not universally accepted as a worthwhile treatment. For the majority of women investigation will exclude these causes.

In a small number the diagnosis will be made of **cervical incompetence.**

Recurrent miscarriage is often attributed to this cause especially if there has been a history of previous trauma such as a second trimester elective termination of pregnancy, or some traumatic incident associated with childbirth. The condition is not a common one and tends to be overdiagnosed. The patient's history is the best guide to diagnosis although even this is limited and the following features may help to differentiate cervical incompetence from other causes of pregnancy loss.

a) Pregnancy ends in mid-trimester or early third trimester.
b) The cervix may dilate silently allowing prolapse of the gestation sac into the vagina and rupture of the membranes.
c) Bleeding is not a feature. If the cervix is seen to be damaged it should be repaired, but often there is no visible or palpable lesion, and the treatment of cervical suture (McDonald Suture: Shirodkar suture: cervical cerclage) is applied empirically.

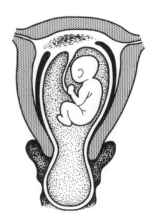

RECURRENT MISCARRIAGE

Technique of cervical suture

Under anaesthesia the cervix is grasped with a vulsellum and four bites of non-absorbable, inert suture are inserted at the level of the internal os. The suture is tightened to resist a No. 6 dilator and is removed at 37 weeks.

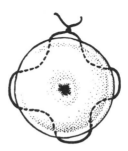

This treatment does not harm but is too often applied irrationally to patients who have suffered recurrent miscarriage not obviously because of cervical incompetence. This arises in part because of the lack of an effective method of confirming the diagnosis.

Difficulties arise when miscarriage becomes inevitable in spite of the suture which must then be removed to prevent further damage to the cervix.

Pregnancy and assisted conception programmes

Pregnancy following in vitro fertilisation and ovulation induction techniques is now commonplace. These women tend to be older and the risk of Down's syndrome and multiple pregnancy are both increased. Being older they are also at increased risk of pre-existing medical disorders and hypertension is a particular concern. Management should be based on conventional obstetric factors but intervention rates (induction of labour and caesarean section) are often increased because of anxiety on the part of the mother (or her attendants!).

CHAPTER 11

NORMAL LABOUR

LABOUR

Labour is the process of birth. In response to uterine contractions the lower segment stretches and thins, the cervix dilates, the birth canal is formed and the baby descends through the pelvis.

UTERINE ACTION

The fibres of the myometrium **Contract** and **Relax** like all muscle.

In labour when the muscle fibres relax they do not return to their former length but become progressively shorter: this is **Retraction.**

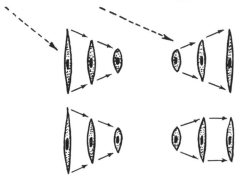

The uterine capacity is thus progressively reduced and the thickness of the uterine wall increased.

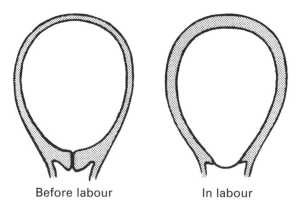

Before labour   In labour

As labour progresses the contractions increase in frequency, strength and duration. The muscle of the lower segment of the uterus (see Chapter 2) is thin and relatively passive, and the cervix consists mainly of fibrous connective tissue.

LABOUR

Cervical effacement

The effect of the progressive retraction of the upper segment muscle is to stretch and thin the lower segment and cause effacement and dilatation of the cervix. The junction of the upper and lower segments is called the physiological retraction ring.

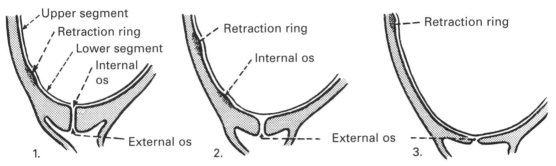

Cervical dilatation

Effacement is most striking in the primigravida. In the parous patient dilatation and effacement usually occur together.

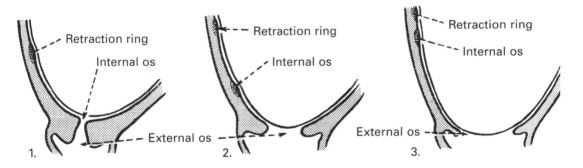

'Show' and formation of forewaters

The effacement and dilatation of the cervix loosens the membranes from the region of the internal os with slight bleeding and sets free the mucus plug or operculum. This constitutes the 'show' and allows the formation of forewaters, the amniotic sac pushing against the cervix.

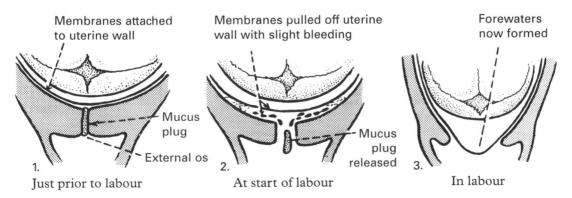

Just prior to labour   At start of labour   In labour   225

LABOUR — THE BIRTH CANAL

Labour is divided into **Three Stages:**
First Stage...   start to full dilatation of the cervix.
Second Stage...   full dilatation to birth of baby.
Third Stage...   birth of baby to delivery of placenta (afterbirth).

AT THE BEGINNING OF LABOUR

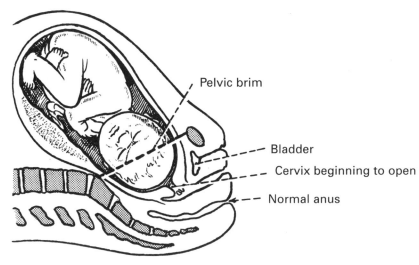

The fetus is descending during first and second stages of labour.
The birth canal is formed by dilatation of the cervix and vagina and by stretching and displacement of the muscles of the pelvic floor and perineum.
The bladder is pulled above the pubis because of its attachment to the uterus; the urethra is stretched and the bowel is compressed.

BIRTH CANAL AT BEGINNING OF SECOND STAGE

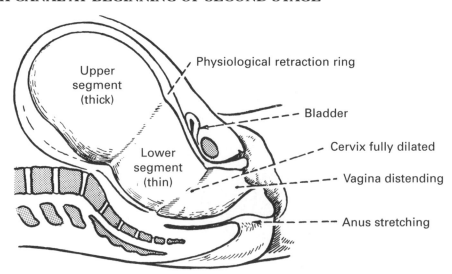

LABOUR – THE BIRTH CANAL

At the **End** of the **Second** stage the birth canal has been fully formed. The outlet of the canal is at right angles to the inlet. The angulation is called the Curve of Carus.

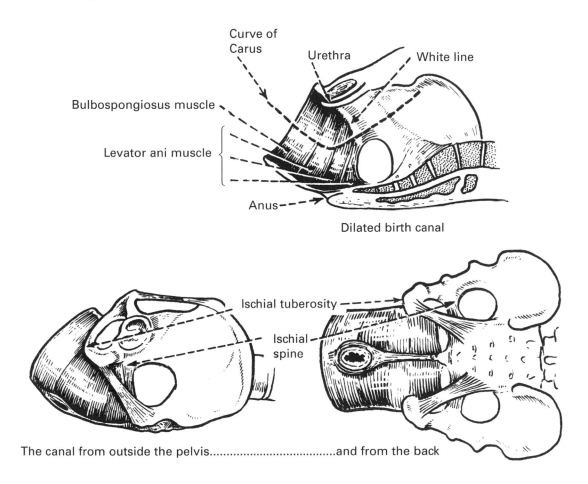

Curve of Carus
Urethra
White line
Bulbospongiosus muscle
Levator ani muscle
Anus
Dilated birth canal

Ischial tuberosity
Ischial spine

The canal from outside the pelvis.....................................and from the back

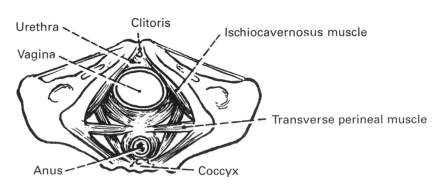

Urethra
Clitoris
Ischiocavernosus muscle
Vagina
Transverse perineal muscle
Anus
Coccyx

Stretching and displacement viewed from below (after delivery)

THE MECHANISM OF LABOUR

The mechanism of labour is the series of passive movements of the baby, particularly its presenting part, as it descends through the birth canal.

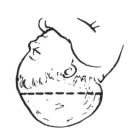

Illustrated is the mechanism of labour where the vertex presents in the left occipito-lateral (LOL) position.

NORMAL MECHANISM

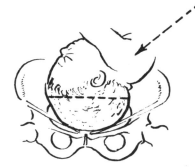

The **head** is presenting in the **transverse** diameter of the pelvic brim with the **Occiput** to the **Left**. There is often **Asynclitism** prior to engagement, i.e. when one or other parietal bone is the leading part.

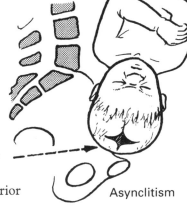

Asynclitism

The diagram shows the posterior parietal bone leading — this is posterior asynclitism. (If the anterior parietal bone is leading there is anterior asynclitism.)

At the **beginning** of **labour** the fetus is in an attitude of **Flexion** but the neck is not yet fully flexed so the **Occipito-Frontal** is the **presenting** diameter.

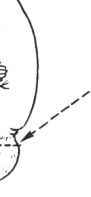

Flexion

As labour progresses the fetus becomes compact. The neck is fully flexed and the **Suboccipito-Bregmatic** becomes the presenting diameter.

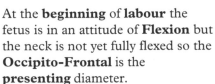

Compaction

THE MECHANISM OF LABOUR

Descent and Engagement occur.

Engagement is the descent of the presenting diameters through the pelvic brim.

The leading part — the vertex — is now near the level of the ischial spines.

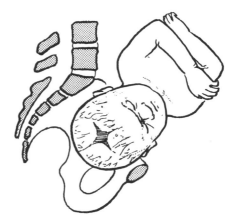

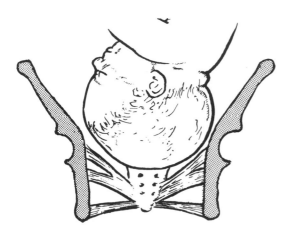

Descent continues and the occiput rotates in the cavity of the pelvis anteriorly to the right oblique diameter bringing the occiput to the left obturator foramen anteriorly.

Now in left occipito-anterior (LOA) position.

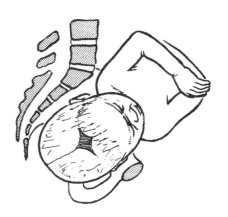

The LOA position is partly attributed to the presence of the sigmoid colon in the left posterior quadrant of the pelvis.

Note how the neck is twisting.

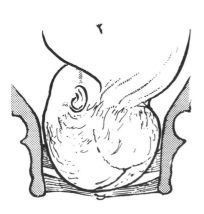

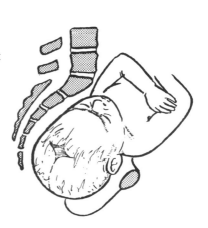

229

THE MECHANISM OF LABOUR

Descent continues and the occiput reaches the pelvic floor.

The occiput rotates to the front. This is **Internal rotation.** The head is now occipito-anterior (OA). Note twisting of the head and shoulders. The shoulders are in the left oblique of the brim.

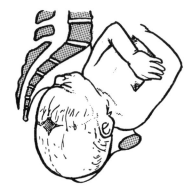

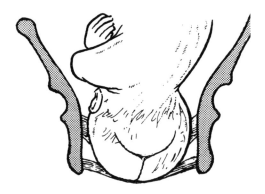

It is a maxim that the fetal part which first comes in contact with the pelvic floor rotates anteriorly (Internal rotation).

Rotation is through 45° from oblique and is called Anterior or Short rotation.

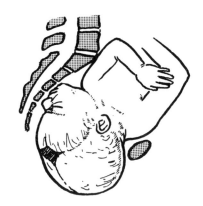

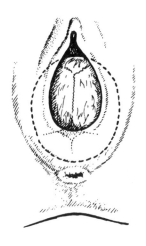

The Occiput is now below the symphysis. Further descent of the fetus pushes the head forwards with a movement of extension and the occiput is delivered.

Increasing extension round the pubis delivers the Bregma, Brow and Face.

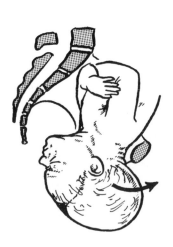

THE MECHANISM OF LABOUR

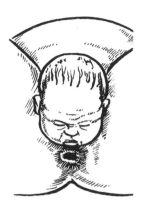

Delivery of head

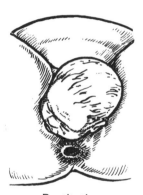

Restitution

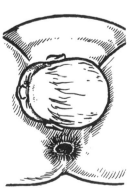

External Rotation

Descent and **Delivery** of the head has brought the shoulders into the pelvic cavity.

The head on delivery is oblique to the line of the shoulders. The bisacromial diameter is in left oblique diameter of the cavity.

The bisacromial diameter is the distance between the acromion processes and is 11 cm.

The head now rotates to the natural position relative to the shoulders. This movement is known as **Restitution.**

Descent continues and the shoulders rotate to bring the bisacromial diameter into the antero-posterior diameter of the pelvic outlet.

This descent and rotation causes the head to rotate so that the occiput lies next to the left maternal thigh. This is **External rotation.**

The anterior shoulder now slips under the pubis and with lateral flexion of the fetal body the posterior shoulder is born. The rest of the body follows easily.

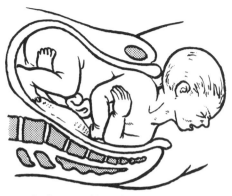

Delivery of head

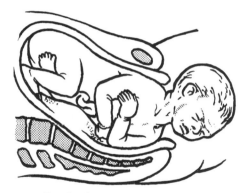

Restitution

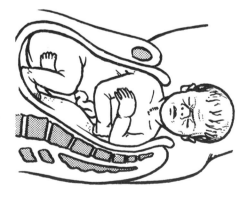

External Rotation

231

DIAGNOSIS OF LABOUR

The point of onset of labour is often uncertain as dilatation and effacement of the cervix may be present before labour, particularly in parous women. 'Show' is not always present and observation over a period of time may be needed to establish the diagnosis.

True labour
Regular contractions.
'Show'.
Progressive dilatation and effacement of cervix.

False or Spurious Labour
Irregular contractions.
No 'Show'.
No progressive dilatation or effacement of cervix.

LABOUR IS RECOGNISED BY:

1. Palpable uterine contractions which are regular in frequency and intermittent in character. The interval between contractions is 10 minutes or less and each contraction may last half a minute or longer.

The uterus becomes firm and rises, altering the abdominal contour. This is due to the rising forwards of the uterus so that it approximates to the direction of the birth canal. This movement is easier if the patient is upright. Ambulation may therefore give mechanical advantage.

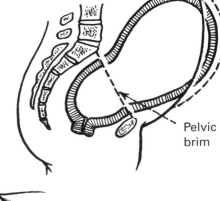

Altered abdominal contour with contraction

Pelvic brim

The discomfort is felt in the upper sacral region and lower abdomen.

2. 'Show'. A little blood and mucus discharged from the vagina. This is from separation of the membranes at the lower pole causing bleeding which mixes with the operculum of the cervix.

3. Dilatation of the Cervix. This is accompanied by the formation of forewaters or bag of waters.

Cervical dilatation is gauged by vaginal examination and is expressed in the diameter across the cervix.

1 finger
2 cm

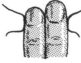

2 fingers
3.5 cm
⅓ DILATED

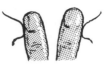

3 fingers
5.5 cm
½ DILATED

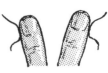

4 fingers
7.5 cm
¾ DILATED

PROGRESS IN LABOUR

PROGRESS IN LABOUR IS GAUGED BY:

1. Increasing strength, frequency and duration of **uterine contractions** — assessed by palpation, external abdominal transducer or intrauterine catheter.

2. **Dilatation of the cervix.** This may be estimated by vaginal examination.

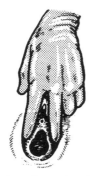

After cleansing the vulva the labia are parted with the gloved hand

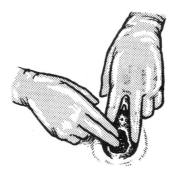

The fingers of the right hand are introduced gently into the vagina

Points to be noted:

i. Degree of dilatation and effacement of the cervix.

ii. Presence or absence of forewaters.

iii. State of the liquor if any (clear? meconium stained?).

iv. Position of the presenting part. This is determined by palpating the suture lines and fontanelles in relation to the pelvic diameters.

v. Level of the presenting part. This is judged by its relationship to the brim or ischial spines.

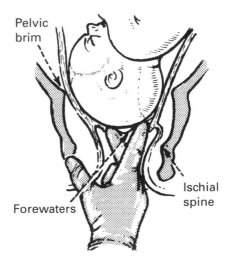

The diagram shows a well-flexed head in the LOL position which is almost engaged (the suboccipitobregmatic diameter is just above the brim), the cervix is about 3 fingers dilated and the forewaters are present.

PROGRESS IN LABOUR

3. Descent of the presenting part

This can be recognised by abdominal palpation or vaginal examination.

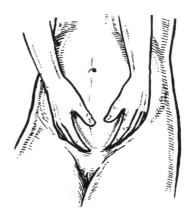

On palpation the amount of head felt above the brim is expressed in 'fifths'.

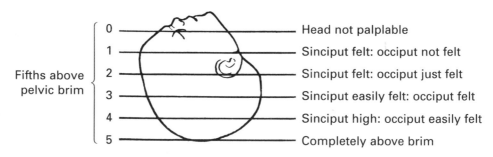

Fifths above pelvic brim		
0	Head not palplable
1	Sinciput felt: occiput not felt
2	Sinciput felt: occiput just felt
3	Sinciput easily felt: occiput felt
4	Sinciput high: occiput easily felt
5	Completely above brim

On vaginal examination descent is judged by zero station notation.

Zero is the level of the ischial spines, that is the mid pelvis, and estimations are in centimetres above and below zero.

The leading part at zero = just engaged.

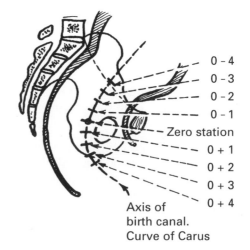

0 - 4
0 - 3
0 - 2
0 - 1
Zero station
0 + 1
0 + 2
0 + 3
0 + 4

Axis of birth canal. Curve of Carus

PROGRESS IN LABOUR

The **First** Stage of labour in a primigravida lasts up to 12 hours and sometimes longer and in a parous woman is usually 4–8 hours.

The effects of the increasing strength of contractions on the mother will be obvious in her appearance. During them she is preoccupied and slips into the breathing pattern she has learned. She may become distressed with the contractions. Commonly spontaneous rupture of the membranes occurs as the first stage proceeds.

The normal **Second** Stage of labour in a primigravida lasts about one hour and is much shorter in the parous woman. It is recognised by a change in the character of the contractions. They become more powerful and expulsive with a desire to bear down, and the secondary forces now come into action. The diaphragm is fixed, the patient holds her breath and the abdominal muscles contract. Sometimes the mother feels nauseated and may vomit. She may have the feeling that the bowel is about to move, due to pressure on the rectum, and this may have an inhibiting effect on her until the reason is explained. The head descends deeply in the pelvis and may be visible or palpable through the perineum.

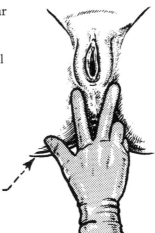

MANAGEMENT OF LABOUR

GENERAL CONSIDERATIONS

The aim should be to provide the mother with a relaxed, friendly atmosphere within which her well-being and that of the baby can be closely supervised. The presence of her husband, partner, mother or friend should be encouraged. The mother's preferences in respect of the conduct of her labour and delivery should be met as far as possible.

The Labour Suite should provide a sitting room furnished with comfortable chairs of various heights and types. Radio/Cassette tape recorder, CD player or television may provide entertainment and distraction. Ideally the atmosphere created should be as near to a 'home within hospital' as much as is compatible with facilities and safety.

There should be a separate delivery room with a bed to which the mother can retire if she wishes.

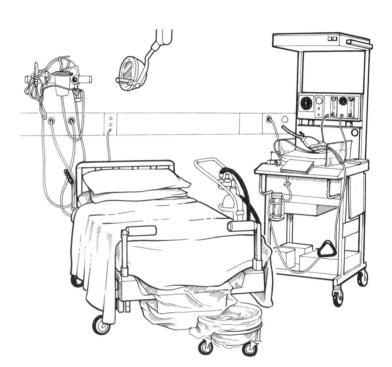

CARE OF THE MOTHER

1. **General.** The mother should not be left alone. Fears can be allayed and confidence engendered by a supportive midwife. Minimal perineal shaving may be done in case an episiotomy is required. If the rectum is full a suppository is given to reduce the risk of faecal soiling in late labour. Access to a bath or shower should be available.
2. **Diet** is withheld because delayed gastric emptying leads to the danger of inhalation of stomach contents should a general anaesthetic be required. The routine administration of antacids has now been stopped in many hospitals but H_2-antagonists such as cimetidine may be given intramuscularly if surgical intervention seems likely.
3. **Pulse rate,** blood pressure and urinary output are measured regularly and if ketosis or dehydration develops this is treated by intravenous fluids.
4. Progress in labour is assessed as already described.

MANAGEMENT OF LABOUR

CARE OF THE MOTHER *(continued)*

5. **Analgesia** is given as required. The method chosen depends on the mother's preference, her reaction to her contractions and the likely length of her labour.

(a) Inhalation — Entonox is a 50/50 mixture of oxygen and nitrous oxide. It may be used near the end of the first stage or during the second stage of labour.

The device is designed for self-administration by inhalation through a mask or mouthpiece attached to a cylinder.

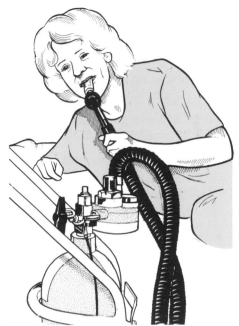

(b) TENS (transcutaneous electrical nerve stimulation)
This is a technique by means of which an electrical stimulus is applied to the mother's skin over her back by means of electrodes connected to a battery powered device. The position of the electrodes is in the dermatome corresponding to the pain. The strength of the stimulus may be controlled by the mother. Many women find it helpful in the early first stage of labour.

(c) Narcotic drugs
Pethidine 100–200 mg, morphine 10–20 mg or diamorphine 5–10 mg by intramuscular injection are the mainstay for women in established labour. Pethidine, for so long the drug of choice because it causes less depression of the fetal respiratory centre, has given way to some extent in recent years to diamorphine with its better analgesic and anxiolytic effect. These may all be combined with an anti-emetic to reduce the incidence of nausea. The aim is to avoid their use within 2–3 hours of delivery, but if there is any evidence of respiratory depression in the baby this can be countered by the IV administration of Naloxone (Narcan neonatal).

(d) Continuous epidural anaethesia
Local anaesthetic (0.25% or 0.5% bupivacaine) is instilled at 3–4 hour intervals through a catheter inserted into the epidural space. This gives the patient complete freedom from pain of labour. Most obstetricians consider epidural anaesthesia justified if the patient asks for it and it is the method of choice in some cases e.g. hypertension, premature labour.

Its use has transformed the management of difficult or prolonged labour and it has been of great benefit to many women. The absence of maternal distress must not mislead the obstetrician into ignoring signs of obstructed labour and the effect of prolonged contractions on the mother and fetus.

MANAGEMENT OF LABOUR

(d) Continuous epidural anaethesia (continued)

It may also lead to prolongation of the second stage of labour by abolishing involuntary expulsive efforts and thus lead to a higher incidence of operative vaginal delivery. This is by no means inevitable where weaker concentrations of bupivacaine are used and midwives are used to managing such labours. Operative delivery, including caesarean section, can be done under epidural block.

Epidural anaesthesia should be administered by an experienced anaesthetist, and supervised by him throughout labour even if the 'top-ups' are given by the midwives.

The epidural space is about 4 mm wide and lies between the dura and the periosteum of the vertebral canal. It is limited above at the foramen magnum where dura and periosteum fuse, and below by the ligament covering the sacral hiatus.

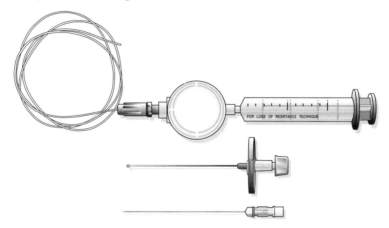

Local anaesthetic can be injected into this space through a fine catheter introduced through a specially designed needle, which is traversed by the spinal nerves, and produces the same effect as a spinal block without the risk of headache, meningism or nerve root trauma.

Complications

i.   Mild hypotension (about 20%).
ii. Sepsis (a bacterial filter should be attached to the syringe).
iii. Needle inserted into cerebrospinal space. (This is a failure of the technique.)
iv. Bladder atony and increased need for catheterisation (about 40%).
v.   Total spinal block. This occurs if the local anaesthetic is injected into the cerebrospinal space. Respiration is paralysed and there is hypotension. This is an acute anaesthetic emergency.

6. Second stage

The mother is allowed to make involuntary expulsive efforts provided full dilatation of the cervix has been confirmed. Premature pushing can make the cervix oedematous and delay progress.

Organised pushing should not be started until the baby's head is visible. This is hard work and the mother will tire quickly.

MANAGEMENT OF LABOUR

CARE OF THE BABY

Assessment of the baby's condition in labour depends essentially on observations of the fetal heart rate. The presence of **Meconium** in the liquor should always be noted but is, at best, only a warning that there may be a problem. It is postulated that fetal hypoxia leads to an increased output by the vagus, stimulating the fetal gut and resulting in the passage of meconium.

(a) FETAL HEART RECORDINGS

The traditional method of recording the fetal heart intermittently, between contractions, by the Pinard stethoscope suffers from the grave drawback that changes in the heart rate are first seen in association with uterine contractions, and must be related to them in time.

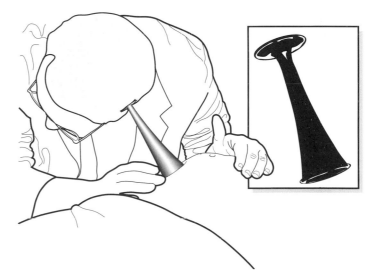

Continuous fetal heart recording, as presently established, however, has the marked disadvantage of limiting the mother's mobility in labour restricting her to bed. While its use is mandatory in high risk labours, it can be used intermittently in normal labour by detaching the ultrasound transducer, or fetal scalp electrode if used, from the monitor to facilitate mobility or when the woman wishes to be seated in a chair. The increasing availability of telemetric monitoring will make some of these conflicts obsolete.

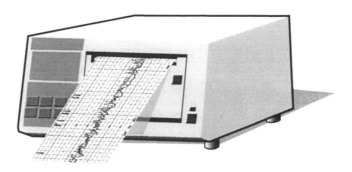

MANAGEMENT OF LABOUR

Continuous Fetal Heart Rate Monitoring

The fetal monitor provides a continuous printed record of the fetal heart rate and uterine contractions. The fetal heart rate is also displayed on a screen as is the intra-uterine pressure. The FHR may be recorded through an ultrasonic transducer or through the fetal ECG obtained by an electrode attached to the fetal scalp. Uterine contractions are indicated by an external tocograph, a very delicate pressure gauge, or more accurately by an intrauterine catheter.

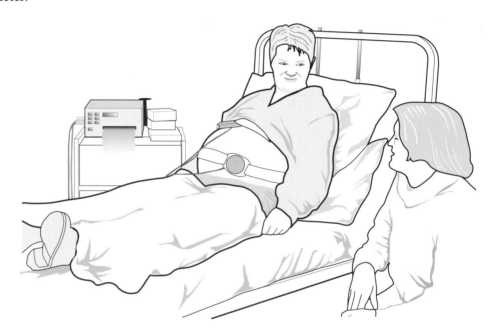

Fetal ECG Recording

The monitor records the rate at which the R wave of the fetal ECG is obtained from the scalp electrode. This gives a technically superior recording but requires that the membranes must be ruptured and the presenting part accessible. In contrast a midwife can set up ultrasound apparatus at any stage in the labour. Furthermore, a scalp electrode should not be used when there is risk of transmission of viral disease, such as HIV or Hepatitis B or C, from mother to fetus.

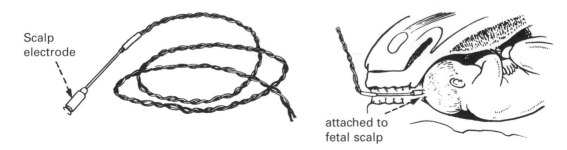

Scalp electrode

attached to fetal scalp

MANAGEMENT OF LABOUR

Interpretation of intrapartum FHR Tracings

1. The average baseline rate should be between 120 and 160 beats per minute. Sustained tachycardia may be a warning of fetal distress and prolonged or severe bradycardia is ominous.

2. Baseline variability. The normal FHR fluctuates by 10 beats/min every 5 seconds or so, evidence of fetal ability to react normally to the stress of labour. Loss of this variability, especially in association with tachycardia, indicates severe hypoxia. (This is sometimes referred to as 'beat-to-beat variation'.)

3. Response of FHR to uterine contractions. The uterine contraction acts as a stress to the fetus, producing a transient reduction in oxygenated blood supply. The normal FHR should be maintained with the contraction or show only a slight deceleration of less than 40 beats/min. If it is greater than this and especially if there is a 'lag phase' or late deceleration occurring after the period of uterine contraction, a pathological degree of hypoxia may be present.

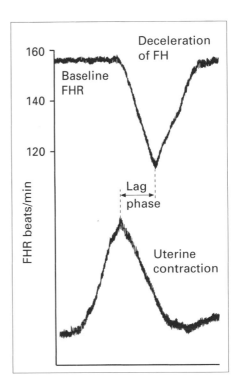

(A promising new development from conventional cardiotocography is computerised analysis of the ST segment of the fetal ECG waveform (ST ANalysis or STAN) which identifies changes reflecting myocardial ischaemia which is a more accurate method of assessing fetal compromise. It is yet to be widely introduced.)

MANAGEMENT OF LABOUR

In conventional cardiotocography decelerations may be classified as:

(a) Early, where the lowest rate of the FH coincides with the peak of contractions. These may be normal in late labour but should not be ignored if persistent or severe.

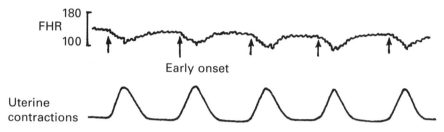

(b) Late, where the lowest rate of the FH follows the peak of contraction. These may indicate hypoxia.

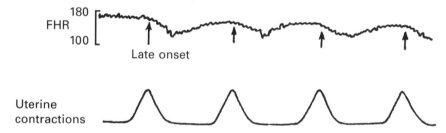

(c) Variable, where the pattern and timing of deceleration varies with contractions. These are thought to be due to cord compression. They are quite common and may be related to the mother's position. They should not however be ignored if persistent or associated with other adverse features.

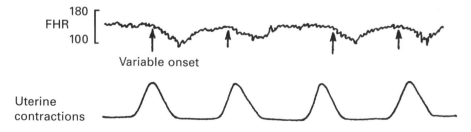

MANAGEMENT OF LABOUR

(b) FETAL BLOOD SAMPLING

During the arduous work of normal labour the mother gradually develops a metabolic acidosis (a depletion of her buffer reserves), but the pH is maintained at 7.38 ± 0.03. In dysfunctional labour the acidosis may be of such degree as to bring about an actual lowering of the pH.

Normal fetal pH is much more acid at 7.30 ± 0.05, but in the presence of hypoxia it compensates by the anaerobic catabolism of its glycogen stores, leading to an accumulation of lactic acid and a fall in pH.

To obtain a sample of fetal blood for pH estimation, a special tube (amnioscope) is passed through the cervix which must be sufficiently dilated. By using a special guarded knife a blob of blood is obtained from the scalp which can be aspirated into a fine pipette and analysed in a pH meter. There is a small risk of scalp haemorrhage which may be difficult to control.

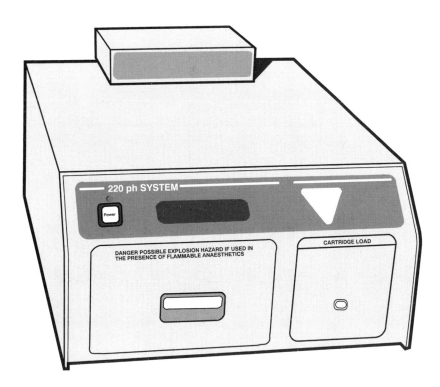

Indications for fetal scalp blood sampling (FBS)

It will be seen that this technique takes time and trouble and may cause discomfort to the mother. However FBS is still the only available test for confirming or excluding fetal hypoxia which may be suggested by FHR monitoring or by the presence of meconium.

pH levels between 7.20 and 7.25 are suspicious and require repeat estimation if the labour is allowed to proceed. Levels below 7.20 are indicative of significant fetal acidosis and delivery is indicated.

PARTOGRAMS IN THE MANAGEMENT OF LABOUR

The partogram, a graphic display of progress in labour, has become widely used in many different situations.

The development and use of graphical representations of cervical dilatation with time have been modified and adapted by many workers, and the partogram now, in addition to illustrating cervical dilatation, will show the descent of the head and is used to record all the routine observations on mother and baby, together with uterine action and drug therapy.

It is recognised that progress in cervical dilatation goes through a **latent phase,** from the onset of labour up to a dilatation of 3–4 cm when the **active phase** begins. There is usually progressive dilatation of the cervix at approximately 1 cm per hour from this point. During the latent phase the cervix and lower segment are gradually changing and this period may last some hours.

PARTOGRAMS IN THE MANAGEMENT OF LABOUR

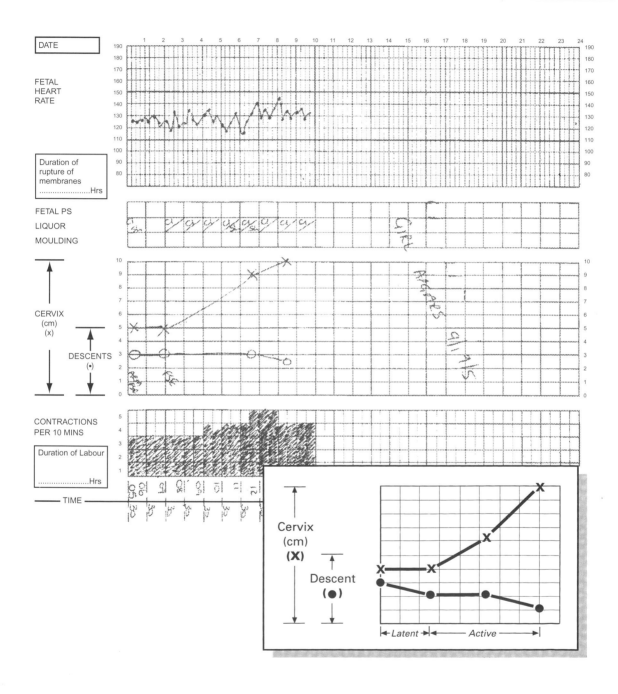

DATE

FETAL
HEART
RATE

Duration of
rupture of
membranes
..................Hrs

FETAL PS
LIQUOR
MOULDING

CERVIX
(cm)
(x)

DESCENTS
(•)

CONTRACTIONS
PER 10 MINS

Duration of Labour
..................Hrs

TIME

Cervix
(cm)
(X)

Descent
(●)

Latent | Active

MANAGEMENT — DELIVERY

As in the rest of her labour the mother will commonly be accompanied by her partner, even at operative delivery.

To help create a more informal and 'homely' atmosphere, many hospitals have abandoned the use of sterile gowns and masks for attendants, only sterile gloves being worn.

Most women are delivered in the dorsal position but the left lateral or an upright position may be preferred. If delivery is conducted in the dorsal position, the mother should be tilted by the use of a wedge to avoid supine hypotension.

For mother
Sterile drapes for legs and thighs. Sterile sheet and pad to go below buttocks and on bed. Sterile towel to cover abdomen.

For episiotomy and repair of perineal wounds
Local anaesthetic syringe and needles. Scissors — for cutting perineum (episiotomy). Sutures and needles for repair.

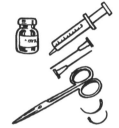

For baby care (see Care of Newborn and Asphyxia.)
Sterile towel — for reception.
Mucus suction catheter.
Oxygen.
Laryngoscope.
Warm cot.
Syringes, needles and ampoules of Naloxone (Narcan).

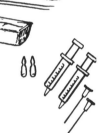

For swabbing and wiping clean
Bowls with lotions.
Swabs and cotton wool.
Gamgee pads.

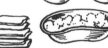

For controlling bleeding
Oxytocic drugs.
Syringe and needles.
Pressure forceps for bleeding points in perineum.
Bowl to collect and measure third stage blood loss and to receive placenta.

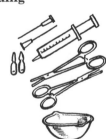

For care of cord
Pressure forceps to clamp cord, or cord clamp or cord ligatures. Scissors to cut cord.

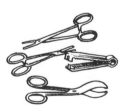

MANAGEMENT — DELIVERY

With the further descent and rotation of the head the perineum distends, the anus dilates and the vagina opens with contractions. There is regression between contractions but each contraction gives further progress and delivery is imminent.

Delivery is a sterile and antiseptic procedure

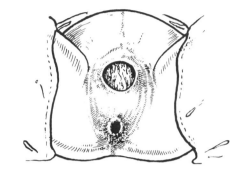

Delivery of the baby may be conducted in the left lateral or in the dorsal position.

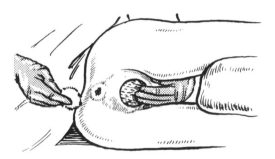

In the left lateral position the right leg is supported.

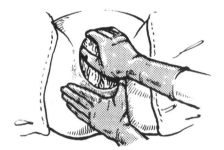

In the dorsal position the anal region is not so well seen.

A sterile pad is placed over the anus. The sinciput may be felt behind the anus at the tip of the sacrum.

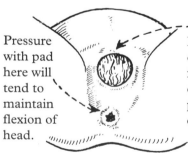

Pressure with pad here will tend to maintain flexion of head. Pressure downwards on head will promote flexion and allow occiput to slip under pubis. The distending diameter is usually the occipito-frontal.

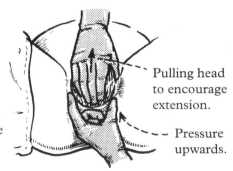

Pulling head to encourage extension.

Pressure upwards.

Crowning of the head is when there is no recession between contractions and is due to the biparietal diameter having passed through the bony pelvis.

When the occiput is free, extension is encouraged and the head is delivered. The neck region is now explored and if the cord is felt it is pulled to give some slack.

MANAGEMENT — DELIVERY

Restitution now occurs and then external rotation as the shoulders descend in the pelvis. The head is now grasped — fingers of the left hand beneath chin and jaw and the right fingers below the occiput.

The head is now taken towards the anus to dislodge the anterior shoulder from behind the pubis.

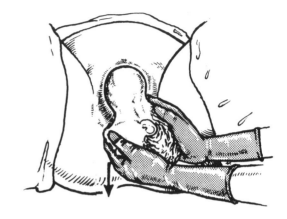

After the birth of the anterior shoulder the head is lifted up over the pubis. This allows the posterior shoulder to slip over the perineum and be delivered.

The perineum is often torn by the birth of the shoulders especially if the delivery is hurried and not allowed to occur with uterine contraction.

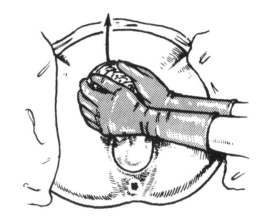

The shoulders are now gripped and the trunk delivered by lifting up over the pubis. This can sometimes be aided by taking the shoulders posteriorly first and then upwards. The trunk and legs are thus delivered.

The baby's mouth and nose are drained by posture and suction. The baby soon cries and is now laid between the mother's legs or on her abdomen and the cord is divided between clamps or ligatures.

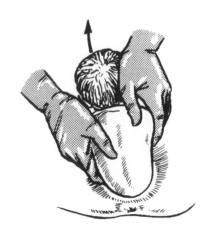

MANAGEMENT — THIRD STAGE

The first and second stages of labour are now complete and the THIRD stage has started. The management of the Third Stage begins during the delivery of the baby. It is almost universal practice, in normal cases, to give Syntometrine (syntocinon 5 units and ergometrine 0.5 mg) intra-muscularly either with the crowning of the head or with the delivery of the anterior shoulder. The Syntocinon acts in 2–3 minutes and the aim is to reduce the risks of post-partum haemorrhage. If the injection is given with the crowning of the head and the rest of the delivery proceeds in an unhurried manner, the drug will be taking effect on the uterus as the delivery of the baby is completed.

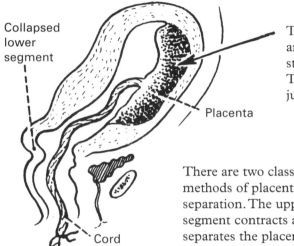

Collapsed lower segment

Placenta

Cord

The placenta is attached to the fundus and anteriorly. The lower segment has been stretched and has no tone so it is collapsed. The upper segment is firm and the fundus is just below the umbilicus.

There are two classical methods of placental separation. The upper segment contracts and separates the placenta and there is usually little bleeding at this time.

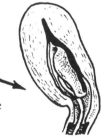
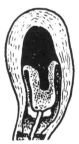

Matthews Duncan
Maternal surface
appears at introitus

Schultze
Fetal surface
appears at introitus

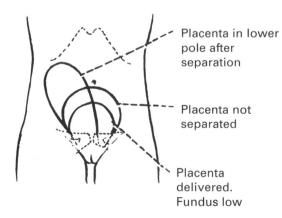

Placenta in lower pole after separation

Placenta not separated

Placenta delivered. Fundus low

The placenta now descends into the lower segment and gives it form. The fundus thus rises above the umbilicus, is hard and, no longer containing the placenta, is narrower and often displaced laterally.

The placenta is then expelled or removed, and as the lower segment is again empty it collapses and the fundus is now narrow, hard and found below the umbilicus.

249

MANAGEMENT — THIRD STAGE

The management of the third stage is now described in the light of this physiological account. It is best conducted in the dorsal position.

1. The height, width and consistency of the fundus may be felt by gentle palpation. Rubbing the fundus may cause irregular uterine activity which partly separates the placenta and causes bleeding.

2. It is useful to put a ligature or clamp on the cord at the vulva. Descent of the placenta will cause the ligature to move away from the vulva. A bowl is placed against the perineum to collect any blood.

3. The signs of placental separation are:
   Narrow, hard, ballotable fundus.
   Slight bleeding.
   Lengthening of the cord.

4. The separated placenta may be removed by traction on the cord while the other hand maintains pressure upwards on the fundus (Brandt-Andrews' method).
   Cord traction has become established as the commonest way of delivering the placenta. Alternatively the mother may be asked to expel it by bearing down once separation has occurred. The risks of cord traction are uterine inversion (see Chapter 13) or avulsion of the cord.

5. When the placenta appears at the vulva it is caught by both hands and the membranes are twisted gently to allow them to peel off completely. The bowl placed against the perineum allows blood loss to be assessed. Normal loss is about 250 ml.

6. The uterine fundus is now rubbed up to assure firm contraction.

7. The vagina, labia and perineum are inspected for tears or other injuries. The vulva is swabbed down and a sterile pad placed over it to collect the lochial discharge.

8. The placenta is now examined. It is suspended by the cord to show the extent of the membranes and any deficiencies. It is then placed maternal side uppermost to see if it is complete. An incomplete placenta is an indication for immediate exploration of the uterus.

CHAPTER 12

ABNORMAL LABOUR

INDUCTION OF LABOUR

Termination of a pregnancy by inducing labour may be indicated because of a suspected or confirmed risk to the mother or baby, or both.

Such indications are:
Hypertensive disorders.
Prolonged pregnancy.
Compromised fetus e.g. growth restriction.
Maternal diabetes.
Rhesus sensitisation.

Hypertensive disease and prolonged pregnancy have long been the largest groups. Induction in such cases has often been carried out on epidemiological data as opposed to established risk in an individual case. Modern methods of fetal assessment aim to establish the risk in an individual and thus avoid needless intervention.

Other indications for induction are:
Fetal abnormality or death — the main reason for intervention is to alleviate distress in the mother.
Social — induction may be requested by a mother for a variety of social or domestic reasons. The obstetrician may reasonably agree to such requests if the findings are favourable for delivery and if there are no features which would make intervention unusually hazardous.

The effectiveness of modern methods of induction may tempt the obstetrician to be over-enthusiastic in their use. Any intervention should carry the implication of delivery by whatever means necessary and must therefore be justifiable.

METHODS OF INDUCTION

As labour approaches, the cervix normally shows changes known as 'ripening' so that it becomes 'inducible' and is then called a 'favourable' cervix. The condition of the cervix is the most important factor in successful induction and, where ripening has not occurred, there is a greater chance of a long labour, fetal hypoxia and operative delivery.

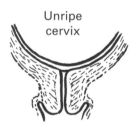

Unripe cervix

An unripe cervix is hard, long, closed and not effaced.

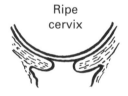

Ripe cervix

A ripe cervix is soft, effaced or becoming effaced and admits the finger.

INDUCTION OF LABOUR

The Bishop score
This is an accepted method of recording the degree of ripeness before labour (cf. the Apgar Score applied to the newborn baby). It takes account of the length, dilatation and consistency of the cervix and the level of the fetal head. A score of 9 or higher is favourable.

Cervical Score

	0	1	2	3	
Dilatation (cm)		<2	2–4	>4	
Length (cm)		>2	1–2	<1	
Consistency	Firm	Average	Soft		
Position	Post.	Mid Anterior			
Level	0–3	0–2	0–1:0	0+	
				Total	

(a) RIPENING THE CERVIX
The collagen fibres of which the cervix is composed can be much softened in consistency by the local application of prostaglandin. A vaginal tablet or gel containing Dinoprostone (Prostin E2) may be inserted into the posterior fornix to soften and efface the cervix. This will permit amniotomy and may even result in the initiation of labour. Increasingly the cheaper alternative of Misoprostol given intravaginally is being used for ripening the cervix and also for induction of labour.

Physical methods such as the introduction of a Foley catheter through the cervical os appear to stimulate local production of prostaglandins and may also ripen the cervix.

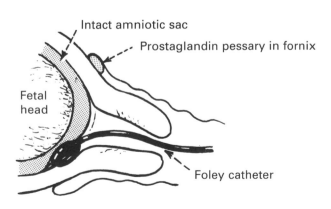

INDUCTION OF LABOUR

(b) AMNIOTOMY (Artificial Rupture of Membranes)

This is done to initiate labour (surgical induction) or, during labour, to try to accelerate the process, or to allow a fetal scalp electrode to be applied or to permit estimation of the fetal pH. Amniotomy appears to release a local secretion of endogenous prostaglandins.

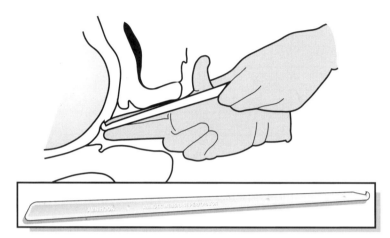

Amniotomy, using a Hollister Amnihook or other device, may be used to rupture the membranes overlying the presenting part. Care must be taken not to damage the fetal tissues. The operation may be done blindly by passing the instrument along the fingers or by direct vision using a speculum.

The procedure is carried out using an aseptic technique and sometimes sedation or even epidural anaesthesia may be required to permit adequate examination. The colour and quantity of the liquor removed should be noted. Prolapse of the umbilical cord should be excluded at the beginning and end of the procedure.

Complications of Amniotomy
Failure to induce effective contractions
Labour may not become established after amniotomy alone and it is usual to stimulate the uterus further by intravenous oxytocin after an interval of 3 hours or so if contractions are inadequate.

Placental separation (Abruption)
This may be caused by the sudden reduction in the volume of liquor where there has been polyhydramnios.

Bleeding
This is not uncommon. The usual source is maternal blood from an element of forced dilatation of the cervix by the examining fingers. Occasionally it may come from fetal vessels running in the membranes (velamentous insertion of the cord). The best method of identifying the source of blood is by Kleihauer's test, a laboratory procedure, by which a blood slide is so stained as to show the fetal cells standing out in a field of 'ghost' maternal cells (see Chapter 8).

Prolapse of the cord
This will only happen with an ill-fitting presenting part. Cord prolapse, occult or frank, should give warning signs on the Fetal Heart Rate monitor.

INDUCTION OF LABOUR

Infection

The uterus may become infected if the interval from amniotomy to delivery is excessive, and both mother and child are at risk. Infection may perhaps be delayed by observing careful antiseptic techniques, and by exhibiting antibiotics whenever delay is anticipated.

Pulmonary embolism of amniotic fluid

This rare condition presents as severe shock of rapid onset, with intense dyspnoea and often bleeding. It is associated with amniotomy and strong uterine contractions, and must be distinguished from eclampsia, abruption, ruptured uterus, and acid aspiration. Treatment must include positive pressure ventilation, and correction of the inevitable coagulation defect. Post mortem examination of the maternal lungs will show fetal cells and lanugo.

(c) I.V. OXYTOCIN

Synthetic oxytocin by continuous intravenous infusion is commonly used after amniotomy to stimulate uterine contraction. It is also used occasionally with intact membranes e.g. to help stabilise the fetus with a variable lie prior to amniotomy. In this circumstance care should be taken to prevent excessive uterine action which can cause amniotic fluid embolism. Like amniotomy, intravenous oxytocin is also used to augment or accelerate labour.

Synthetic oxytocin is a powerful drug and sometimes unpredictable, as uterine sensitivity can show a wide variation. It must be administered with great care by the doctor or midwife who should be present throughout.

Effect on uterine activity

This varies with time and the progress of labour. Since too little oxytocin is useless and too much may cause fetal hypoxia or uterine rupture, it is necessary to adjust the dosage to the individual patient's response.

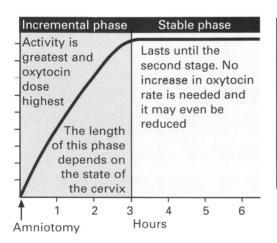

Units of Syntocinon in 500 ml Hartmann's solution	Drops per minute				
	10	20	40	60	80
	Dose of Syntocinon (mU/min)				
2	2.66	5	11		21
8		21	43		85
16			85		85
32			171	256	341

The best method of administration is by a suitable semi-automated infusion system incorporating an accurate drop counter. A solution of 2 units of syntocinon in 500 ml of Hartmann's solution is used beginning at a dose of 2.66 mU/minute). This is increased every 15 minutes until satisfactory contractions are established.

INDUCTION OF LABOUR

Complications of oxytocin

Poor uterine action

This may occur where amniotomy has been carried out in spite of an unfavourable cervix. Ripening of the cervix with prostaglandin should be used first in these circumstances. Sometimes, in spite of apparently satisfactory uterine action, little dilatation of the cervix occurs and labour has to be terminated by caesarean section. This is due to incoordinate uterine action resulting in dysfunctional labour.

Abnormal fetal heart rate patterns

Prolonged or excessive oxytocin administration can cause fetal hypoxia by over-stimulation of the uterus. Continuous fetal heart rate monitoring is required for all patients undergoing oxytocin stimulation.

Hyperstimulation

Overdosage can cause excessive, painful contractions and even a prolonged spasm (tetanic contraction). If hyperstimulation becomes evident the infusion should be stopped to allow the uterus to relax.

An intra-uterine pressure transducer may be used in women who are difficult to assess e.g. the obese.

Rupture of the uterus

The possibility of rupture must be borne in mind when using oxytocin. It is unlikely in a primigravida but has been reported. It is more to be expected in the parous woman or in the patient who has had a previous caesarean section or hysterotomy. The use of an intra-uterine pressure transducer may be advisable in such patients. Epidural anaesthesia does not mask the pain of uterine rupture but it should be used with caution.

Water intoxication

This may result from the prolonged administration of high doses of oxytocin in large volumes of electrolyte-free fluid. This should not be an issue in labour using normal dosage of oxytocin in an agent such as Hartmann's solution.

ACCELERATION OF LABOUR

The progress of spontaneous labour can be speeded up by amniotomy and oxytocin infusion. By using these techniques most women can be delivered within 12 hours. Prolonged labour is thus avoided together with its possible accompaniment of maternal exhaustion, fetal distress and intra-uterine infection. Such interventions should not, however, be automatic and their indiscriminate application has aroused hostility in some mothers. If acceleration is considered desirable the reason for this should be explained and discussed with the mother.

FAILURE TO PROGRESS IN LABOUR

Failure of the cervix to dilate and for the presenting part to descend is a common event but it is important to appreciate that it is a clinical observation and **not** a diagnosis.

CAUSES OF FAILURE TO PROGRESS IN LABOUR

1. Incorrect diagnosis. Patient not in labour.
2. Dysfunctional uterine activity. Common in primigravidae, rare in multiparae. Associated with occipito-posterior malposition.
3. Malposition/malpresentation.
4. Cephalopelvic disproportion.
5. Rare causes e.g. cervical stenosis from previous cervical surgery or pelvic tumour such as fibroid or ovarian cyst.

Dysfunctional Labour

Dysfunctional labour occurs when the cervix does not dilate despite the presence of uterine contractions. The cervix should dilate at a rate of between 1 and 2 centimetres per hour in the active phase. Progress is more rapid in parous women and dysfunctional labour is much commoner in primigravidae.

Treatment consists of escalating doses of oxytocin. This should only be used in parous women when there is no evidence of malpresentation and even then only with caution. The dose of oxytocin should be titrated against the quality and frequency of uterine contractions.

Malposition/Malpresentation

Malposition means incorrect positioning of the vertex. This includes occipito-posterior (OP) positions and deflection of the head short of brow presentation.

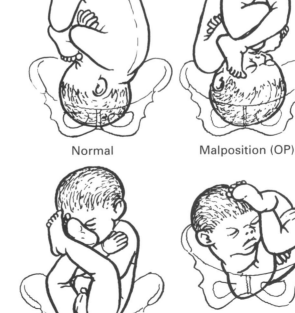

Normal   Malposition (OP)

Malpresentation means the presence of any presenting part other than the vertex — face, brow, breech, shoulder, compound presentation.

Breech   Shoulder

MALPOSITION/MALPRESENTATION

Dangers

1. Ill-fitting presenting part. The forewaters are not protected from the forces of uterine contractions, and are forced through an incompletely dilated cervix.

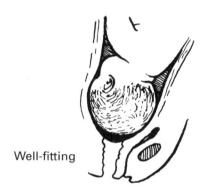

Well-fitting

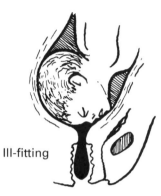

Ill-fitting

2. Membranes rupture early and the cord may prolapse past the presenting part.

3. Contractions may be irregular and poorly sustained. If moulding occurs, when the skull bones overlap, the presenting part may become a better fit and the labour will perhaps progress more normally; otherwise dilatation of the cervix is likely to cease temporarily after the forewaters have ruptured.

4. In parous women labour may proceed quickly in spite of an ill-fitting presenting part.

With a malpresentation such as brow or shoulder there is a danger of obstructed labour and uterine rupture if unrecognised.

DIAGNOSIS OF MALPRESENTATION

1. ABDOMINAL EXAMINATION
a) A lie other than longitudinal will lead to malpresentation.
b) If the lie is longitudinal the presentation is either head or breech.
c) If the head presents the leading part is either vertex, face or brow. The last two may be suspected by recognising unusual width of the head.

2. VAGINAL EXAMINATION
The **mouth** and **anus** may be mistaken.

Mouth

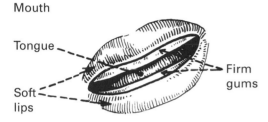

The mouth may be mistaken for the anus because of oedema masking laxity of the orifice.

Anus

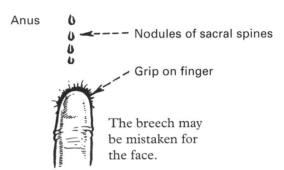

The breech may be mistaken for the face.

If in doubt do not use force as other tissues such as eyes or genitalia may be damaged.

Sacrum
The sacrum is recognised by the shape, nodular ridge of the spines and possibly the foramina and the posterior portion of iliac crest. The spine nodules are continuous with the vertebrae above.

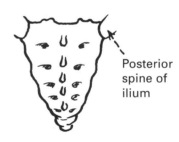

Supra-orbital ridges
Supra-orbital ridges are recognised by double curve, root of nose, orbits and frontal suture. All may be partly obscured by caput.

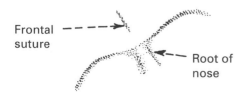

Nose
The nose is recognised by the 'saddle', and its firm elasticity.

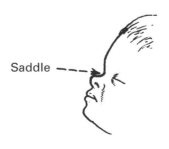

DIAGNOSIS OF MALPRESENTATION

2. VAGINAL EXAMINATION *(continued)*

The **foot** and **hand** may be mistaken.

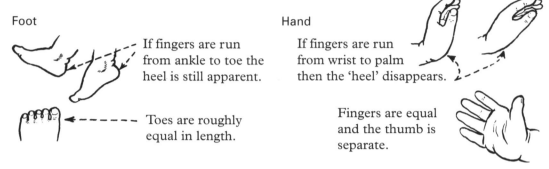

Foot

If fingers are run from ankle to toe the heel is still apparent.

Toes are roughly equal in length.

Hand

If fingers are run from wrist to palm then the 'heel' disappears.

Fingers are equal and the thumb is separate.

Right or left is identifiable by the position of the great toe or thumb.

Shoulder

The shoulder is identified by the humerus, scapula, acromion process, coracoid process, clavicle and ribs. All of these cannot be palpated at once.

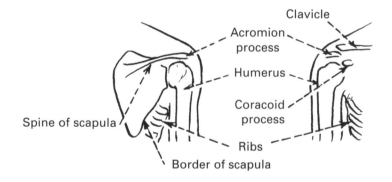

Clavicle

Acromion process

Humerus

Coracoid process

Spine of scapula

Ribs

Border of scapula

The **knee** and **elbow** may be mistaken.

The knee has a hollow as the knee cap is not yet formed.

The elbow has the point of the olecranon process.

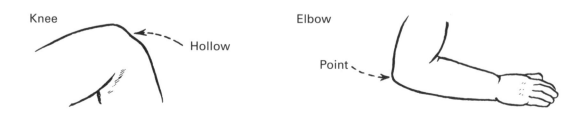

Knee

Hollow

Elbow

Point

OCCIPITO-POSTERIOR POSITION

Occipito-posterior position is a malposition of the head and occurs in 13% of vertex presentations. The presenting part is the vertex and the denominator is the occiput.

Postulated Causes

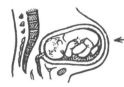

Pendulous Abdomen — This is found in Multiparae.

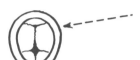

Anthropoid pelvic brim — This favours direct O.P. or direct O.A.

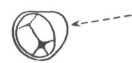

Android pelvic brim — The transverse diameter of the brim being near the sacrum encourages the biparietal diameter to accommodate posteriorly.

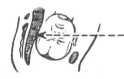

A flat sacrum with a poorly flexed head leads to further deflexion and O.P.

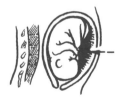

The placenta on the anterior uterine wall tends to encourage the fetus to flex round it.

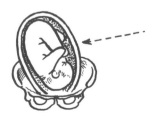

R.O.L. position of the head and the normal right obliquity and dextro-rotation of the uterus favours deflexion of the head and R.O.P. descent. There is some assistance from the pelvic colon in the left posterior pelvic quadrant.

Chance is clearly an important cause.

OCCIPITO-POSTERIOR POSITION

DIAGNOSIS
Palpation

A.
The fetal back is found to one side or may be difficult to identify.

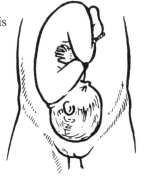
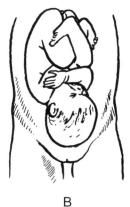

A   B

B.
The fetal head is postero-lateral and will be free above the brim in late pregnancy, even in a primigravida. The limbs are to the front and give hollowing above the head. This may be particularly noticeable after rupture of the membranes.

Auscultation
The fetal heart is heard best well out in the flank but descends to just above the pubis as the head rotates and descends.

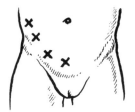

Vaginal examination
The membranes tend to rupture early, often before labour is established. If the membranes are intact they may protrude through the cervix giving finger-like forewaters, or may fill the upper vagina and obscure the presenting part. The presenting part is the vertex, but there is deflexion (incomplete flexion) so the anterior fontanelle is readily felt in the anterior part of the pelvis near the ileo-pectineal eminence. The sagittal suture aims towards the sacro-iliac joint. The posterior fontanelle is not readily felt till the head is in the lower pelvic cavity.

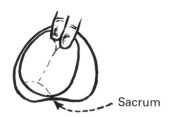

Sacrum

OCCIPITO-POSTERIOR POSITION

MECHANISM

Two types of occipito-posterior (O.P.) are described.

A. Flexed O.P. with suboccipito-frontal and biparietal diameter engaging, 10 cm x 9.5 cm.

B. Deflexed O.P. with occipito-frontal and biparietal diameters engaging 11.5 cm x 9.5 cm.

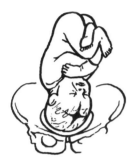

Engagement occurs in the transverse or the right oblique diameter of the brim. Descent occurs in the right oblique diameter of pelvis giving the right occipito-posterior position (R.O.P.). Descent continues to pelvic floor.

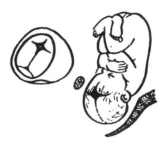

Further progress depends on flexion of the head.

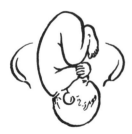

A. If flexion of the head increases in descent then the occiput strikes the pelvic floor first and rotates anteriorly through the right occipito-lateral (R.O.L.) position — and then to the R.O.A. position and to the direct O.A. position.

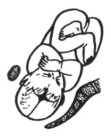

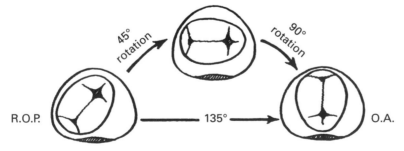

The occiput has thus rotated through the angle of 135° to bring the occiput to the symphysis pubis. This is known as Long rotation. The mechanism is thereafter the same as for the occipito-anterior position.

OCCIPITO-POSTERIOR POSITION

MECHANISM *(continued)*

B. If flexion of head remains incomplete in descent then rotation of the occiput anteriorly on the pelvic floor may not occur; but rotation of the occiput posteriorly may occur bringing the occiput into the hollow of the sacrum. This is known as SHORT rotation (45°) and gives the persistent occipito-posterior (P.O.P.) position or direct O.P. position.)

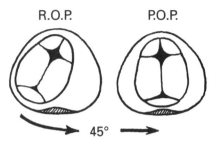

R.O.P.   P.O.P.

45°

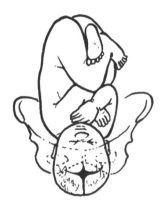

The mechanism now is difficult for flexion of the head is restricted by the fetal chest though the brow is pressed to the pubis and some flexion occurs. The soft tissues are stretched more than in O.A. and the fetus is delivered face to pubis.

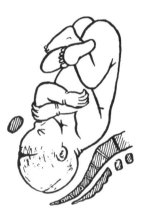

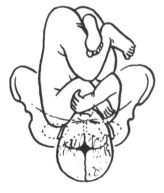

If this does not occur then an impasse is reached and labour becomes obstructed.

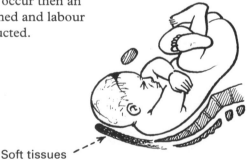

Soft tissues

Sometimes the long rotation of the O.P. is arrested and the head is left in the occipito-lateral position in the cavity of the pelvis. This is one form of transverse arrest of the head.

OCCIPITO-POSTERIOR POSITION

MANAGEMENT IN LABOUR

Occipito-posterior positions may lead to dysfunctional labour especially in primigravidae. Contractions may be painful and accompanied by troublesome backache, but uterine action is incoordinate and progress slow. Good analgesia is necessary and an epidural block is ideal. Accurate assessment of the quality of uterine action by an intra-uterine catheter may be helpful and syntocinon can be employed.

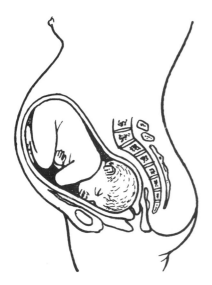

Retention of urine is common in such labours and catheterisation may be required. The mother may feel an urge to bear down before the second stage is reached, probably due to pressure on the sacrum and rectum. Premature expulsive efforts can delay progress by causing oedema of the cervix and an epidural is again helpful in this situation.

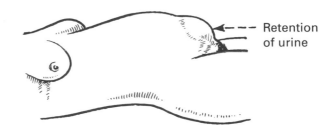

Retention of urine

DELIVERY

Two thirds of the cases will deliver spontaneously as O.A. 12% will deliver spontaneously face to pubis. The perineum is distended by the occipito-frontal diameter, and a large episiotomy may be required.

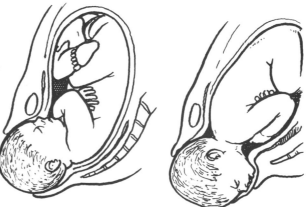

Internal rotation may be interrupted by prominent ischial spines or be restricted by reduced pelvic diameters as in the android pelvis. Delivery then has to be completed by section or, if full dilatation has been reached, by manual or forceps rotation, or by the use of the ventouse (see Chapter 14).

FACE PRESENTATION

This occurs around once in every 300 pregnancies. The presenting part is the face and the denominator is the mentum or chin.

High parity, fetal abnormality and fetal thyroid enlargement form the commonest causes.

MECHANISM

The engaging diameters in a face presentation are the submento-bregmatic followed by the biparietal. The submento-bregmatic and suboccipito-bregmatic are the same size (9.5 cm at term), therefore the engaging diameters are the same size as in a normal vertex presentation.

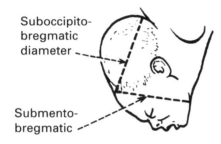

Suboccipito-
bregmatic
diameter

Submento-
bregmatic

In a normal vertex presentation the suboccipito-bregmatic and the biparietal diameters are in the same plane.

In a face presentation the submento-bregmatic and the biparietal diameters are in different planes. The submento-bregmatic and bitemporal diameters engage together.

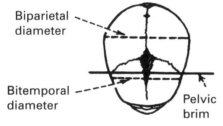

Biparietal
diameter

Bitemporal
diameter

Pelvic
brim

In a normal vertex presentation the engaging diameters enter the plane of the pelvic brim together.

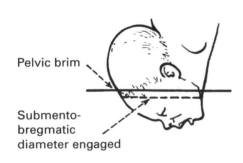

Pelvic brim

Submento-
bregmatic
diameter engaged

In a face presentation the submento-bregmatic diameter enters the plane of the brim and is followed by the other engaging diameter.

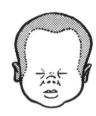

The pale areas
engage first,
followed by the
shaded areas

Engagement is usually in the transverse diameter of the brim giving a right or left mento-lateral position. The left mento-lateral (L.M.L.) is the more common.

Vaginal delivery is possible if the chin is anterior (mento-anterior) but mento-posterior positions require delivery by caesarean section in appropriately grown babies.

MALPRESENTATIONS

BROW PRESENTATION

A brow presentation is unstable and tends to convert to a vertex or face presentation. The aetiology is similar to that of face.

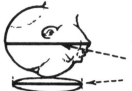

Vaginal delivery is not possible unless the baby is very small since the presenting diameter is the mento-vertical diameter (14 cm) and the largest pelvic diameter is 12.5 cm.

A Brow presentation should be suspected when a parous woman has unexpectedly prolonged labour with failure to progress.

Delivery is by caesarean section if conversion to a vertex presentation does not occur.

COMPOUND PRESENTATION

This means the prolapse of a limb alongside the presenting part. It is a rare complication and head and arm are most often seen although head and foot and breech and hand have been described.

Treatment

Usually nothing need be done. If the hand is palpated in front of the head and appears to be causing delay, it should be pushed up out of the way. It is important to distinguish hand from foot by identifying the presence or absence of the heel.

SHOULDER PRESENTATION

Shoulder presentation occurs in 1 out of 250–300 cases. It is more common in multipara than in primipara and in preterm than in term labours.

Aetiology

This is similar to other malpresentations. Twins, polyhydramnios, placenta praevia, contracted pelvis, anything preventing engagement of the head in the pelvis may encourage shoulder presentation. Unusual fetal shape (due to some abnormality) or an abnormal uterine shape, e.g. subseptate uterus, are occasional causes. The commonest cause, however, is laxity of the uterine and abdominal wall muscles in parous patients. Delivery is by caesarean section.

In early labour, if the membranes are intact, external version to a longitudinal lie can be attempted. If the membranes have ruptured and the liquor drained, the uterus wraps around the fetus and manipulation is very dangerous. Caesarean section is therefore the treatment of choice, even with a dead baby. The lower segment may be poorly formed and classical section may occasionally be required.

CEPHALOPELVIC DISPROPORTION (CPD)

Cephalopelvic disproportion occurs when the fetal head is too large to pass through the pelvis. This may occur when the head is large as in cases of hydrocephalus, or when the pelvis is abnormally small or of an unusual shape. A small pelvis may result from conditions such as childhood rickets. Orthopaedic disorders in childhood may also result in an abnormally shaped pelvis. The most common form of CPD results from an Occipito-Posterior malposition. In such cases the fetal and pelvic dimensions are not abnormal but the presenting diameter of a deflexed O.P. malposition is greater than an occipito-anterior position and labour may become obstructed. In such cases the term **Relative Disproportion** is used and in subsequent pregnancies vaginal delivery might reasonably be allowed.

Diagnosis

In the absence of any gross abnormality such as marked hydrocephalus, cephalopelvic disproportion may only be reliably diagnosed during labour. Typically the first stage of labour will be prolonged. There is failure of descent of the head, apparent on both vaginal and abdominal examination. Moulding will occur and is the process in which the fetal skull bones override each other. The parietal bones override each other commonly and both overlie the frontal bones. This occurs in normal labour but in cases of CPD the moulding is irreducible i.e. the bones will not separate.

Caput formation, in which the subcutaneous tissue and skin of the vertex become oedematous is a feature of the duration of labour rather than CPD. A diagnosis of CPD necessitates delivery by caesarean section.

BREECH PRESENTATION

The breech is a malpresentation and occurs once in about 2.5% of cases of labour at term.

AETIOLOGY

The breech is the presenting part in 25% of cases before 30 weeks, therefore prematurity is an important factor.

The legs of the fetus may be extended and interfere with flexion of the body so breech with extended legs is common especially in primigravidae. Multiple pregnancy will interfere with spontaneous version.

Other related factors are: fetal malformation, hydramnios, lax uterus and pendulous abdomen, abnormal shape of pelvic brim or uterus, placenta praevia.

Three types of presentation are described:

Fully flexed fetus

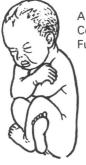

A
Complete or
Full Breech

Not fully flexed fetus
with legs extended

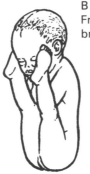

B
Frank
breech

One or both thighs extended

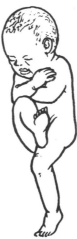

C
Footling or
Incomplete
breech

MECHANISM

The denominator is the sacrum; the leading part the anterior buttock.

The bitrochanteric diameter (transverse diameter between the great trochanters of the fetus) is 10 cm. The most common position is the left sacro-anterior (L.S.A.). With labour there is compaction, descent and engagement of the breech (bisiliac diameter).

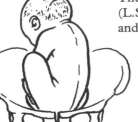

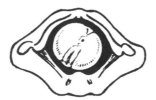

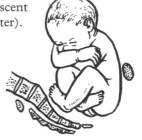

BREECH PRESENTATION

MECHANISM *(continued)*

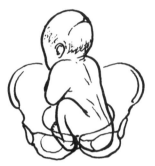

Descent continues until breech reaches pelvic floor. The anterior buttock rotates forward under the pubis (internal rotation).

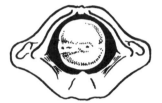

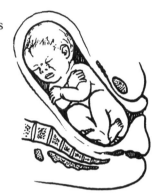

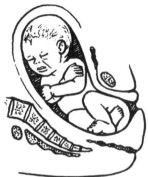

Lateral flexion of the fetal body round the pubis allows the anterior buttock to slip forward under the pubis and the posterior buttock to slip over the perineum. The breech is delivered followed by the legs.

A movement of restitution of the hips takes place.

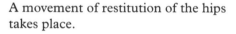

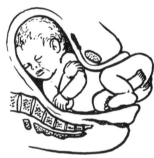

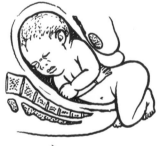

The shoulders now engage in the same pelvic diameter as the hips — the left oblique. (The bisacromial diameter of the shoulder is 11 cm.)

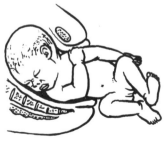

As descent continues internal rotation of the shoulders occurs in the pelvic cavity bringing one shoulder beneath the pubis and the other into the hollow of the sacrum. The anterior shoulder and arm are born first.

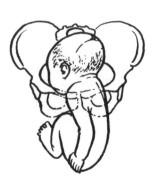

BREECH PRESENTATION

MECHANISM *(continued)*

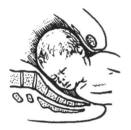

As the shoulders are being born the head enters the pelvic brim either in the transverse or left oblique of the brim. The engaging diameters of the head are the biparietal and the suboccipito-bregmatic or suboccipito-frontal.

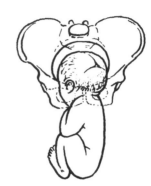

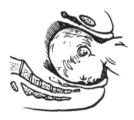

The head descends into the pelvic cavity and rotates to bring the occiput under the pubis.

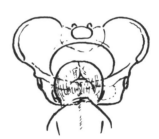

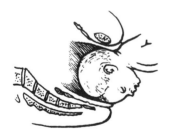

The occiput is arrested at the pubis and the head is born by flexion. The chin, face and brow are born first, and then the occiput.

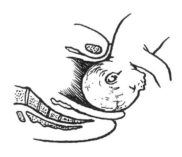

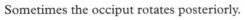

Sometimes the occiput rotates posteriorly.

If the head is flexed the root of the nose is arrested behind the pubis and the occiput and vertex are born first followed by the face.

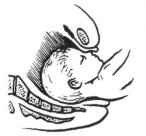

If the head is extended the chin is arrested above the pubis and the occiput and vertex are delivered and the face follows.

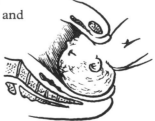

271

BREECH PRESENTATION

DIAGNOSIS
Palpation

1. Longitudinal lie.
2. Firm lower pole.
3. Limbs to one side.
4. Hard head at fundus.

(Head may not be palpable at fundus because it is under the ribs — always confirm by pelvic examination or ultrasound scan.)

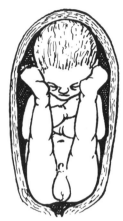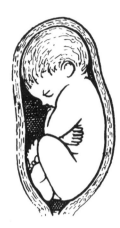

Frank breech   Full breech

Auscultation
The fetal heart (FH) is best heard above the umbilicus.

Vaginal examination
No head in pelvis. Soft buttocks felt and hard irregular sacrum. Feet may be in pelvis as leading part.

Ultrasound
Differentiation of head and breech is not always easy but the head will be readily detected by a scan.

DANGERS
(a) Ante-natal

As with other malpresentations there is an increased risk of premature rupture of the membranes and cord prolapse. This applies least to the extended breech which is a well-fitting presenting part.

(b) Delivery

The main danger in breech delivery is the speed with which the head descends through the pelvis. Rapid compression and decompression can cause intracranial injury.

Conversely, undue delay in the delivery will lead to asphyxia due to cord compression, at least from the time of delivery of the shoulders.

Traumatic injuries may occur if intervention in the delivery is required.

BREECH PRESENTATION

Risks to the fetus

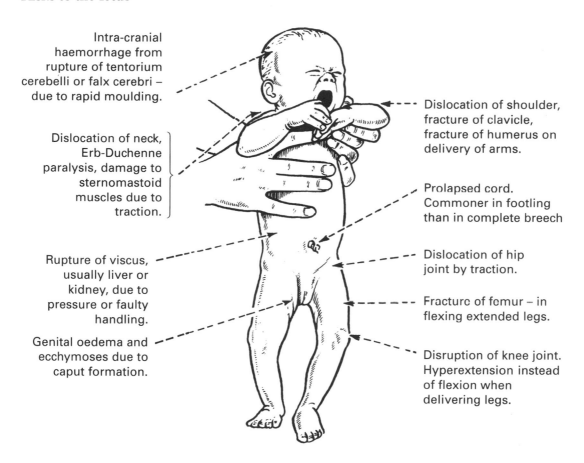

Intra-cranial haemorrhage from rupture of tentorium cerebelli or falx cerebri – due to rapid moulding.

Dislocation of neck, Erb-Duchenne paralysis, damage to sternomastoid muscles due to traction.

Rupture of viscus, usually liver or kidney, due to pressure or faulty handling.

Genital oedema and ecchymoses due to caput formation.

Dislocation of shoulder, fracture of clavicle, fracture of humerus on delivery of arms.

Prolapsed cord. Commoner in footling than in complete breech

Dislocation of hip joint by traction.

Fracture of femur – in flexing extended legs.

Disruption of knee joint. Hyperextension instead of flexion when delivering legs.

The placenta separates frequently in the second stage of labour as the active uterus contracts and the fetal head is in the pelvis. Apnoea is therefore a danger.

Manual assistance to complete delivery of the baby is essential and may be a sudden need. Episiotomy is desirable to permit sudden interference, or complete perineal tear may result.

A large multicentre study of breech delivery at term concluded that caesarean section was the safest route of delivery for the newborn.

In this study perinatal mortality, neonatal mortality, or serious neonatal morbidity was significantly lower for the planned caesarean section group than for the planned vaginal birth group.

Although there was no significant difference in early morbidity between vaginal delivery and section for the mothers, there was a reduced incidence of urinary incontinence for mothers delivered abdominally at three months post natal.

BREECH PRESENTATION

MANAGEMENT (Antenatal)

As already noted, many babies present by the breech at 30 weeks. Most undergo spontaneous version by 32–34 weeks. If this does not occur the possible causes should be considered and an ultrasound scan carried out for localisation of the placenta and to exclude major fetal abnormality.

External cephalic version, in which the breech is elevated from the pelvis may be undertaken at any time from 34 weeks gestation. Technically this is easier earlier in pregnancy but spontaneous version is likely before this stage.

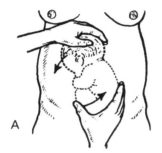 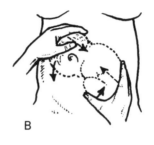 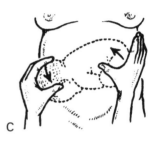

A. The breech must be eased away from the pelvis.
B. Pressure is applied to encourage flexion of the fetus to allow it to slip round. If the legs are flexed the baby may kick round at this point.
C. Once past the transverse the hands simply push the fetus into position.

Complications
1. The placenta may be partly separated. The fetal heart must be checked on completion and the vagina examined for bleeding.
2. There may be unsuspected complications such as an abnormal uterus or short umbilical cord.
3. Excessive force may rupture the uterus.

Contra-indications
1. Pre-eclampsia (as predisposing to placental bleeding).
2. Previous scar on the uterus.
3. Multiple pregnancy or fetal abnormality.

The commonest causes of failure are too large a fetus or too little liquor, or 'splinting' of the fetus by extended legs.
Version should not be performed in pregnancies complicated by twins, hypertension and when caesarean section is already planned.

As a result of the findings of the term breech trial mentioned earlier, planned vaginal delivery of a term singleton breech may no longer be appropriate. In those instances in which breech vaginal deliveries are conducted, great caution should be exercised. Patients with persistent breech presentation at term in a singleton gestation should undergo a planned caesarean section.

A planned caesarean delivery does not apply to patients presenting in advanced labour imminent delivery or to patients whose second twin is in a nonvertex presentation.

BREECH PRESENTATION

VAGINAL BREECH DELIVERY

There will still be situations when vaginal breech delivery is appropriate, particularly if the woman presents in advanced labour. Labour should proceed normally in the breech with extended legs. In flexed and footling breeches there is an increased risk of early rupture of the membranes and cord prolapse. In these cases also, especially if premature, the breech may slip through the incompletely dilated cervix and precipitate delivery.

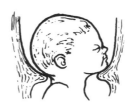

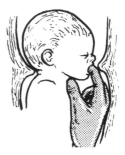

In these circumstances there is no alternative to attempting to complete the delivery by passing a hand up the fetal abdomen and inserting a finger into the baby's mouth. Traction on the jaw is applied to promote flexion and passage through the cervix.

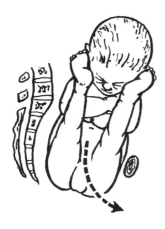

Where labour is proceeding normally analgesia is best provided by an epidural block which will prevent premature expulsive efforts and permit controlled delivery of the head. Delivery should be in the lithotomy position to allow the baby to hang over the perineum.

Once the breech reaches the pelvic floor lateral flexion of the trunk is required to allow progress. This will be facilitated by episiotomy when the posterior buttock distends the introitus.

If the legs are flexed they will fall out but if they are extended they should be lifted out once access can be gained to the popliteal fossa. Pressure is applied to aid flexion of the legs.

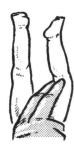

Pressure to the popliteal space to flex the knee and displace it to the side of the trunk.

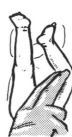

Fingers are worked along leg towards ankle to encourage further flexion of knee.

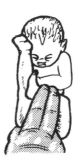

The ankle is grasped and the foot swept down over the other leg.

A loop of cord is pulled down as soon as is practicable to prevent possible tearing of it later.

BREECH PRESENTATION

DELIVERY *(continued)*

When delivery of one leg is complete the delivery of the second follows quickly.

The delivery proceeds spontaneously and, as the anterior shoulder blade appears, the arm is delivered (1) by placing two fingers of the appropriate hand (right if right shoulder) over the clavicle and sweeping them round the point of the shoulder and down the humerus to the elbow and carrying the forearm free. (2) The ankles are then grasped and swung upwards. This permits the posterior arm being freed in a similar way. (3) The body is now allowed to hang till the head descends into the pelvis and the hair line shows.

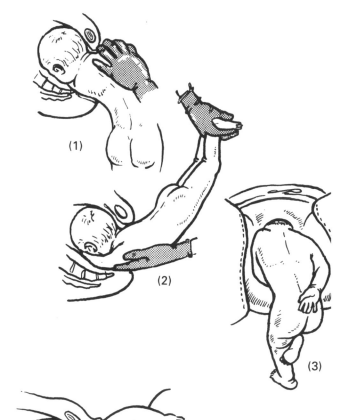

The head may then be delivered using forceps applied to the aftercoming head

or

Laying the child along the arm, the middle finger is placed in the mouth, the index and ring fingers catch the cheek bones. Traction by these fingers will tend to promote flexion of the head. The index finger and thumb of the other hand grasp one shoulder, the middle finger presses on the occiput and the other two fingers grasp the other shoulder. Traction of the two hands will deliver the head and keep it flexed. (The Mauriceau–Smellie–Veit manoeuvre.)

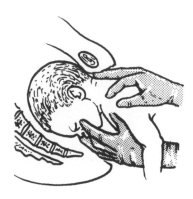

BREECH PRESENTATION

DELIVERY *(continued)*

or

The Burns–Marshall method

The feet are grasped and with gentle traction are swept in an arc over the maternal abdomen. Thus the mouth is freed and the delivery is completed slowly by further swinging over the abdomen.

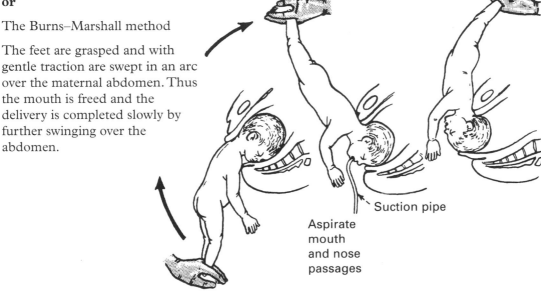

Suction pipe

Aspirate
mouth
and nose
passages

In all cases the delivery of the head should be as slow as possible to decrease the risk of damage to skull membranes by sudden compression and release. The air passages should be cleared as quickly as possible by aspirating the nose and mouth. Delivery thereafter can be slow without fear of asphyxia and it can also allow slow release of pressures and tensions on the skull. The method used to deliver the head is unimportant; what matters is the operator's experience and the achievement of a controlled delivery.

BREECH PRESENTATION

Delivery may be complicated by extension or nuchal displacement of the arms.

These complications are best managed by LØVSET's MANOEUVRE. This makes use of the inclination of the pelvic brim, the short anterior wall and the long posterior wall of the cavity. The anterior shoulder is above the symphysis while the posterior is below the promontory and if these are now reversed in position the posterior shoulder will keep below the brim and be just below the symphysis and can be easily delivered.

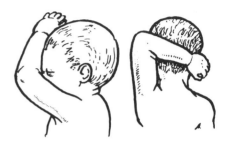

The Løvset manoeuvre is done by grasping the fetus by the pelvis and pulling gently while rotating to bring the posterior shoulder to the front. The direction of rotation is so that the posterior arm trails towards the chest (anti-clockwise rotation with back to mother's left and clockwise rotation with back to mother's right).

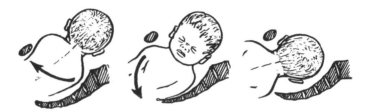

The arm is then lifted out and the rotation reversed, using the delivery arm for traction, so that the original anterior arm, which became posterior below the promontory is now swept round in the cavity to be easily picked out below the symphysis. (Often the second arm can be extracted easily without further rotation when the first arm has been delivered.)

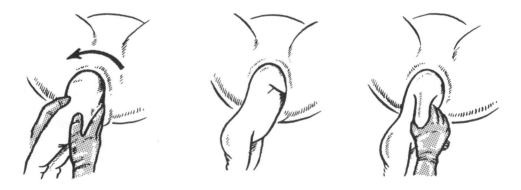

The delivery described, where most of the baby is delivered by maternal effort and the obstetrician delivers the head (with or without Løvset's manoeuvre) is classified as an **Assisted Breech Delivery.**

BREECH PRESENTATION

BREECH EXTRACTION is the process whereby the obstetrician places a hand inside the uterus and grasps a foot. The baby is then delivered by traction on the foot. This procedure is now restricted to delivery of a second twin. The twin will most commonly be lying transversely and the membranes will be ruptured. If the membranes are intact external cephalic version may be possible.

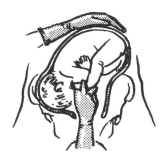

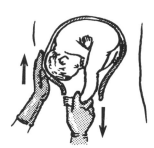

1. A hand is introduced into the uterus and the anterior foot is grasped by the heel. (Pulling on the posterior limb tends to turn the baby into a sacro-posterior position: if possible both feet should be grasped.)

2. Downward traction is made on the leg and the outside hand presses the head upwards.

3. Gentle traction is made on the delivered leg until the breech is fixed, then the other leg is extracted and the delivery completed by the obstetrician.

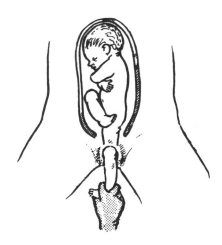

The arms will invariably extend as a result of traction and Løvset's manouvre is applied, followed by delivery of the head as described.

Complications

There is a risk of uterine rupture, of injury to the fetus, and of infection.

Internal version should never be attempted when the uterus has contracted down on an impacted fetus and the lower segment is thin. In this situation delivery by caesarean section is the method of choice.

LABOUR IN WOMEN PREVIOUSLY DELIVERED BY CAESAREAN SECTION

Women who have previously delivered once by lower segment caesarean section might reasonably be allowed to labour if that delivery were for a non-recurring cause e.g. fetal distress. Previous cephalopelvic disproportion is an indication for repeat operation. Although there is evidence that some women with two previous caesarean sections may safely deliver vaginally, most obstetricians would undertake elective caesarean section.

The conduct of labour in a woman previously delivered by section is sometimes referred to as 'Trial of Scar.' Such a trial must be undertaken under careful supervision in an obstetric unit equipped for immediate repeat caesarean section. The principal danger is of uterine rupture in which the fetus is extruded into the peritoneal cavity with catastrophic results. Uterine rupture presents as severe pain, often described as 'tearing' and with evidence of fetal distress and maternal haemorrhage. If this is suspected laparotomy and delivery are indicated.

'Trial of Labour' is a term which is currently misused but in its original sense meant an attempt to achieve vaginal delivery in a woman in whom cephalopelvic disproportion was suspected antenatally on the basis of small stature or known abnormal pelvic anatomy e.g. in rickets.

In both cases prolonged labour should not be permitted and careful observations of the fetal and maternal condition made. Labour must be progressive, that is, there must be evidence of progressive cervical dilatation and descent of the presenting part. Any delay should raise suspicion and delivery by section considered.

CHAPTER 13

ABNORMALITIES OF THE THIRD STAGE OF LABOUR AND OF THE PLACENTA AND CORD

RETAINED PLACENTA

The Third Stage of Labour, from the delivery of the child until the expulsion of the placenta, remains the most unpredictable and dangerous stage of labour from the mother's point of view.

The first part of this chapter describes two relatively common third stage complications, retained placenta (1–2%) and primary postpartum haemorrhage (PPH 3–4%) and the rare, but very grave, complication of inversion of the uterus. The chapter concludes with an account of some of the commoner abnormalities of the placenta and cord.

RETAINED PLACENTA

When Syntometrine has been given as described in Chapter 11, with the crowning of the head or the delivery of the anterior shoulder, separation of the placenta will usually occur within a few minutes of the delivery of the baby. Certainly, if the placenta is undelivered at 20 minutes it should be considered to be 'retained'.

CAUSES

1. Placenta separated but undelivered

In such cases there have usually been signs of placental separation – bleeding, alteration of the shape of the uterus, lengthening of the cord. If the signs have been missed, bleeding into the uterine cavity will occur because the uterus cannot retract fully until it is empty. The fundus will therefore appear broad and boggy, thus disguising the fact that separation has occurred. Failure to recognise the signs of separation is one of the commonest forms of mismanagement of the third stage.

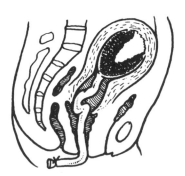 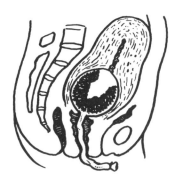

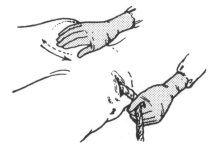

In this situation the fundus should be rubbed up to make it contract and the placenta removed by the Brandt–Andrews method. The cord is pulled gently, and the other hand presses the uterus upwards so as to prevent inversion. A slight see-sawing motion is imparted by both hands, and provided separation has occurred the placenta should be delivered. It is likely to be accompanied by a considerable volume of accumulated blood.

RETAINED PLACENTA

CAUSES *(continued)*

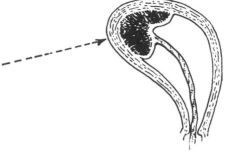

2. Placenta partly or wholly attached

If the placenta fails to separate at all there will be no bleeding. A cornual implantation of the placenta may cause this.

Partial separation will cause bleeding but the fundus will remain broad because the placenta still occupies the upper segment. Needless handling of the uterus during the third stage is thought to encourage partial separation.

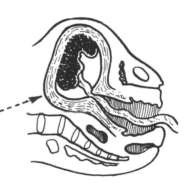

Where oxytocics have been given an hour glass constriction may develop in the lower segment and the cervix begins to close down.

3. Placenta Accreta is a rare cause of retained placenta. There is abnormal adherence of the placenta to the uterine muscle due to a defect of decidual formation. It is usually partial, and presents by partial separation accompanied by bleeding. On rare occasions it is complete, and bleeding is absent. Attempts at manual removal open the blood sinuses causing severe bleeding, and hysterectomy may be necessary.

Placenta accreta should be suspected when the operator has difficulty in finding the plane of cleavage when attempting manual removal. The placenta may be left in utero if there is no bleeding, but infection is inevitable. Probably, in this rare condition, hysterectomy is the safest course.

RETAINED PLACENTA

TREATMENT

Intervention becomes necessary either because of bleeding or when 20 minutes have elapsed. An attempt should be made to remove the placenta by rubbing up a contraction and applying cord traction as described previously. If the placenta remains adherent the cord may break. If this occurs, or the attempt is unsuccessful, manual removal of the placenta under anaesthesia should be performed.

This should not be delayed because of the risk of haemorrhage from partial separation. The procedure itself, however, is not without risk from infection and damage to the uterus.

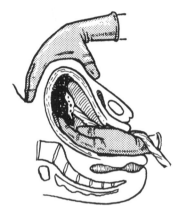

1. The hand covered with antiseptic cream is introduced into the vagina, following the cord.

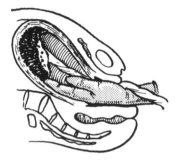

2. The fingers begin to separate the placenta from the uterine wall. Never grasp the placenta until it is separated.

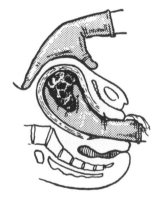

3. Note that the abdominal hand presses the uterus into the placenta and prevents tearing of the lower segment.

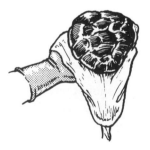

4. The placenta is inspected at once to see that it is complete and, if there is any doubt, the uterus is re-explored. Ergometrine or oxytocin is then given and the uterus rubbed up to make it contract.

PRIMARY POST-PARTUM HAEMORRHAGE

Primary Post-Partum Haemorrhage is blood loss from the birth canal of 500 ml or more within 24 hours of delivery. After 24 hours, abnormal bleeding is classed as Secondary Post-Partum Haemorrhage.

CAUSES

1. Uterine Atony – the uterus, although empty, fails to contract and control bleeding from the placental site. This is the commonest and potentially most dangerous cause.

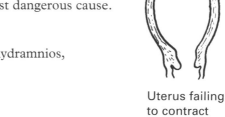

Uterus failing to contract

Predisposing Causes

(a) Excessive uterine distension (twins, polyhydramnios, large baby)
(b) Multiparity (fibrosis in uterine muscle).
(c) Prolonged labour (uterine inertia).
(d) Labour augmented with Syntocinon.
(e) General anaesthesia.
(f) Placenta praevia — lower segment does not contract well enough to stop bleeding.
(g) Placental abruption — the Couvelaire uterus may not contract. In addition a coagulation defect may develop and fibrin degradation products (FDPs) discourage uterine contraction.

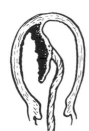
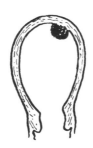
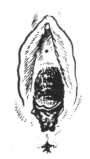

2. Partial Separation of the Placenta — uterus is prevented from contracting.

3. Retention of Placental Fragments

4. Trauma (uterus, cervix, vagina, episiotomy).

CONSEQUENCES OF PPH

1. Bleeding may be very rapid causing circulatory collapse leading to shock and death.
2. Puerperal anaemia and morbidity.
3. (Very rarely) damage to the pituitary blood supply leading to pituitary necrosis — Sheehan's syndrome.
4. Fear of further pregnancies. Haemorrhage is terrifying for the mother.

PRIMARY POST-PARTUM HAEMORRHAGE

TREATMENT

1. Measurement of blood loss

Blood spilt on bed linen and dressings is often ignored and only blood actually collected in a bowl is measured. The estimated loss is therefore invariably lower than the actual loss. The mother's response will be governed by her haemoglobin level.

2. Use of oxytocic drugs

Two are used: ergometrine 0.5 mg and oxytocin 5 units. Syntometrine is a proprietary combination of both these drugs.

Ergometrine produces tonic contractions of the uterus and is also a vasoconstrictor. It may therefore cause elevation of the blood pressure especially if given intravenously. Its action affects the uterus for 2–3 hours.

Synthetic oxytocin produces rhythmic contractions of the uterus. It is virtually free from systemic effects in therapeutic dosage and its action lasts for 20–30 minutes. In an emergency either can be given intravenously with almost immediate effect.

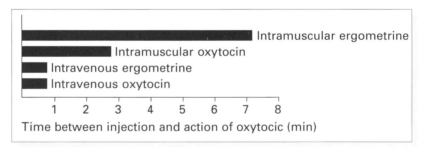

Intramuscular ergometrine
Intramuscular oxytocin
Intravenous ergometrine
Intravenous oxytocin

Time between injection and action of oxytocic (min)

3. Plan of treatment

The aim is to stop the patient bleeding.

(a) Give an oxytocic intravenously (as above).
(b) Rub up a contraction of the uterus to control bleeding and if the placenta is undelivered attempt removal by cord traction.
(c) Rapid assessment of the mother's condition; set up an I.V. line and send blood for cross-match.
(d) Treat the cause
   (i) If the placenta has been delivered check for completeness. If in doubt exploration of the uterus must be carried out.
   (ii) If the uterus appears well-contracted and bleeding continues, damage to the cervix or vagina should be suspected. Proper assessment of this will require exploration under anaesthesia.
   (iii) If both these causes have been excluded uterine atony is diagnosed.

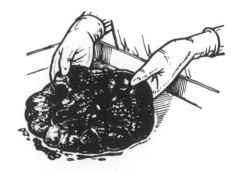

Placenta examined on a flat surface to demonstrate any missing lobe

PRIMARY POST-PARTUM HAEMORRHAGE

Treatment of Uterine Atony

A recent Report on Confidential Enquiries into Maternal Deaths in the United Kingdom (published 1994) contains guidelines for the management of massive obstetric haemorrhage. These are of great value and should be referred to by all departments in preparing their local protocol.

1. Prostaglandins

If the uterus continues to fail to contract in spite of the above measures, the next step is to employ the prostaglandin Carboprost (Hemabate). It is given by intramuscular injection in a dosage of 250 micrograms and this may be repeated.

2. Bi-manual compression of the uterus

Having excluded an incomplete placenta and trauma to the genital tract by thorough exploration, the uterus is compressed between the hands to control bleeding and stimulate contraction.

The fingers of one hand are pressed into the anterior fornix.

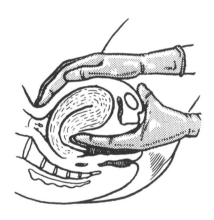

If satisfactory pressure is not obtained, vaginal laxity permits insertion of the whole fist.

3. Uterine packing

Occasionally it may still be necessary to resort to packing the uterus firmly with gauze.

The packing usually remains in position for at least 12 hours. If contraction is still not obtained hysterectomy must be carried out. By this time the patient is likely to be in a serious condition and a decision to operate, difficult as it is, must not be made too late. In cases of persistent bleeding the presence of a clotting defect should be excluded.

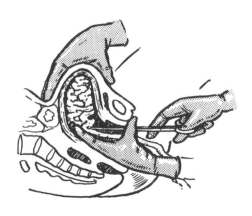

287

ACUTE INVERSION OF THE UTERUS

Acute inversion of the uterus is a very rare condition in modern practice but important because of its serious consequences.

First Degree (Incomplete)
The inverted fundus reaches the external os. – – – – –▶
Diagnosis is made by vaginal examination
and difficulty feeling the fundus abdominally.

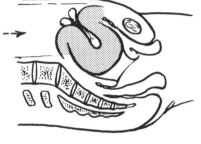

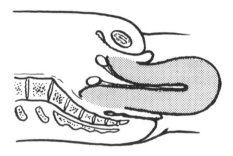

◀– – – – – – **Second degree** (Complete)
The whole body of the uterus is inverted
as far as the internal os and protrudes into
the vagina.

Third Degree
Prolapse of inverted uterus, cervix – – – – – –▶
and vagina outside the vulva.

CAUSATION
1. Most commonly due to a too vigorous attempt to deliver the placenta by cord traction in the presence of an uncontracted uterus.
2. It is favoured by laxity of the uterine muscles as in women of high parity, and by fundal attachment of the placenta. It can be brought on by any sudden bearing down effort.

CONSEQUENCES
1. Usually very severe shock and perhaps bleeding. Death may follow if untreated.
2. Sepsis is common and the shock may be followed by anuria and renal failure.
3. Inversion may become chronic.
4. The uterus may strangulate and slough off.

ACUTE INVERSION OF THE UTERUS

TREATMENT

If the doctor is present when inversion occurs he should at once attempt to replace the uterus by hand. He must not use too much force, and if not immediately successful, he should simply replace the inverted uterus in the vagina and institute treatment for shock. It is probably safer to leave the placenta if it is attached; removal might precipitate severe haemorrhage.

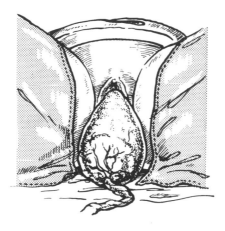

Reduction by taxis

Under general anaesthesia an attempt is made to reduce the inversion by gradual replacement of the uterus, pressing first on that part of the corpus which was inverted last. The most difficult part to reduce is the retraction ring between upper and lower segments. Once reduced, the hand is kept inside the uterus until ergometrine or oxytocin has produced a firm contraction.

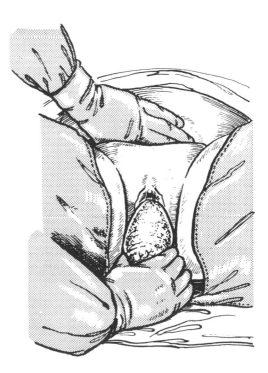

ACUTE INVERSION OF THE UTERUS

Reduction by hydrostatic pressure

If taxis fails, O'Sullivan's hydrostatic method should be attempted. A douche nozzle is passed into the posterior fornix, and an assistant closes the vulva around the operator's wrist. Warm saline is run in (up to 10 litres) until the pressure gradually restores the position of the uterus.

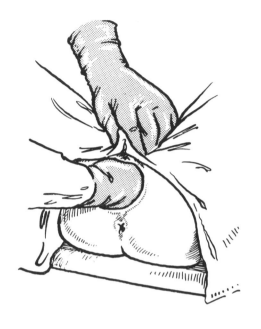

Reduction by the abdominal route

If other methods fail, the abdomen should be opened.

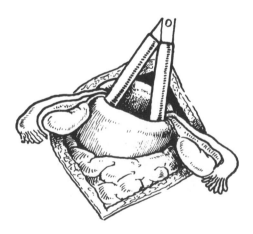

The constricting ring is stretched. Then the posterior part of the ring is divided and the fundus hooked up and resutured.

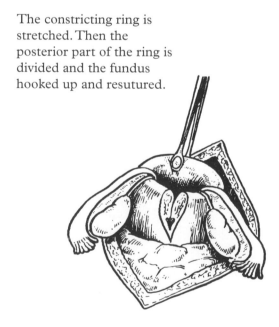

ABNORMALITIES OF THE PLACENTA

Various abnormalities of placental development are seen and may have clinical significance.

Bipartite Placenta

The placenta is partly divided into two lobes with connecting vessels.

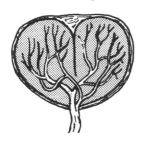

Duplex Placenta

The placenta is completely divided into two lobes, with vessels uniting to form the cord.

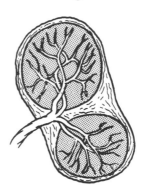

Succenturiate Placenta

Sometimes the placenta is partly or completely divided into two or more lobes.

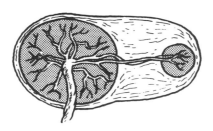

In succenturiate placenta there is a vascular connection between the main and accessory lobes. If, during labour, the rupture in the membranes (spontaneous or induced) lies between the two lobes, then these blood vessels may be torn and cause antepartum haemorrhage in which the blood is of fetal origin. This is difficult to diagnose and carries a high fetal mortality rate once bleeding has occurred. Following delivery, torn vessels may be seen at the edge of the membranes. In such cases the accessory lobe is retained and must be manually removed.

ABNORMALITIES OF THE PLACENTA

Circumvallate Placenta

The membranes appear to be attached internally to the placental edge, and on the periphery there is a ring of thick whitish tissue which is in fact a fold of infarcted chorion. This abnormality has an association with antepartum and postpartum haemorrhage.

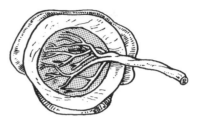

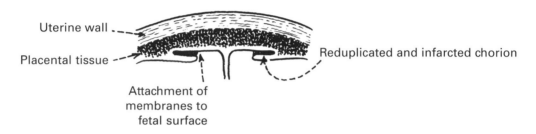

Uterine wall

Placental tissue

Attachment of membranes to fetal surface

Reduplicated and infarcted chorion

Battledore Placenta

Sometimes the cord has a marginal instead of a central insertion. This has no clinical significance.

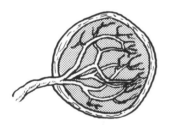

Velamentous Insertion of the Cord

The placenta has developed some distance away from the attachment of the cord and the vessels divide in the membranes. If they cross the lower pole of the chorion a condition arises called vasa praevia. Rupture of the membranes will then precipitate haemorrhage which will exsanguinate the fetus.

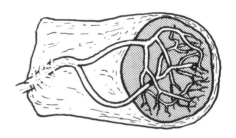

Placental Infarcts are areas of degeneration showing hyaline and often calcareous change. Their aetiology is unknown and they have no clinical significance unless so large as to interfere with fetal nutrition.

Placental Tumours are exceedingly rare and the haemangioma is the only one of any significance. It is often accompanied by polyhydramnios.

ABNORMALITIES OF THE CORD

Cord Round the Neck

One or two loops of cord are quite often seen round the baby's neck at vertex delivery and normally do no harm. As soon as the neck is visible at the vulva the loop should be clamped and divided before delivery of the shoulders and trunk.

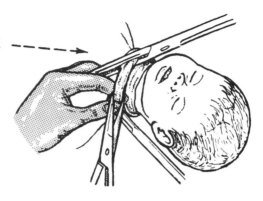

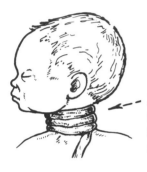

Much less frequently six or seven loops are drawn tightly round the neck. As the fetus descends the cord tightens, the blood supply is interrupted and fetal distress may occur. Fetal death may occur if not treated appropriately.

Abnormal Length of Cord

The average length is 50 cm but extremes of 15 cm and 150 cm have rarely occurred. Prolapse and looping round the neck seem more likely with lengthy cords, while delayed fetal descent and premature placental separation may occur with very short ones. A cord of normal length may become relatively short because of multiple looping round the neck.

Knots in the Cord

True knots are seen quite often, but Wharton's jelly usually prevents actual obstruction by kinking. False knots are protuberances of connective tissue matrix, sometimes containing varices.

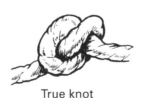

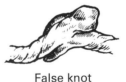

True knot   False knot

Single Umbilical Artery

This finding is sometimes associated with congenital abnormalities in the fetus, particularly renal abnormalities.

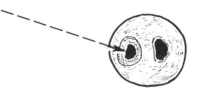

CHAPTER 14

OBSTETRICAL OPERATIONS AND MATERNAL INJURIES

EPISIOTOMY

EPISIOTOMY (Greek A CUTTING OF THE PUBIC REGION)
Making an incision in the perineal body at the time of delivery.

Indications
1. To prevent a perineal tear or excessive stretching of the muscles. A tear is less controllable and may involve the anal sphincter, and overstretching will predispose to prolapse in later years.
2. To protect the fetus if it is premature or is being forced repeatedly against an unyielding perineum which is obstructing delivery.
3. To prevent damage from an abnormal presenting part — occipitoposterior positions, face presentations, after-coming head in breech deliveries, all instrumental deliveries. In such cases it may be done before the perineum is distended. The obstetrician must himself put the tissues on the stretch before cutting.

Types of Incision
1. The median incision is easiest to make and to repair, but in the event of extension it does not give any protection to the anal sphincter.
2. The posterolateral incision is more difficult to repair as the edges retract unequally. Anatomical apposition is, therefore, sometimes difficult to achieve. It gives the best protection against sphincter damage, and best answers the purpose of the operation.
3. The 'J-shaped' incision is a theoretical compromise which becomes a postero-lateral incision in practice.

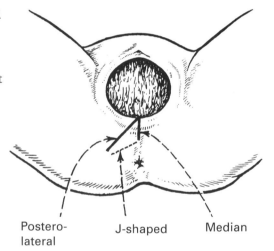

Postero-lateral   J-shaped   Median

Episiotomy incisions

EPISIOTOMY

Anaesthesia

In the conscious patient the best method is to inject 10 ml of lignocaine 1% along the track of the proposed incision. Time should be allowed for this to take effect.

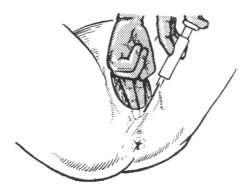

Technique

Two fingers are placed as shown to protect the fetal head, and a long clean cut is made with scissors. It is important to start from the fourchette, otherwise anatomical apposition will be difficult when the repair is undertaken. Too long an incision will open up the ischiorectal fossa and fatty tissue will be seen, but provided there is no infection this does not affect healing.

The timing of an episiotomy must be learnt by experience. If done too soon, blood loss will increase, if delayed too long, a tear of the vagina or deep perineal muscles will occur.

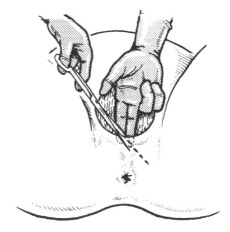

Repair

The repair is done in 3 layers using absorbable material:

1. Vaginal skin — a continuous suture starting at (1) and ending at the hymen, bringing together points (2a) and (2b).
2. Muscle — interrupted sutures, burying the knots under the muscle layer.
3. Perineal skin — continuous or interrupted sutures burying the knots under the surface.

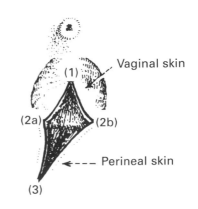

FORCEPS DELIVERY

This remains a common procedure in British obstetric practice, although the incidence has tended to fall in recent years. A forceps delivery rate of approximately 15% is common in many British centres.

Indications for the use of forceps

1. Delay in the second stage of labour. This may be due to:
   Poor contractions.
   Poor maternal effort.
   Malrotation of the head.
   Perineal rigidity.
   The use of epidural anaesthesia. (When epidurals are employed some obstetricians will allow the second stage to last much longer than normal.)
2. Fetal distress.
3. Maternal distress.
   Hypertension.
   Cardiac disease.
   Maternal exhaustion.
   Over-stressed emotionally.

Conditions for forceps delivery

1. The cervix must be fully dilated.
2. A suitable presenting part.
   Vertex.
   Face.
   After-coming head in breech.
3. Head *at least* engaged and no significant mechanical problem.

These are fundamental requirements and failure to observe them will lead to fetal and/or maternal injury. To them may be added:

4. The bladder should be empty,
5. Suitable anaesthesia.

OBSTETRIC FORCEPS

The obstetric forceps is designed to grasp the fetal head when it is in the vagina and effect delivery by traction and guidance without causing injury to mother or fetus.

A forceps consists of two arms which can be articulated.

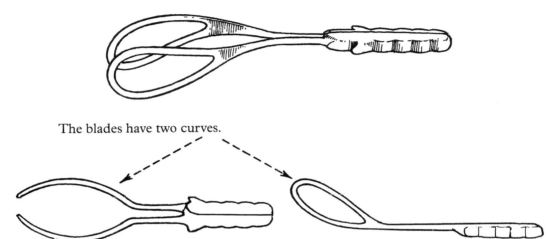

The blades have two curves.

The cephalic curve is adapted to provide a good application to the fetal head.

The pelvic curve allows the blades to fit in with the curve of the birth canal.

There are several kinds of lock:

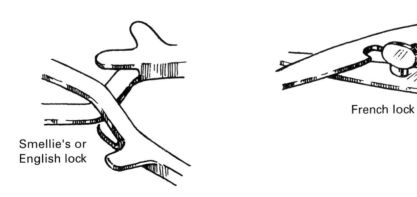

Smellie's or English lock

French lock

OBSTETRIC FORCEPS

Forceps operations are of two kinds:

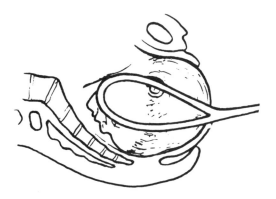

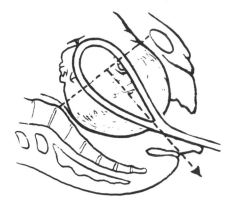

Low Forceps
The fetal head has reached the perineal floor and is visible at the vulva.

Mid Forceps
Engagement has taken place and the leading part of the head is below the level of the ischial spines.

Application of the forceps when the head is not engaged is known as 'high forceps'. In this situation the pelvic axis necessitates traction 'round the corner', so some forceps have detachable handles on rods which allow traction in the correct direction. Although high forceps delivery has been abandoned in favour of caesarean section, 'axis traction forceps' are still favoured by some obstetricians.

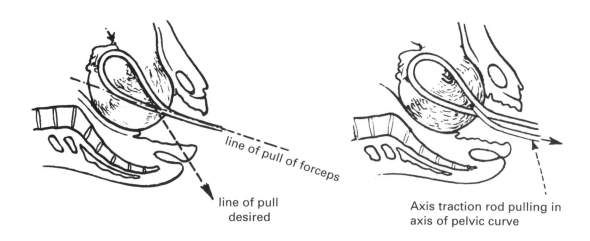

line of pull of forceps

line of pull
desired

Axis traction rod pulling in
axis of pelvic curve

OBSTETRIC FORCEPS

There are very many different patterns. The forceps shown here are all well known and are identified with the three main operations — the low forceps, the mid forceps, and the rotation-extraction forceps delivery.

Wrigley's Forceps
Wrigley's Forceps is designed for use when the head is on the perineum and local anaesthesia is being used. It is a short light instrument with pelvic and cephalic curves and an English lock.

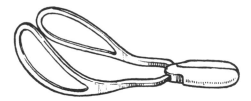

Anderson's (Simpson's) Forceps
This forceps is suitable for a standard mid-forceps delivery with the sagittal suture of the head in the antero-posterior axis. It has cephalic and pelvic curves but the shanks and handle are longer and heavier than Wrigley's.

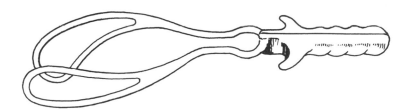

OBSTETRIC FORCEPS

Kielland's Forceps

This forceps was originally designed to deliver the fetal head at or above the pelvic brim, lying in the transverse axis of the pelvis and rotating it when it had reached the pelvic cavity. The forceps is used today for rotation and extraction of the head which is arrested in the deep transverse or occipito-posterior position.

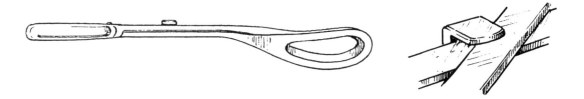

The blades have very little pelvic curve and are virtually an axis traction forceps. A large episiotomy is needed. The shallowness of the curve allows safe rotation in the vagina. Downward traction encourages rotation of the head.

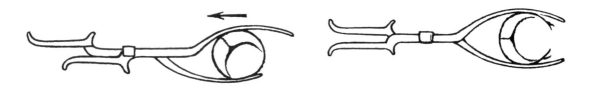

The claw lock allows the blades to slide on each other and correct or encourage asynclitism of the fetal head as required.

This range of movement allowed by the lock makes it possible to apply lethal compression to the fetal head if the instrument is used improperly.

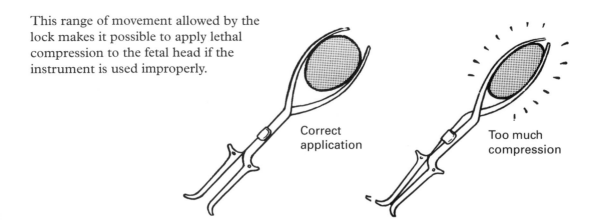

Correct application

Too much compression

FORCEPS DELIVERY

Preparations

1. The patient will usually be in the lithotomy position although some operators prefer the left lateral position.
2. The vulva should be cleaned and draped and aseptic precautions observed.
3. An anaesthetist should be present unless the delivery is to be conducted with only local perineal infiltration or pudendal nerve block.
4. Facilities and personnel for the resuscitation of the baby, if necessary, should be available.

Anaesthesia

1. Low forceps delivery, using Wrigley's blades, requires only the *local infiltration* necessary to make an episiotomy.
2. Anaesthesia for mid-cavity forceps delivery is usually a combination of *local infiltration* and *pudendal nerve block.* Lignocaine 1% without adrenaline is satisfactory and up to 50 ml may be used with safety.

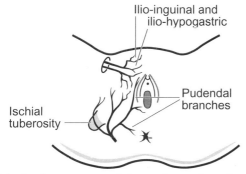
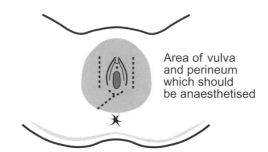

Principal nerves supplying vulva and perineum.

Pudendal Nerve Block

The forefinger is placed on the ischial spine (behind which runs the pudendal nerve) and a long needle is passed via the ischiorectal fossa. When needle point, spine and finger are in conjunction, 5 ml of lignocaine are injected. It is advisable to withdraw the plunger before injecting to make sure that the needle is not in a blood vessel. The needle, preferably a guarded one, can be passed per vaginam if the operator finds it easier.

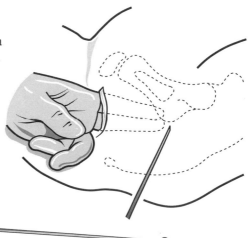

A transvaginal guided needle

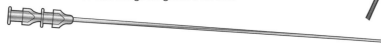

3. *Epidural block* is widely used and suitable for all types of vaginal delivery (see Chapter 11).

303

FORCEPS DELIVERY

4. *Spinal anaesthesia* may sometimes be used for speed, when a full block is needed and an epidural is not already in situ.

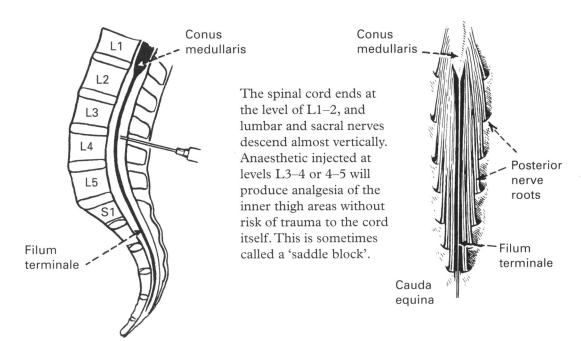

The spinal cord ends at the level of L1–2, and lumbar and sacral nerves descend almost vertically. Anaesthetic injected at levels L3–4 or 4–5 will produce analgesia of the inner thigh areas without risk of trauma to the cord itself. This is sometimes called a 'saddle block'.

Physiology of Spinal Anaesthesia
The effect is that of 'chemical sympathectomy'. The pre-ganglionic autonomic fibres are blocked first, followed by those serving temperature, pain, touch, motor and proprioceptive function in that order. Skeletal muscle action may still be possible when sensory blockade is complete.

Circulatory Effects
Paralysis of the pre-ganglionic fibres lead to arterial dilatation with a fall in venous return and cardiac output. Blood loss at operation may aggravate this and cause an acute and serious fall in blood pressure.

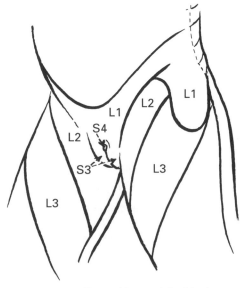

Areas affected by saddle block

FORCEPS DELIVERY

LOW FORCEPS DELIVERY

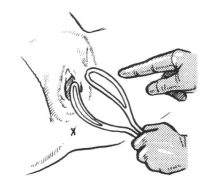

1. Choosing the left blade.

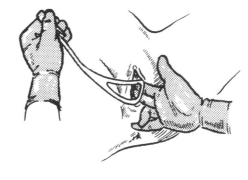

2. Applying the left blade.

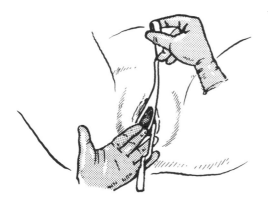

3. Applying the right blade.

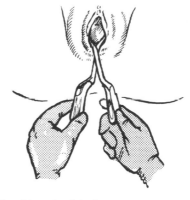

4. Locking the blades.

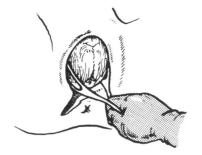

5. Gentle traction with an episiotomy at crowning.

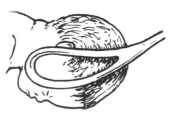

6. The correct cephalic application (in the mento-vertical line).

FORCEPS DELIVERY

MID FORCEPS DELIVERY

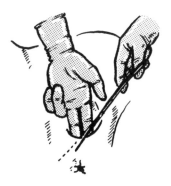

1. Making a large episiotomy before starting.

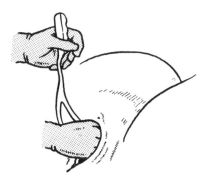

2. Applying the left blade. Hand protects vagina from damage by careless insertions of blade.

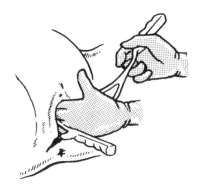

3. Applying the right blade.

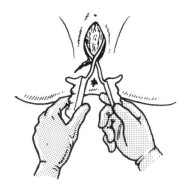

4. Locking the handles.

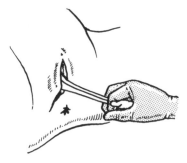

5. Traction, maintaining downward pressure to keep in the line of the birth canal.

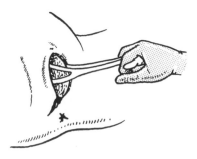

6. As the head crowns the handles of the forceps rise and the head is lifted over the perineum.

FORCEPS DELIVERY

DELIVERY WITH KIELLAND'S FORCEPS

The position of the occiput must be known and is here taken as R.O.L.

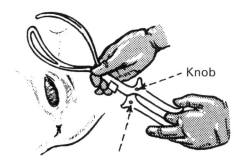

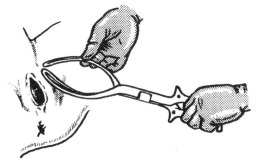

1. Holding forceps with the knobs directed towards fetal occiput.

2. The anterior blade is selected to be applied first (some obstetricians prefer to apply the posterior blade first).

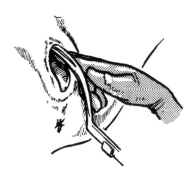

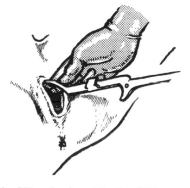

3. **The Direct Method** The anterior blade is guarded by the finger and slipped into the correct position (see 5) on the side of the head.

4. **The Wandering Method** The guarded blade is applied laterally (over the face) and then gently eased round to lie on top of the head.

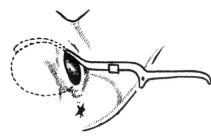

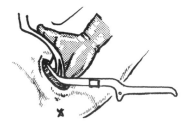

5. It now lies with the concavity of the blade applied to left (uppermost) side of the fetal head.

6. The posterior blade is applied directly to the right (lower) side of the head. The vagina is protected by the guiding hand.

307

FORCEPS DELIVERY

DELIVERY WITH KIELLAND'S FORCEPS *(continued)*

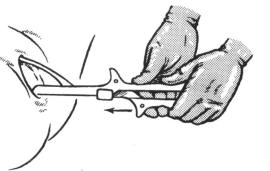

7. The forceps are locked. Note how their position shows asynclitism.

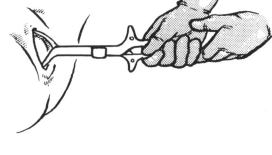

8. Asynclitism is corrected and the forceps blades are opposite each other.

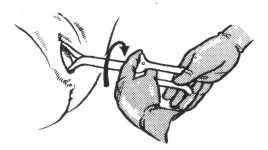

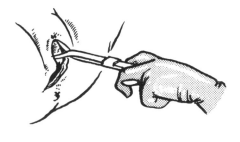

9. The head is gently rotated to the OA position. Varying asynclitism and gentle traction help to rotate into the pelvic axis. A large episiotomy is needed.

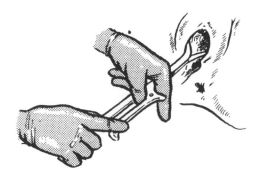

10. To prevent over compression of the baby's head, a thumb is kept between the handles.

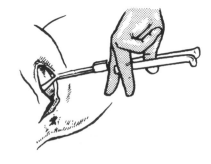

11. As the head extends, the direction of pull must be altered upwards.

FORCEPS DELIVERY

MANUAL ROTATION

This may be used as an alternative to rotation with forceps and delivery is then completed with Anderson's blades.

First determine the exact position by palpating the anterior fontanelle. This may be extremely difficult to detect if there has been much moulding or caput formation.

An ear may be palpable. The root of the pinna must be identified to distinguish left from right.

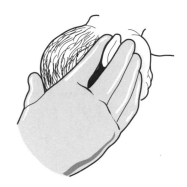

The right hand then grasps the head, while the left hand through the abdominal wall pushes the shoulder forward. The head may have to be dislodged slightly to achieve this, and once round it must be held in position until the forceps blades are applied.

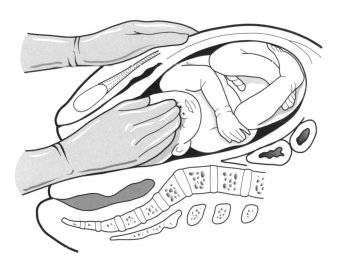

FORCEPS DELIVERY

OTHER APPLICATIONS OF FORCEPS

1. Delivery of the head in the occipito-posterior position.

This may be the easiest and best method of delivering a fetus with the head in the direct OP position, provided the head is low in the pelvis. Little traction should be required and the fetus is spared the risk of manipulation. A large episiotomy is necessary.

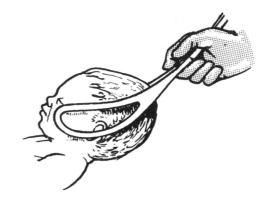

2. In a breech presentation the forceps can be applied to the head once it has entered the pelvis. Anderson's blades are preferred because of their length.

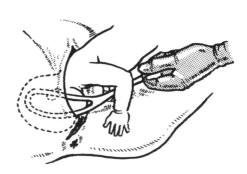

3. In a face presentation (mento-anterior) the forceps may be applied direct. (Mento-posterior positions must be rotated.)

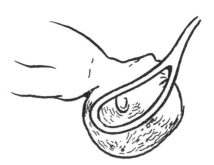

FORCEPS DELIVERY

COMPLICATIONS OF FORCEPS DELIVERY

Lacerations

1. Perineal tears are inevitable unless episiotomy is done at the right time.
2. Vaginal wall may be split, especially if compressed between ischial spine and fetal head or forceps inserted carelessly.
3. Cervical and vaginal tears may be caused during a Kielland's rotation. After delivery the vagina and cervix should be carefully inspected and all damage repaired.

Haemorrhage

Except from lacerations, haemorrhage is no more likely than after spontaneous delivery. Many obstetricians give an intravenous oxytocic with the delivery of the anterior shoulder of the baby when conducting a forceps delivery. This allows speedy completion of the third stage of labour by cord traction.

Injury to baby

If the blades have been properly applied, the fetal head should be protected by the rigid case of the forceps blades. Where excessive traction force has been applied, there may be bruising, facial nerve palsy or depression fracture of the skull.

TRIAL OF FORCEPS

This term is used when delivery is indicated but the obstetrician remains uncertain whether safe vaginal delivery is mechanically possible.

The procedure requires the presence of an experienced operator and the delivery is conducted in an operating theatre with the staff and facilities to proceed to caesarean section. Careful re-examination in theatre may convince the operator that delivery is not possible. If still uncertain, however, he may proceed to apply the forceps blades and even exert traction. If application of the blades is difficult or no descent of the head occurs with reasonable traction, caesarean section is performed. The operator's mental approach to the procedure is important, that is to say the possibility of caesarean section being required has been clearly acknowledged.

VACUUM EXTRACTOR (VENTOUSE)

The vacuum extractor is a traction instrument used as an alternative to the obstetric forceps. It adheres to the baby's scalp by suction and is used in the conscious patient to assist maternal expulsive efforts. The suction cup obtains its grip by raising an artificial caput. The original instrument consisted of a metal cup and a hand pump but this has now largely been replaced by a new extractor with a malleable silicone cup and electrical pump. The advantages of the new instrument are that it produces a much less marked 'chignon' on the fetal scalp and the speed with which the vacuum can be raised. The traditional ventouse still has a place and is associated with *fewer failures to achieve vaginal birth*.

The patient is usually in the lithotomy position and the same precautions are observed as for forceps operations. Probably the most convenient anaesthetic is a pudendal nerve block, but sometimes only inhalational analgesia or sufficient local anaesthetic for an episiotomy is required.

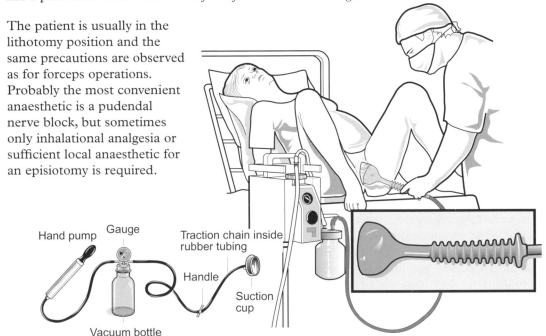

Hand pump Gauge Traction chain inside rubber tubing Handle Suction cup Vacuum bottle

The Place of the Vacuum Extractor

1. This instrument was introduced as a means of avoiding difficult forceps delivery or even caesarean section in patients in whom there was delay in labour with the cervix not quite fully dilated. It may still occasionally be used for this purpose, but it is mainly used as the instrument of choice by obstetricians who prefer it even when forceps delivery would be easy.
2. Like the forceps, it should normally be applied only when the head is engaged and there is no question of disproportion. An exception to this rule may be in the case of a second twin where the head remains at a relatively high level. In these circumstances the application of the vacuum extractor may be simpler and safer than the use of forceps.

Precautions in Use

1. Care should be taken, in applying the cup to the fetal scalp, to exclude vaginal skin from the edges of the cup.
2. Prolonged or excessive traction should not be used. Traction for more than 10 minutes will increase the risk of scalp damage, cephalhaematoma or more serious sub-aponeurotic bleeding.

SYMPHYSIOTOMY

Symphysiotomy means the cutting of the fibres of the symphysis pubis to allow vaginal delivery in the presence of moderate disproportion. The procedure has a place in obstetrical practice in developing countries when facilities for caesarean section are not available, or in order to avoid the risk of rupture of a caesarean section scar in a subsequent pregnancy in women being confined by unskilled attendants in remote areas.

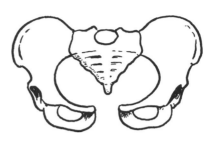

The transverse diameter can be enlarged up to 3 cm and the pubic angle widened, but there is little increase in AP diameters.

Principles of Operation

1. The head should be two-fifths or more in the pelvis.
2. The cervix should be at least 8 cm dilated in a primigravid or 6 cm in a multipara.
3. The legs are held in abduction by assistants (stirrups are not used) to prevent excessive stretching of the vaginal tissues when the joint is divided.
4. A catheter is placed in the bladder and one finger in the vagina pushes the urethra to the side to protect it from injury.
5. The symphysis pubis and perineum are infiltrated with local anaesthetic.
6. A stab incision with a scalpel is made into the centre of the joint. The blade is moved to divide the fibres of the symphysis.
7. The baby is then delivered spontaneously or by vacuum extractor aided by an episiotomy.
8. The mother's legs are strapped together for 12 hours post-operatively and ambulation is gradually introduced.

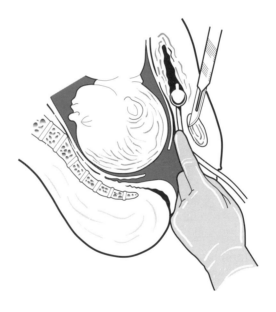

Complications

1. Soft tissue damage and fistula during operation and later stress incontinence.
2. Subsequent pelvic joint pain and difficulty in walking. The incidence of these complications will obviously be reduced by an experienced surgeon, but very few obstetricians in the United Kingdom are familiar with the operation which has been completely replaced by lower segment section.

CAESAREAN SECTION

Caesarean section means the delivery of the baby through incisions in the abdominal wall and uterus. The operation has been performed more frequently in the United Kingdom in the last decade and rates of 15% or even higher are now common in British hospitals. Caesarean section has replaced complicated operative vaginal delivery and it is used increasingly in the management of the 'at risk' fetus, especially if premature.

It must be remembered, however, that the morbidity and mortality of caesarean section are considerably greater than for vaginal delivery, and the patient's management in a subsequent pregnancy is likely to be dominated by the fact that her uterus is scarred.

INDICATIONS

The decision to deliver by caesarean section will often be based on a combination of factors or circumstances. The following list gives the common indications for caesarean section but should not be regarded as comprehensive:

In Labour

Fetal distress in the first stage of labour,
Delay in the first stage of labour due to disordered uterine action or suspected disproportion.

Other Emergencies

Cord prolapse, Fulminating pre-eclampsia,
Abruption of the placenta where the baby is alive.

Elective

Placenta praevia,
2 previous caesarean sections,
and in some cases:
Intra-uterine growth restriction,
Bad obstetric history,
Maternal diabetes,
Breech presentation (especially if premature).

ANAESTHESIA

Epidural block has become the preferred method of anaesthesia for caesarean section in many hospitals.

Advantages

Avoids the dangers of general anaesthesia (failed intubation, inhalation of gastric contents).
Improved retraction of the uterus.
Permits the mother (and her partner) to see and hear the baby at birth.
Rapid post-operative recovery.
The preparation of an epidural anaesthetic for caesarean section may be time-consuming, and, if time is short and it is wished to avoid general anaesthesia, a spinal anaesthetic may be given.

General anaesthesia is still used, however, especially in cases where there may be severe haemorrhage e.g. placenta praevia. Some women may be frightened by the prospect of abdominal delivery while remaining awake and request a general anaesthetic.

CAESAREAN SECTION

LOWER SEGMENT SECTION

In this procedure a transverse incision is made in the lower uterine segment. It is the operation of choice. Although slightly more complicated to perform, repair of the uterus is usually simple, the scar heals well and subsequent rupture is uncommon.

The lower segment may be approached through either a midline sub-umbilical abdominal incision or a transverse suprapubic incision.

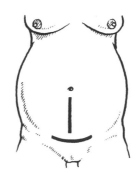

Technique of Lower Segment Section

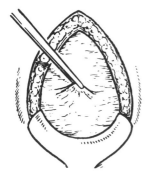

The loose uterovesical peritoneum is picked up.

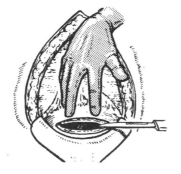

Peritoneum is cut to expose lower segment, and a small transverse incision is made.

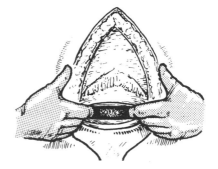

The uterine incision is widened with the fingers.

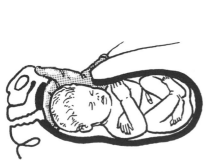

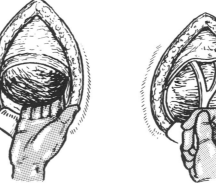

The operator's right hand is passed into the uterus to lift the baby's head, while the assistant presses on the fundus to push the baby out.

Sometimes it is necessary to extract the head with forceps.

CAESAREAN SECTION

Lower Segment Section *(continued)*

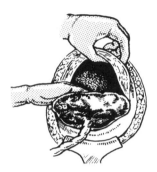 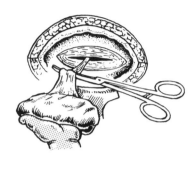 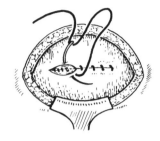

Ergometrine or synthetic oxytocin is given and the placenta and membranes removed.

Uterine wound is closed with 2 layers of polyglycolic acid sutures. The peritoneum need not be closed unless there is evidence of infection.

CLASSICAL CAESAREAN SECTION

This means a longitudinal incision in the upper uterine segment.

The operation is quick and easy but it is an abdominal procedure rather than a pelvic one and more often followed by peritonitis and ileus. The involution of the uterus may not allow sound healing and the scar may rupture in a subsequent pregnancy.

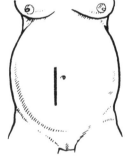

The operation is still, however, occasionally indicated:
1. Some cases of placenta praevia with an ill-formed lower segment.
2. Transverse or unstable lie with poorly formed lower segment.
3. Fibroid distorting the uterus.
4. When an inexperienced surgeon is operating in an emergency.

Technique of Classical Section

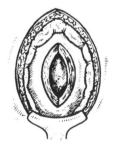 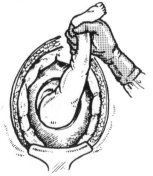

Abdominal contents are packed off and the uterus is opened in the midline. If the placenta is anterior (30 to 40% of cases) it is cut through or pushed aside at once. Bleeding is ignored.

The easiest way to deliver the baby is to pull it out gently by the legs.
The placenta is delivered as before and the wound closed in 3 layers.

CAESAREAN SECTION

COMPLICATIONS

Haemorrhage

Caesarean section is a vascular operation and the blood loss is commonly between 500 and 1000 ml. Cross-matched blood should, therefore, always be available and an intravenous drip set up. Increased bleeding is to be anticipated in cases of placenta praevia or multiple pregnancy where there may be impaired retraction of the placental site.

If the lower segment incision tears at the angles during the extraction of the baby, the large uterine vessels may be torn and haemorrhage will be severe. The patient can very quickly become shocked. The blood loss can usually be controlled by suturing, but if this proves impossible the operator may need to resort to removal of the uterus. Identification of the cervix is not always easy and a sub-total hysterectomy may be carried out.

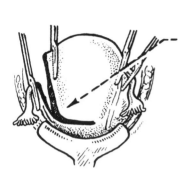

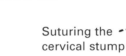

Suturing the cervical stump

Post-operative distension

Gaseous distension of the bowel is common after caesarean section, but the lax condition of the abdominal muscles, although it accentuates the swelling, reduces the pain of distension. There may be reduced bowel sounds and an absence of flatus for the first 24–48 hours. If this 'incipient ileus' does not resolve quickly, gastric suction and parenteral fluids should be started.

Wound dehiscence and infection

Because of the abdominal distension a longitudinal sub-umbilical incision is under tension and dehiscence is commoner than after other abdominal operations. A transverse abdominal incision is therefore much to be preferred. A Pfannenstiel incision rarely dehisces but haematoma formation is relatively frequent and careful attention to haemostasis is important. To reduce the risk of infection prophylactic antibiotics are now recommended routinely at the time of emergency caesarean section.

CAESAREAN SECTION

Pulmonary embolism

The risk of this serious complication is increased with caesarean section compared with vaginal delivery. The risk is reduced by early ambulation and this is further aided by the use of epidural anaesthesia.

Routine prophylaxis with subcutaneous heparin is now commonplace and its widespread introduction has led to a dramatic reduction in the incidence of thromboembolic disease and pulmonary embolism in particular. Low molecular weight preparations are more easily monitored and have a lower side effect profile.

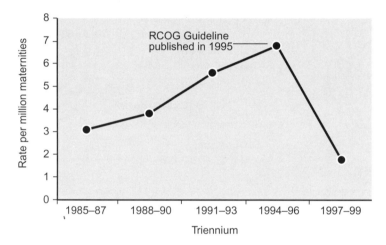

Pulmonary embolism reduction follows increased use of heparin

The publication of guidelines on the use of heparin produced by the Royal College of Obstetricians and Gynaecologists has contributed to this reduction.

DESTRUCTIVE OPERATIONS

These procedures were designed to reduce the bulk of dead or grossly abnormal fetuses to allow vaginal delivery. Nowadays caesarean section will usually be preferred.

The only procedure likely to be employed in practice today is perforation of the head of a hydrocephalic fetus. This may be done in the second stage of labour to allow vaginal delivery.

CRANIOTOMY — Perforation of the skull to allow drainage of CSF and collapse of the skull. Any pointed instrument will serve, such as a wide-bore trocar and cannula.

Head Presentation
The skull sutures are perforated per vaginam, and an assistant must press the head downwards to prevent rupture of the lower segment as the operator forces the trocar upwards.

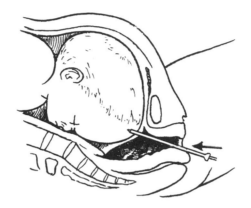

Breech Presentation
The trocar is passed through the abdominal wall. If a meningocele is present it is possible to drain a hydrocephaly by passing a straightened male catheter up the spinal canal.

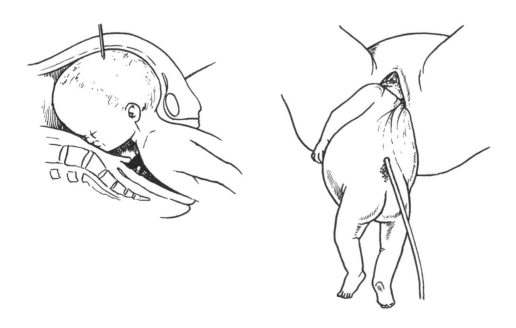

STERILISATION

Too often contraceptive practice remains the responsibility of the female partner. Vasectomy is vastly preferable in terms of morbidity and mortality as well as reliability.

Notwithstanding this, sterilisation of the female is commonly requested. In practice this means the interruption of the continuity of the fallopian tubes. The patient's convenience is best suited by doing it in the immediate post-natal period, but the operation has a slight but recognised association with thromboembolism and a higher failure rate when performed at this time. It is wiser to delay the procedure for at least two months. A further reason for delay is to allow the patient time to reconsider her decision, free from the pressures of pregnancy and also to recognise the possibility of an abnormality in the baby which is not apparent at the time of delivery.

Tubal Ligation
This is the technique most commonly employed when sterilisation is carried out at the time of caesarean section or where there is an open approach to an interval procedure.

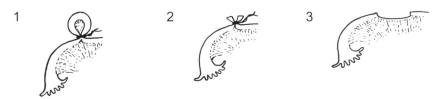

A loop of tube is ligated with PolyGlycolic Acid (PGA) sutures and the top of the loop is excised.

When the PGA absorbs, the divided areas will separate leaving a defect in the tube. This is known as the Pomeroy method of sterilisation.

The patient should understand that the operation is designed to be permanent, and, although patency can sometimes be restored, normal function leading to conception can by no means be guaranteed.

There is a very small risk of failure with the method — 3–4 per thousand — and this may be higher when the operation is done at the time of caesarean section or early in the puerperium. Ectopic pregnancy is also a recognised complication. Ligated tubes can become patent through a fistulous opening or by recanalisation.

INDUCTION OF ABORTION

Abortion may be induced under the terms of the Abortion Act or following a diagnosis of non-continuing pregnancy.

MEDICAL METHODS

a) First trimester

Abortion may be induced up to 63 days' gestation by a combination of the anti-progesterone Mifepristone and the prostaglandin Gemeprost. Mifepristone 600 mg is given (under supervision) orally and 48 hours later Gemeprost 1 mg is given as a vaginal pessary. In the majority of cases abortion will occur within 4 hours of the prostaglandin administration.

b) Mid trimester

Gemeprost pessaries, 1 mg given into the posterior fornix 3 hourly for up to five pessaries, may be used. As in the first trimester, pre-treatment with Mifepristone 600 mg 48 hours earlier may be employed to facilitate the process.

Complications of prostaglandin administration are nausea, vomiting or diarrhoea. Palpitations and mild pyrexia may occur and there have been reports of uterine rupture and cervical damage, usually in parous women or those with a previous Caesarean section.

Occasionally prostaglandins may still be given by the extra-amniotic route, using a solution of Dinoprostone. This may be employed where a patient finds difficulty in using pessaries or where there has been no response to Gemeprost.

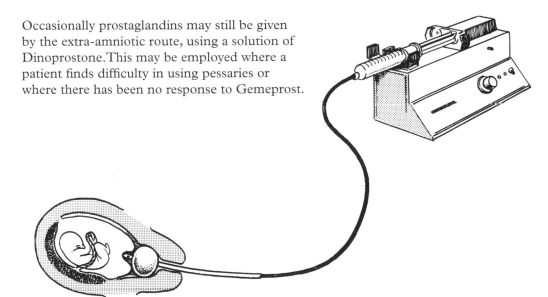

INDUCTION OF ABORTION

SURGICAL METHODS

a) Vacuum aspiration

This is the commonest method of uterine evacuation in pregnancies up to 12 weeks' gestation. It is usually preceded by cervical ripening to facilitate dilatation of the cervix and thus avoid damage. Usually this will be done by Gemeprost 1 mg vaginally, 1–3 hours before evacuation. Alternatively Mifepristone 600 mg 48 hours before surgery may be used.

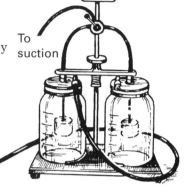

To suction

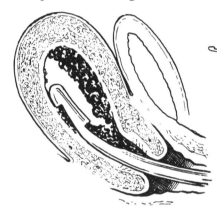

After dilatation, usually under a general anaesthetic, the products of conception are removed by suction using a plastic curette.

Complications include cervical trauma, perforation of the uterus and incomplete evacuation leading to sepsis.

b) Abdominal hysterotomy

This operation, the emptying of the uterus by the abdominal route before fetal viability, is rarely performed now but may still occasionally be needed where there is no response to prostaglandin stimulation.

The main disadvantages of the procedure are the risks of any abdominal operation — general anaesthesia, sepsis and thrombosis and a slight risk of rupture in subsequent pregnancy.

A small suprapubic incision is made and a finger, hooked through a stab wound, delivers the uterus. Quite a large uterus can be delivered through a small incision.

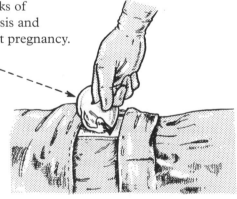

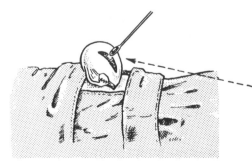

After removal of the fetus and placenta the cavity should be confirmed to be empty. Spillage of the decidua should be avoided as there is a well-recognised risk of implantation endometriosis in the abdominal scar.

MATERNAL INJURIES

INJURIES TO THE VULVA
Haematoma of the Vulva

Rupture of vaginal veins (after prolonged or operative delivery) may produce a very large effusion of blood, extending downwards into the labium major. If acute and extensive, it causes great pain and this, with blood loss, soon causes shock.

Haematoma may not develop until after perineal repair.

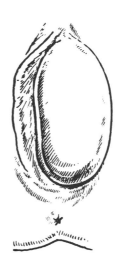

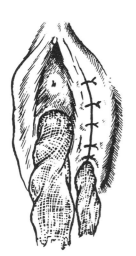

Treatment
1. Analgesia and blood transfusion as required.
2. The haematoma may contain itself but if it continues to extend it will require evacuation under general anaesthesia. The cavity will require suture and possibly packing.
3. Antibiotics may be given.

Tears of the Vestibule

These are not common and arise from over-distension during delivery (see Perineal tears). They may bleed freely, especially if the clitoral artery is approached, and should be sutured. If the tear passes close to the urethral meatus a catheter should be inserted and continuous drainage with antibiotic cover continued for 48 hours.

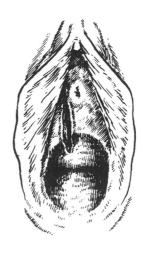

MATERNAL INJURIES

PERINEAL TEARS

These are more common in primigravid patients where the perineum is more rigid. Probably the most important factors are the width of the pubic arch (and hence the amount of room available) and the size and position of the fetal head. All malpresentations increase the amount of distension of the perineum.

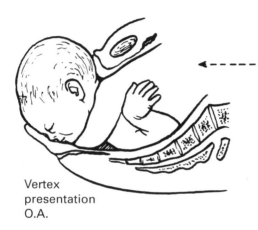

In the normal O.A. position the suboccipito-frontal diameter (10.0 cm) distends the vulva, and the widest part of the head is under the bony arch.

Vertex presentation O.A.

When the position is O.P. the occipito-frontal diameter (11.5 cm) distends the vulva, and the widest part of the head distends the perineum.

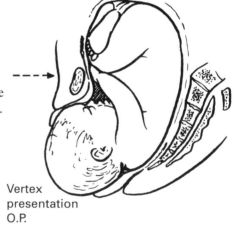

Vertex presentation O.P.

Face presentation M.A.

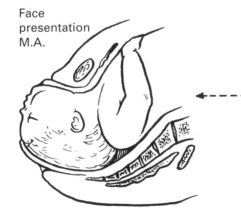

When the face is presenting, once the chin is delivered, the submento-vertical diameter (13.5 cm) will distend the vulva, and again the widest part of the head passes over the perineum.

MATERNAL INJURIES

PERINEAL TEARS *(continued)*

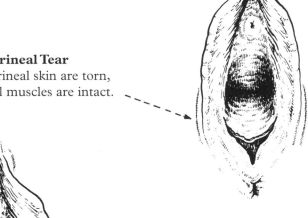

1st Degree Perineal Tear
Vaginal and perineal skin are torn, but the perineal muscles are intact.

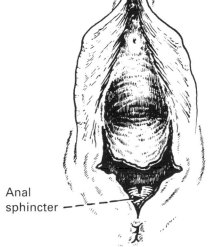

2nd Degree Perineal Tear
The perineal body is torn right down to (and sometimes partly involving) the anal sphincter. The vaginal tears often extend up both sides of the vagina.

Anal sphincter

3rd Degree Tear
The tear involves the internal and external anal sphincters (the anal sphincter complex).

The injury in **4th Degree Tears** involves the anal sphincter complex and rectal mucosa.

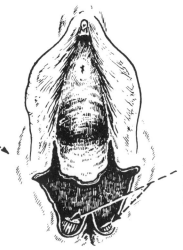

Torn ends of anal sphincter

MATERNAL INJURIES

PERINEAL TEARS — REPAIR

Perineal damage should be repaired very soon after delivery. Blood loss will be lessened and the chance of infection reduced.

First and Second Degree Tears

The repair is done under aseptic conditions with the patient in the lithotomy position under a good light. 20–30 ml of 1% lignocaine are injected into the muscles and under the skin.

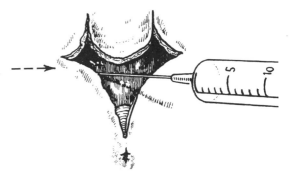

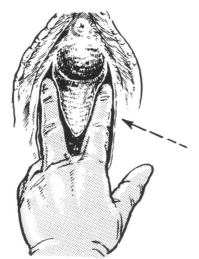

Correct anatomical apposition is essential and swabs used freely to expose the tissues. The upper limits of the tear must be demonstrated by stretching apart with the fingers so that suturing may begin there.

1. Close vaginal tears with continuous polyglycolic acid (PGA) suture.
2. Suture perineal muscles together with interrupted PGA sutures.
3. Close skin over muscles with 2/0 PGA or non-absorbable sutures.

Care should be taken that the vagina is not narrowed by tightening sutures inappropriately.

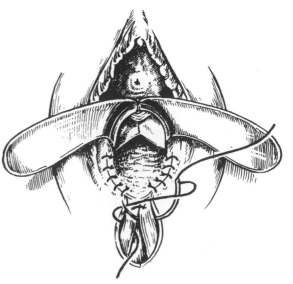

MATERNAL INJURIES

3rd and 4th Degree Tears

All third and fourth degree tears should be managed by clinicians with sufficient expertise in the management of perineal tears.

The operation is best performed under regional or general anaesthesia in an operating theatre.

1. The rectal wall is repaired with fine PGA sutures with the knot tied inside the rectum.
2. The two ends of the anal sphincter (which are often markedly retracted away from each other) should be grasped in tissue forceps and brought together so that one end overlaps the other giving a 'double layer' at the site of the muscle disruption. A fine monofilament suture, Polydioxanone (PDS), should be used for sphinter repair.
3. The repair is then continued as for a 2nd degree tear. The skin around the anal margin is closed with fine PGA.
4. Broad spectrum antibiotics are given intra-operatively.

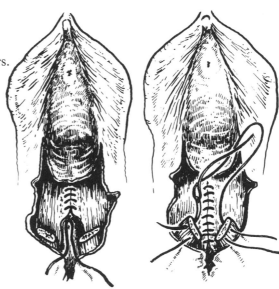

Post-operative Treatment

1. Laxatives reduce wound breakdown rates.
2. Broad spectrum antibiotics, incorporating metronidazole, are continued post-operatively and appear to reduce wound breakdown and fistula rates.
3. The patient must be reviewed at her post-natal visit by an obstetrician and specific enquiry made about continence of both faeces and flatus.

Any plans for future deliveries should take into account the final result of the repair and the woman's attitude to future births. Caesarean section may be considered.

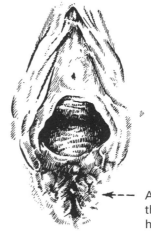

A complete tear that has failed to heal

MATERNAL INJURIES

VAGINAL TEARS
Colporrhexis (Rupture of the vaginal wall)
This is an uncommon but serious injury. The
most usual site is the posterior or lateral fornix
and the cervix may be involved. Tearing may
result from obstructed labour but it is more often
due to improper application of the forceps,
especially when attempts at delivery have been
made before the cervix is fully dilated.

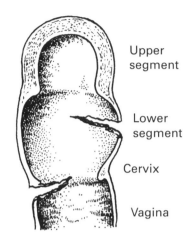

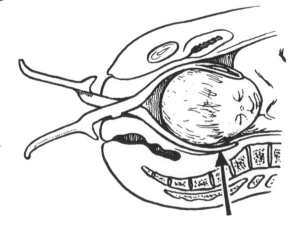

In obstructed labour the pathological
retraction ring (Bandl's ring) is a sign of
excessive traction on lower segment and
cervix. Rupture may occur in the lower
segment or at the cervico-vaginal
junction (see Uterine rupture).

If the posterior blade of
Kielland's forceps is not
properly guided by the
hand, the tip of the
blade may perforate and
tear the posterior fornix.

Treatment
If the examining finger passes completely through the vaginal tear, laparotomy is necessary to
check on the extent of the damage. The symptoms are those of rupture of the uterus, and
bleeding is usually considerable. A blood transfusion will probably be needed and
hysterectomy may be the quickest and easiest way of stopping the haemorrhage.

MATERNAL INJURIES

VAGINAL FISTULAE
Vaginal fistulae are uncommon injuries in present day obstetrics.

Vesicovaginal Fistula
This is caused by direct trauma e.g. in operative delivery or by prolonged compression of the vaginal wall and bladder between the fetal head and maternal symphysis pubis as may occur in obstructed labour.

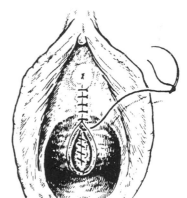

If a fistula is due to trauma, urine appears at once. Sloughing of necrotic bladder tissue, following untreated obstructed labour, takes about 5 days, and a fistula may not be obvious until then.

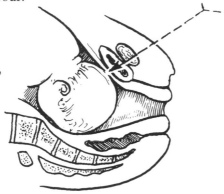

Repair of Vesicovaginal Fistula
If observed at delivery it should be closed forthwith, using PGA (interrupted through-and-through, then a continuous suture).
Continuous catheter drainage is instituted for a week and antibiotic cover provided.
Fistulae caused by obstructed labour must be repaired some weeks after delivery and may be closed by the vaginal or abdominal route. The assistance of a urologist may be valuable.

Rectovaginal Fistula
This type of fistula nearly always occurs after the imperfect healing of a repair of a complete tear.

Repair
No attempt at re-repair should be made for at least 3 months. It is usual to break down the perineum to some extent so that the rectum may be mobilised before suture.

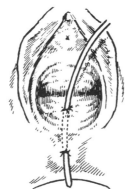

329

MATERNAL INJURIES

INJURIES TO THE CERVIX
Lacerations

The cervix is always torn to some extent during delivery. This causes the appearance of the parous os. Severe tears may follow strong contractions on a rigid cervix, or arise from a previous cervical operation. The commonest cause is surgical trauma following forceps or breech delivery.

A tear is suspected when bleeding is heavy although the uterus is firmly contracted. The cervix must be examined and this may be difficult because of the bleeding and friability of the tissues.

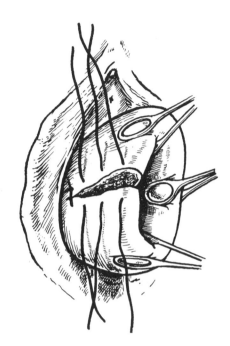

Several pairs of ring forceps and at least one assistant are needed and, once demonstrated, the tear should be sutured with PGA sutures. By the time the operation is completed, if not before, the patient may need a blood transfusion.

Annular detachment of the cervix

This rare laceration usually occurs in a primigravida in whom strong contractions are driving the vertex against a rigid cervix. The cervix gradually develops a pressure necrosis, and the sloughed cervix separates and is delivered in front of the head. There is little bleeding and the cervical stump heals well.

MATERNAL INJURIES

RUPTURE OF THE UTERUS

Rupture of the uterus is an uncommon injury in the United Kingdom and it is nearly always due to rupture of a previous caesarean section scar. It may however arise, particularly in a parous patient, from obstructed labour due to cephalopelvic disproportion or malpresentation.

Rupture of a classical caesarean scar

This may occur in late pregnancy or early labour. Bleeding is often slight because the fetus and placenta are extruded into the peritoneal cavity and the uterus retracts. There is acute abdominal pain and this may be accompanied by shock.

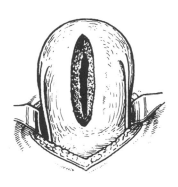

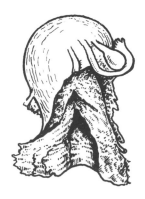

Rupture of lower segment scar

This may not be clinically obvious initially and the first indication of a problem may be fetal distress identified on cardiotocography. The presenting part will no longer be in the pelvis on vaginal examination.

Dehiscence of a lower segment scar may cause little bleeding and may be found only when repeat section is undertaken for poor progress in labour. If, however, the tear extends there will be significant intraperitoneal haemorrhage.

Spontaneous rupture

The patient is typically of high parity, and labour has been obstructed by malpresentation or disproportion. Contractions have been strong and rupture begins in the lower segment and is accompanied by pain, bleeding, haematuria and collapse.

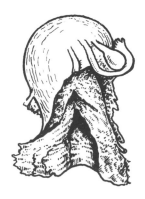

MATERNAL INJURIES

Diagnosis and treatment

The diagnosis is sometimes obvious but may be impossible without laparotomy. Persistent abdominal pain, a rise in pulse rate and fresh vaginal bleeding should be looked for. Rupture is followed by cessation of contractions. If the fetus is wholly or partly extruded into the abdominal cavity the uterus will contract and may be detectable as a separate mass in the abdomen. Vaginal examination reveals an empty pelvis.

Once the diagnosis is reached, laparotomy must be carried out with blood transfusion set up.

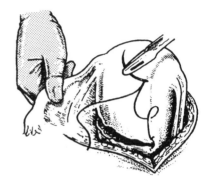

Hysterectomy may be the safest treatment, but this decision will depend on the extent of the damage and the patient's parity. If the tear is small it can be repaired with conservation of the uterus.

If hysterectomy is decided on, the tear will in most cases have half completed the operation. Subsequent steps in the operation are indicated below. If bleeding is severe this will be an operation in which speed is of importance.

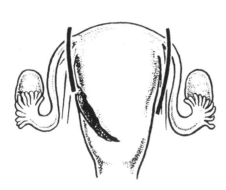

Division of the fallopian tubes and broad ligaments, leaving behind the ovaries and part of the tubes.

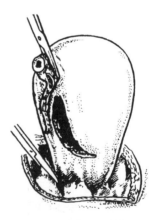

After incision of the peritoneum at the site of rupture the bladder is stripped from the uterine wall. It may be difficult to identify the cervico-vaginal junction and sub-total hysterectomy is performed.

MATERNAL INJURIES

HAEMATOMA OF THE RECTUS SHEATH

This is an uncommon condition occurring mostly in multiparous women as a result of coughing or sudden expulsive effort. Muscle fibres and branches of the deep epigastric veins are torn. If rupture occurs below the umbilicus, blood can track anywhere along the transversalis fascia and is virtually retroperitoneal. If above the umbilicus the haematoma is more likely to be localised.

The condition is most likely to be diagnosed on the history of sudden effort followed by pain. There may be peritonism and a vague abdominal swelling. If the blood loss is large there may be collapse. The condition must be distinguished from placental abruption, rupture of the uterus or bleeding from an ovarian cyst.

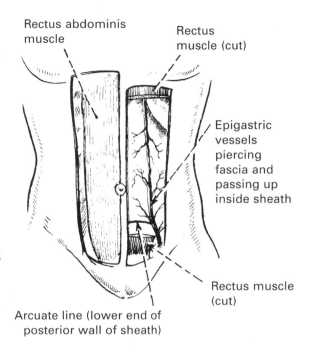

Rectus abdominis muscle

Rectus muscle (cut)

Epigastric vessels piercing fascia and passing up inside sheath

Rectus muscle (cut)

Arcuate line (lower end of posterior wall of sheath)

Treatment

If small and localised, the haematoma may be left to absorb, but usually operation is required with evacuation of clot, ligation of any bleeding points and closure with drainage.

PELVIC FLOOR NEUROPATHY

This term has been used in recent years to describe ano-rectal and/or urinary incontinence after childbirth. It seems to be diagnosed more commonly than previously but this may be because women are less embarrassed to raise these difficulties than formerly. Such complications seem to be particularly associated with a prolonged second stage of labour and operative vaginal delivery, both of which are seen commonly in patients with epidural anaesthetics. The symptoms seem to result from damage to the innervation of the pelvic floor sphincter muscles. Recovery usually occurs spontaneously within two months but occasionally the condition persists and expert urological or surgical help should be sought.

TRAUMATIC NEURITIS (OBSTETRIC PALSY)

This is a rare condition which may result from compression of the lumbo-sacral trunk, as it crosses the sacro-iliac joint, by the fetal head or obstetric forceps. Occasionally there may be disc prolapse or direct pressure on the popliteal nerve when the legs are in the lithotomy position. There may be pain, sensory impairment, muscle weakness and footdrop.

Backache, from sacro-iliac strain, can follow childbirth and cause limping without any evidence of a lower motor neurone lesion.

Treatment

Where disc prolapse or footdrop are diagnosed or suspected, the usual supportive measures should be employed and an orthopaedic opinion sought.

333

CHAPTER 15

PUERPERIUM — NORMAL AND ABNORMAL

THE PUERPERIUM

Obstetricians consider the puerperium as that time taken for a woman to have returned, physiologically, to her non-pregnant state. This is usually considered as six weeks, though for the purposes of notification of infections the puerperium is defined, in law, as the 14 days (England and Wales) or 21 days (Scotland) following confinement.

A midwife is required to attend a puerperal woman for a period of not less than 10 days after her confinement.

The uterus contains a raw bleeding surface — a wound. Infection must be prevented.

The newborn baby requires careful nursing and observation.

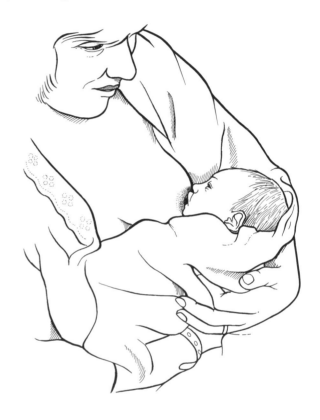

Breastfeeding must be initiated. If artificial feeding is recommended, for example, if the mother is HIV positive, then the breasts should not be stimulated and a well fitting bra should be worn.

Muscles are of poor tone and ligaments slack after pregnancy and labour. Systematic exercises should be given to help prevent chronic postural defects, hernia and prolapse.

Motherhood is accompanied by dramatic effects on the psychology of women. Anxiety and lack of confidence are common and support must be offered.

Better physical and emotional preparation for childbirth, shorter and less tiring labours and early ambulation have led to a decrease in puerperal morbidity. Less nursing care is needed and many women can return to their families after only a short period of recovery in hospital. This is a desirable situation and requires an effective and well-integrated community midwifery service.

THE PUERPERIUM

The process by which the uterus returns almost to its pre-gravid state is known as *Involution* — a dramatic example of the effect of withdrawal of the support of the placental hormones. The uterus is half of its weight on the seventh postnatal day compared with immediately after delivery.

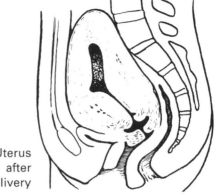

Uterus after delivery

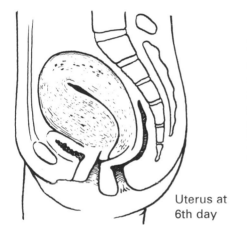

Uterus at 6th day

Involution is caused by the phenomenon of **Autolysis** — enzymatic digestion of excess cytoplasm — and thrombosis and hyaline degeneration of vessels; but traces of fibroelastic tissue remain as evidence of pregnancy. The endometrium is regenerated by the 10th day, except at the placental site, where it takes 6 weeks.

The Lochia (the discharges of childbirth) consist mainly of blood and necrotic decidua. They persist for about 2–3 weeks gradually becoming colourless and scanty. They are sterile to begin with but by the 3rd–4th days the inside of the uterus is said to be colonised by vaginal commensals (non-haemolytic streptococcus, *E. coli*, etc.).

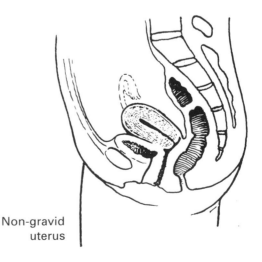

Non-gravid uterus

337

THE PUERPERIUM

Muscle fibres
from uterus

Pregnant

Puerperal

Non-pregnant

The uterus reduces to about one twentyfifth of its size in about 6 weeks although it never returns exactly to its nulliparous proportions.

This reduction in size is achieved partly by the removal of blood and blood vessels, and partly by digestion of a large part of the cell cytoplasm. The number of muscle cells is probably not much diminished, but the individual fibres are very much shorter and thinner than during the pregnancy.

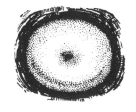

$\frac{5}{8}$

$\frac{2}{3}$

Body

$\frac{3}{8}$

$\frac{1}{3}$

Cervix

Nulliparous uterus

Parous uterus

The cervix never returns to its pristine appearance and although completely healed will always give evidence of parturition.

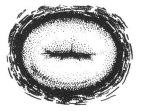

Nulliparous cervix

Parous cervix

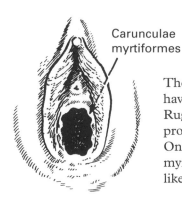

Carunculae
myrtiformes

The vagina and vulva, considerably stretched during labour, have returned almost to their pre-gravid size by the 3rd week. Rugae appear in the vagina, and the labia regress to a less prominent and fleshy state than in the nulliparous condition. Only small sessile tags of hymen are left (carunculae myrtiformes — 'pieces of flesh in the shape of myrtle') and, like the parous cervix, are evidence of previous pregnancy.

CLINICAL ASPECTS

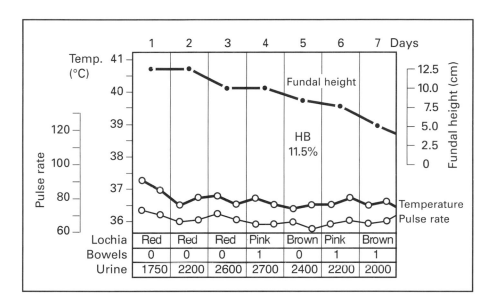

Fundal height is measured each day. The bladder must be empty and the uterus is rubbed up to contract and the height of the fundus above the symphysis is measured. Failure of involution suggests retained placental tissue.

Pulse tends to be slower, about 60–70 per minute, probably because the woman is resting after the exertion of labour.

Temperature may be slightly elevated during the first 24 hours, but thereafter should remain within normal limits. Persistent pyrexia requires investigation.

Constipation is the rule for some days. Progesterone continues to inhibit smooth muscle motility. Haemorrhoids are a common, troublesome complication.

Urine — There is a diuresis during the 2nd to 5th days and urinary nitrogen is much raised. The body is getting rid of the excess fluid retained during pregnancy, and the high nitrogen excretion is a direct result of the autolytic process at work in the uterus. Urinary retention is relatively common especially after instrumental delivery. It may be due to oedema of the bladder neck as a result of stretching or bruising or due to the pain of perineal sutures.

Lochia should gradually change colour from red to pale yellow over 10 days. There are great variations in this due to the fluctuations in the amount of blood being lost during this period. Excess fresh lochia suggest retained products.

Blood — The haemoglobin level is important and should be stable by the 5th day, when normal haemoconcentration is approached.

FEEDING THE NEWBORN

ADVANTAGES OF BREAST MILK
Breast feeding confers many benefits on both the baby and its mother:

1. Chemical Composition
All mammalian animals feed their young on unique milk adapted by nature to their needs. Human milk fats are much better absorbed than the butter fat in unmodified cow's milk which combines with calcium in the gut to reduce the absorption of calcium. Neonatal hypocalcaemia is associated with convulsions and perhaps with dental enamel hypoplasia and subsequent caries. The long chain fatty acids, naturally occurring in breast milk, play an important role in brain development.

2. Protection against Infection
Human milk contains a large amount of immunoglobulin (IgA) including specific antibodies to *E. coli* and respiratory syncytial (RSV) virus. IgA is resistant to digestion in the stomach and reaches the intestine undamaged where it acts on pathogenic organisms and inhibits their multiplication.

Human milk also supplies, from the lactiferous sinuses of the breast, the bacillus bifidus which colonises the baby's gut and, together with the lactobacillus which is the other organism principally found in the alimentary tract of breast fed infants, reduces the pH level so that the growth of pathogens is inhibited in the same manner as in the adult vagina.

The action against bacteria is strengthened by the high proportion of lactoferrin (an iron-binding protein) in human milk. Once in the intestine the lactoferrin reduces the amount of free iron below the level necessary for the growth of iron-dependent bacteria.

Breast milk will also supply smaller amounts of IgM and IgG.

3. Energy
Bottle fed babies may ingest more calories and are more often overweight than breast fed babies. If the feed is too highly concentrated the excessive sodium content makes the baby cry from thirst, and this is mistaken for hunger and more milk may be given. If rehydration does not occur, very high plasma sodium levels (hypernatraemia) may cause brain damage. This is avoided by the use of appropriately prepared modified cow's milk formula.

FEEDING THE NEWBORN

1. PHYSIOLOGY OF LACTATION

At delivery, when the placenta is delivered, a change in hormone production occurs: PROLACTIN, secreted from the anterior pituitary gland, stimulates milk production from the lacteal glands. Prolactin levels rise in response to feeding demands of the baby.

OXYTOCIN, from the posterior pituitary is responsible for promoting the ejection of milk from myoepithelial cells surrounding the glands to the nipples. Oxytocin levels respond to breast stimulation by the baby or by the mother expressing milk.

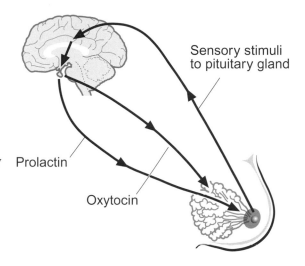

Sensory stimuli to pituitary gland

Prolactin

Oxytocin

The quality of milk and calorie content are controlled by the FEEDBACK INHIBITOR OF LACTATION (FIL). If there is ineffective emptying of the breasts FIL builds up reducing milk production from that breast. Effective emptying encourages more milk production.

All women should have had an opportunity to discuss the benefits of breastfeeding for both mother and baby and have enough information to make a fully informed choice.

FOR MOTHER breastfeeding reduces her risks of premenopausal breast cancer and ovarian cancer. It also reduces the risk of developing osteoporosis and consequent hip fractures in later life.

FOR BABY breast milk has antibacterial and antiviral properties and reduces the incidence of infection. Ear, throat, chest, gastrointestinal, and urinary tract infection are less common in breastfed babies. This reflects the high antibody levels in the early breast milk, colostrum. Breastfeeding also affords protection against asthma, some allergies and eczema. Type 1 diabetes is less common in children who were breastfed.

Expectations of breastfeeding and predisposition to breastfeeding vary between and within different cultures.

Terminology
Supplementary feed: a feed given in place of a breast feed.
Complementary feed: a feed given in addition to regular breastfeeding.

Supplementary and complimentary feeds confer no advantage to the baby and restrict the establishment of effective breastfeeding.

Weaning: a gradual change from exclusive breast milk or breast milk substitute to more solid food. Complimentary weaning foods should be introduced at about six months of age. The World Health Organisation recommends continuing breastfeeding up to the age of two years.

LACTATION AND BREAST FEEDING

PREVENTION OF PROBLEMS

Good positioning and correct attachment of baby at the breast play a crucial role in the prevention of sore nipples and in the successful establishment of breastfeeding. Sore nipples may also result from a candidial infection, but is often later in onset. Miconazole cream for mother and gel for the baby are effective. Treatment should be given to both. If persistent specialist help should be sought.

Understanding the physiology of lactation and being able to express by hand or pump allows women to be in control; the greater the demand from the baby, the greater the supply.

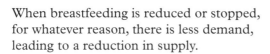

Good positioning and correct attachment of baby at the breast, as shown, are essential for satisfactory feeding.

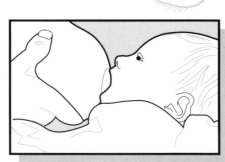

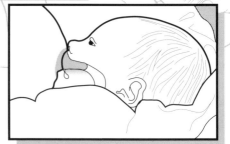

When breastfeeding is reduced or stopped, for whatever reason, there is less demand, leading to a reduction in supply.

With poor attachment there is ineffective milk removal leading to engorgement giving a rise in the FIL levels causing less milk to be produced. Poor attachment may lead to damage to the nipples and mothers may feed less often because it is painful. Again, less demand leads to less production of prolactin and consequently less milk production.

To avoid engorgement it is important to ensure good position and correct attachment. The baby should be fed as often and as long as he or she wants, that is *DEMAND FEEDING*.

All mothers should be taught the technique of hand expressing of milk so that they can be in control of their own breastfeeding.

If a breast is too full then she can express a little to soften the areola so that her baby can attach well.

LACTATION AND BREAST FEEDING

ENGORGEMENT
Engorgement affects the whole of one or both breasts whereas mastitis usually affects part of one breast.

MASTITIS
There are two main causes of mastitis. Non infective. A blocked milk duct causing milk stasis. Infective mastitis. A bacterial infection most commonly gains entry through a cracked nipple though this may occur if there is prolonged milk stasis.

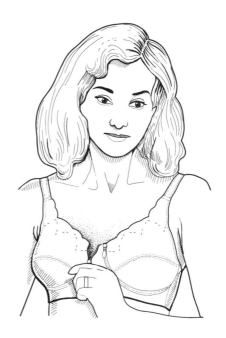

The affected breast needs careful attention to good positioning and correct attachment so that it is emptied. If this is not achieved expressing is an option. Warm baths prior to feeding or expressing are helpful. An anti-inflammatory such as ibuprofen may help by reducing temperature if the mother is feverish.

Cold packs between feeds are soothing and reduce oedema. With an infective mastitis antibiotics are necessary. Usually flucloxacillin or erythromycin are effective in treating infection and preventing recurrence or abscess formation.

LACTATION AND BREAST FEEDING

BREAST ABSCESS

Breast abscesses rarely happen and when they do, they are usually the result of untreated mastitis or delay in treatment or ineffective treatment. If mastitis is not managed actively and breast abscess does occur surgical drainage is required.

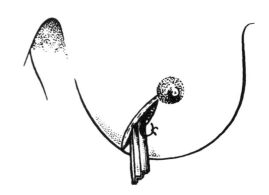

Most mothers can continue to breastfeed their baby from both breasts. Depending on the site of the wound or if it is too painful to feed, expressing milk is an option.

There is no justification in advising a mother to stop breastfeeding. This only compounds the problem.

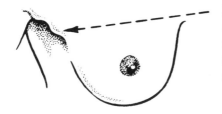

Mammary tissue into the axilla (the axillary tail) may become tender during lactation. Massage and arm exercises to promote drainage are effective.

DRUGS AND LACTATION

Administration of drugs to women who are breastfeeding may be harmful because:
1. The drug suppresses lactation e.g. bromocryptine or the combined oral contraceptive pill.
2. The drug is concentrated in breast milk in toxic levels for the baby e.g. Iodides.
3. The drug suppresses the sucking reflex in the baby by sedation e.g. phenobarbitone.

In many cases an alternative drug without harmful effects could be used. The drug information pharmacist in hospital can advise and the Trent Drug Information Centre has an interest in drugs in lactation and provides an extensive information service.

SECONDARY POST-PARTUM HAEMORRHAGE

Secondary Post-Partum Haemorrhage means abnormal bleeding from the genital tract from 24 hours after delivery until the completion of the puerperium.

Causes
1. Retained placental tissue. This inevitably leads to infection.
2. Intra-uterine infection with or without retained products.
3. Slow involution of the uterus or inadequate drainage of the lochia sometimes lead to fresh bleeding later than expected.

Management
1. Ultrasound scan to detect retained products (see below).
2. Antibiotics (broad spectrum + anti anaerobe e.g. Metronidazole).
3. Evacuation of the uterus if products of conception are seen.

This can be a treacherous condition and bleeding sometimes persists after evacuation. Occasionally packing the uterus and even hysterectomy are required.

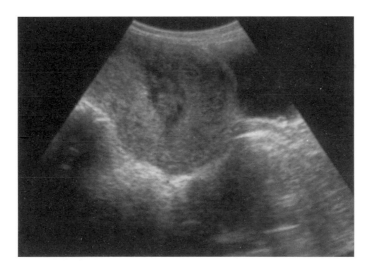

PUERPERAL PYREXIA

Synonyms: Puerperal Fever, Puerperal Sepsis, Childbed Fever.

Puerperal pyrexia means a temperature of 38°C, maintained for or recurring within 24 hours, within 21 days (14 days in England) of childbirth or abortion. This definition derives from the time when notification of puerperal pyrexia (whatever the cause) was a legal obligation.

Puerperal pyrexia may be due to an infection, genital or extra-genital.

1. Genital tract — perineum, vagina, cervix, uterus, adnexa.
2. Breasts.
3. Urinary system.
4. Superficial thrombophlebitis or deep vein thrombosis.
5. Respiratory system — common cold, influenza, after general anaesthesia.

Puerperal pyrexia requires, therefore, a complete physical examination and bacteriological examination of urine specimen, throat swab or sputum, high vaginal swab and in some cases blood culture.

Infection can occur during labour, especially if associated with prolonged rupture of the membranes. Vaginal examination in labour, even with proper care and aseptic precautions, can encourage the transfer of organisms from the vagina to uterine cavity. The most worrying organism, which can be found in the normal, healthy vagina, is the beta-haemolytic streptococcus.

Until the middle of the 20th century infection in childbirth was a major cause of maternal mortality and morbidity. The development of antibiotics provided a means of treating this but better care in labour, the improvements in hospital facilities and the avoidance of overcrowding have all contributed to reduce the incidence of genital tract infection.

In the puerperium infection may enter through one or more of these wounds:

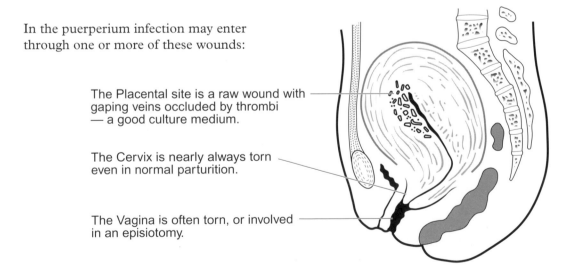

The Placental site is a raw wound with gaping veins occluded by thrombi — a good culture medium.

The Cervix is nearly always torn even in normal parturition.

The Vagina is often torn, or involved in an episiotomy.

In the puerperium the mother should be encouraged to be mobile as quickly as possible and to bath or use a bidet at least twice daily.

GENITAL TRACT INFECTION

1. ENDOMETRITIS

Endometritis is the most common and usually mildest form of genital infection.

Four Classical Signs:

1. Pyrexia 37.8°–38°C.
2. Pulse 100–120.
3. Fundal height not falling — poor involution.
4. Lochia remain red and have characteristic offensive smell.

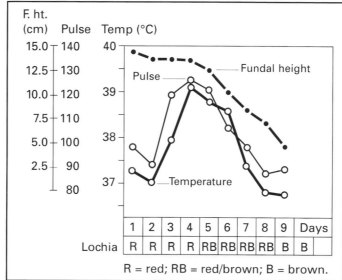

R = red; RB = red/brown; B = brown.

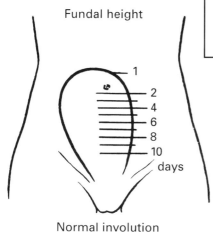

Fundal height

Normal involution

Investigations

Vaginal and cervical swabs are taken via a sterile speculum. If the diagnosis is uncertain, a throat swab and MSSU are also sent.

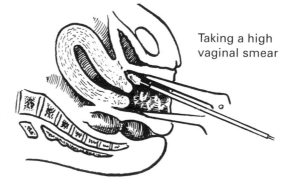

Taking a high vaginal smear

Treatment

A broad spectrum antibiotic such as a Cephalosporin, together with Metronidazole to treat anaerobic infections is given while awaiting the bacteriology reports. Treatment should be maintained for at least 5 days. Blood culture may be advisable.

GENITAL TRACT INFECTION

2. PARAMETRITIS (Syn. Cellulitis)

Infection may spread from the uterus, from a cervical laceration, or even from thrombophlebitis or peritonitis into the loose areolar connective tissue, setting up a *Parametritis*. The infection may extend retroperitoneally in any direction, commonly between the leaves of the broad ligament, round the vagina or rectum, or even up to the loin. Sometimes infection spreads along the round ligament and might then point above the inguinal ligament, near the inguinal ring.

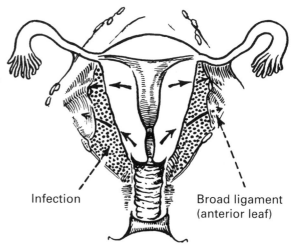

Infection

Broad ligament (anterior leaf)

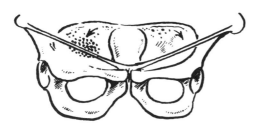

The condition occurs later than endometritis, usually in the second week and presents with fever and malaise. Pelvic examination reveals a large, often very hard mass and the lochia are red and heavy. Pain is less than might be expected.

Treatment

The appropriate antibiotic is given usually for 2 or more weeks, until the pelvis feels normal. If collections of pus appear they must be drained. A poor response to treatment calls for a search for spread. The possibility of subphrenic abscess must be remembered.

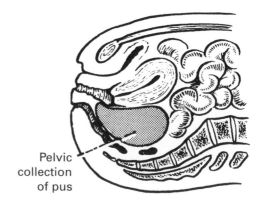

Pelvic collection of pus

GENITAL TRACT INFECTION

3. PERITONITIS AND SALPINGITIS

These two conditions are almost indistinguishable and neither is common. The pelvic peritoneum may be involved in the same way as the parametrium and also be spread along the fallopian tubes. A generalised peritonitis may occur with the development of paralytic ileus; and very rarely the infection is so acute and fulminating that the condition of 'septic' or 'irreversible' shock is met with.

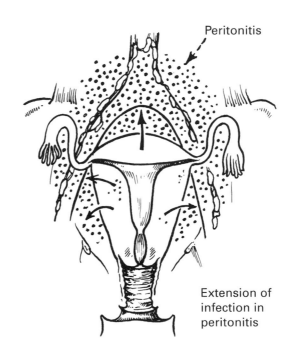

Peritonitis

Extension of infection in peritonitis

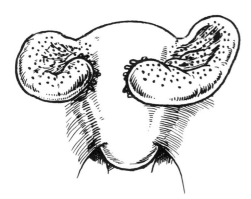

If untreated, salpingitis may produce tubal blockage

Diagnosis and Treatment

In some cases it may be impossible to exclude acute appendicitis without an exploratory laparotomy but otherwise treatment is along the same lines as described for parametritis. If laparotomy is carried out and only acute salpingitis found, the abdomen should be closed without drainage.

MENTAL ILLNESS IN THE PUERPERIUM

Of every 1000 pregnant women around 17 will already be attending the psychiatric services. Fifty percent will have a mild depressive mood disturbance in the first week after delivery (post-partum 'blues') and two will develop puerperal psychosis. Between 10 and 15% will develop postnatal depression.

Post-partum 'Blues'

This occurs in around 50% of women within 4 to 5 days of delivery. It is usually a self limiting condition though in rare circumstances progresses to postnatal depression. Generally support provided by the midwife and/or general practitioner is all that is required.

Postnatal Depression

Postnatal depression is a relatively common disorder with onset between one and six months after delivery and may last six months or longer. A family history of previous depressive illness in the patient or her relatives is commonly found.

The clinical features are of sleep disturbance, depressed mood, social withdrawal and lack of worthiness about being a mother. Suicidal thoughts or concerns that she may intentionally harm her baby are also found.

Diagnosis may be difficult in some women particularly if they withdraw from the support services. The use of screening tests, such as the Edinburgh Postnatal Depression Scale, has been advocated.

Management consists of social support, use of self help groups and, on occasion, antidepressant medication.

Specialist mother and baby units and the involvement of a psychiatric team with an interest in maternal mental health are invaluable.

Referral for psychiatric or psychological care is mandatory if there is evidence of child harm or suicidal intent.

Puerperal Psychosis

Psychotic illness occurs in 0.2% of mothers and the onset is earlier than postnatal depression. This is a serious condition and requires expert psychiatric evaluation and treatment.

Effect on the Mother–Child Relationship

Anything but the most short-lived depressive illness will interfere with the development of this relationship and with the relationship with the woman's partner. There is evidence of an increased incidence subsequently of abuse and of impaired intellectual ability in the child.

Substance abuse may continue or commence in the puerperium. The community midwives, health visitors and general practitioner should be involved in the management.

POSTNATAL PHYSIOTHERAPY

Each woman should be assessed individually to determine her needs and offered advice and initial exercise. This rehabilitation concentrates on back care, strengthening of abdominal and pelvic floor muscles.

When necessary, ice packs or electrotherapy may be required for the traumatised perineum. Modalities commonly used are ultrasound and pulsed electro-magnetic energy.

PELVIC FLOOR
The physiotherapist should make a subjective assessment of pain, awareness of contraction, and bowel and bladder function.

The women should be encouraged to start pelvic floor tightenings as soon as possible following delivery. These done, little and often to begin with, will help to reduce pain and promote healing by producing a pumping action on the local circulation.

It is very important that all women are encouraged to regain muscle strength. Exercises taught should address both type I and type II fibres to recover maximum strength, endurance and power.

The basic exercise: Squeeze and lift as if preventing the escape of flatus and urine. Breathing should be normal and contraction of the adductors, gluteal and unnecessary abdominal muscles should be avoided so that the woman is conscious of the pelvic floor contracting.

To promote endurance (type I fibres) she has to hold the contraction for as long as possible, rest for four seconds and repeat holding to that initial length for up to a maximum of ten contractions.

Type II fibres are activated by doing one second contractions as powerful as possible. This exercise can be done in standing, sitting or lying positions. The mother should be encouraged over the months ahead to increase the strength and length and number of repetitions of the contractions.

At the six-week Postnatal check up, the examining doctor or midwife should check the strength of a contraction during a vaginal examination and emphasise the importance of continuing the pelvic floor exercises.

Some obstetric physiotherapy departments will review identified 'at risk' traumatised pelvic floor after six week postnatal.

ABDOMINAL MUSCLES
Weak abdominal muscles may predispose to lumbo-pelvic instability, leading to back pain. Initial rehabilitation should be to Transversus Abdominus. Progression of abdominal exercises will depend on the degree of diastasis of the rectus muscles. A diastasis greater than 2 cm contraindicates progression as it is thought to cause a shearing effect on the rectus sheath. Any woman presenting with back pain will be assessed and treated.

POST NATAL EXERCISE SESSIONS
Most units offer a short course of exercise to music classes following the six week post natal check. This class gives the physiotherapist the opportunity to reinforce pelvic floor strengthening and general back care whilst providing an overall conditioning programme. These sessions also provide a support group for new mothers.

THE POSTNATAL EXAMINATION

This is usually undertaken at around six weeks by the general practitioner although this function may be delegated by some to midwives and practice nurses. If the pregnancy or delivery has been complicated then review by the obstetrician is valuable.

The functions of the postnatal examination are:
1. To determine that the mother is well and that she has returned to her pre-pregnant state of health.
2. To determine that the baby is well and has not developed any perinatally related problems.
3. To review the pregnancy, if complicated, and discuss the implications of any complications for future pregnancies.
4. To discuss contraceptive requirements.

RETURN OF MENSTRUATION
In lactating women menstruation is suppressed for about three months after which it may return even if breast feeding is continued. If menstruation is occurring, so probably is ovulation. Ovulation may return before menstruation and has been reported as early as 7 weeks.

In the non-lactating women endogenous oestrogen builds up in the endometrium. When it falls irregularly, as it does in the puerperium, the endometrium cannot be maintained and breaks down. This may be reported as continuation of the lochial discharge.

Wide variations in this pattern are met with. On rare occasions, a new pregnancy may be diagnosed at the postnatal visit.

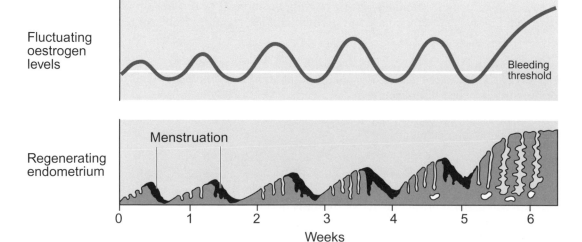

CLINICAL EXAMINATION

The role of vaginal examination at the postnatal visit is limited. In asymptomatic women with no pre-existing abnormality vaginal examination should be carried out only if a cervical smear is required.

A speculum is passed and the cervix examined. An Aylesbury spatula is applied over the transformation zone and smeared onto a glass slide. Fixing solution should be applied immediately.

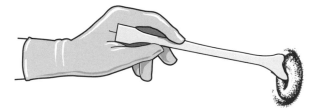

The cervix may show an ectopy in which the squamo-columnar junction of the cervix appears on the ectocervix. This requires no action unless producing symptoms e.g. excessive discharge. Any action (cryocautery, diathermy) should be delayed to allow squamous metaplasia to occur spontaneously.

If an operative vaginal delivery has been undertaken then the episiotomy wound should be checked. Similarly women who are symptomatic, either of dyspareunia or of prolonged vaginal bleeding, should be examined to exclude local abnormalities.

Discharge

Slight discharge is the rule at 6 weeks postpartum. If profuse and irritating, bacteriological specimens must be taken and treatment instituted.

Cervical ectopy

CHAPTER 16

THE NEWBORN BABY

THE NORMAL NEWBORN BABY

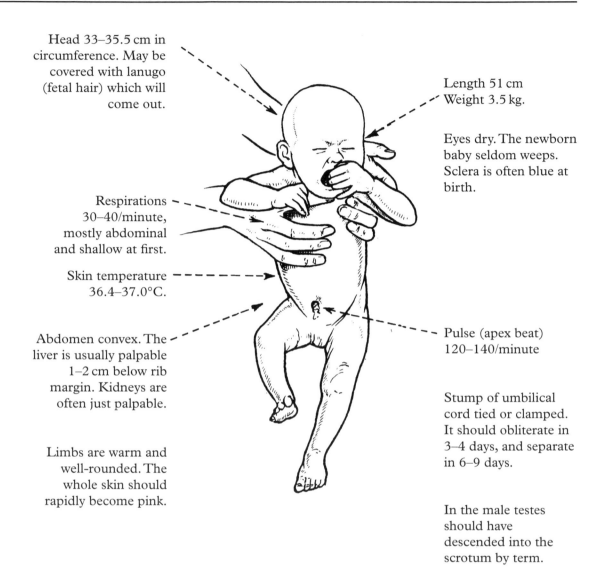

Head 33–35.5 cm in circumference. May be covered with lanugo (fetal hair) which will come out.

Length 51 cm Weight 3.5 kg.

Eyes dry. The newborn baby seldom weeps. Sclera is often blue at birth.

Respirations 30–40/minute, mostly abdominal and shallow at first.

Skin temperature 36.4–37.0°C.

Abdomen convex. The liver is usually palpable 1–2 cm below rib margin. Kidneys are often just palpable.

Pulse (apex beat) 120–140/minute

Limbs are warm and well-rounded. The whole skin should rapidly become pink.

Stump of umbilical cord tied or clamped. It should obliterate in 3–4 days, and separate in 6–9 days.

In the male testes should have descended into the scrotum by term.

The baby is covered in utero with a sebacous secretion called 'vernix caseosa' (L., *a cheese-like coating*). This protects the skin against maceration while in the liquor amnii and has antibacterial properties.

MANAGEMENT OF THE NEWBORN BABY

CLAMPING AND LIGATING THE CORD

The cord is clamped and divided as soon as pulsations have ceased. If ligation is done carelessly, the baby may lose a great deal of blood very quickly. The cord is ligated with a special clamp or rubber bands or tapes. The blood volume of a term newborn infant is 80–100 ml per kg body weight.

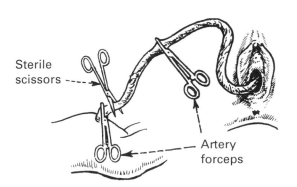

Sterile scissors

Artery forceps

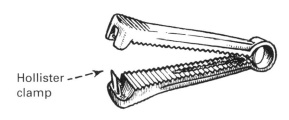

Hollister clamp

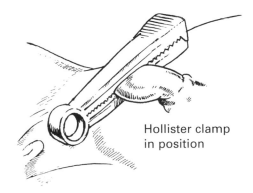

Hollister clamp in position

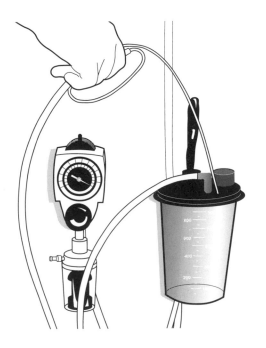

All mucus, blood and meconium must be sucked out of the pharynx before the baby has a chance to inhale them. This should be done using mechanical suction to minimise the risk of virus transmission.

MANAGEMENT OF THE NEWBORN BABY

ASSESSMENT OF THE BABY'S CONDITION AT BIRTH

The Apgar scoring system is universally accepted, and evaluation is made at one minute after birth and again at five minutes. A score above 7 indicates good condition. A score of three or less at one minute indicates the need for active full resuscitation which may include external cardiac massage, intubation and ventilation. A score of six or less at five minutes suggests perinatal asphyxia but is a poor prognostic indicator. Most infants will establish respiration within three minutes of birth.

Sign	0 points	1 point	2 points
Skin colour	Cyanosis pallor	Peripheral cyanosis	Pink
Muscle tone	Flaccid	Moves limbs	Good
Resp. effort	None	Gasps	Good
Heart rate	None	<100	>100
Response to stimulus	None	Slight	Good

NEONATAL APNOEA

There are two sources of stimuli to which the fetal respiratory centre responds, *provided that the period of hypoxia is not prolonged.*

1. Blood gas changes (high CO_2, low O_2 and rising Hydrogen ion concentration) which develop during the second stage and delivery.
2. Sensory stimuli brought about by the change from the warm watery conditions in the uterus to the colder temperature of the outside world in which the fetus is at once touched and handled.

A relatively high negative pressure is required to overcome lung resistance to expansion, but lung compliance increases thereafter, and progressively less effort is needed. The first breath is all-important, and if it does not occur within one minute of delivery a state of apnoea is considered to exist.

DEGREES OF APNOEA
1. Primary Apnoea
Cyanosed, with some muscle tone and a heart beat over 100. Efforts at breathing are made and gasping occurs.

2. Secondary Apnoea
This is sometimes called terminal apnoea because if not soon corrected brain damage or death will follow. The skin is greyish-white, there is no muscle tone and the heart beat is less than 100. There is associated hypotension which is poorly tolerated by the newborn infant.

It is often difficult in practice to decide on the degree of apnoea, especially when drug-induced depression is present.

CAUSES OF APNOEA
Antenatal
Any condition leading to fetal hypoxia, such as placental insufficiency, pre-eclampsia, placental abruption.

Intrapartum
Prolonged hypoxic labour, traumatic delivery, opiate drugs, anaesthesia. (Even epidural anaesthesia if prolonged).

Postnatal
Immaturity, cerebral trauma, congenital abnormalities such as diaphragmatic hernia.

NEONATAL APNOEA

MANAGEMENT OF PRIMARY APNOEA

1. Any liquor, mucus, meconium etc. must be gently sucked out of the nose and mouth. This is unlikely to relieve any obstruction in the airways if one exists, but it often provides sufficient stimulus to make the baby gasp.
2. The baby is gently dried to reduce heat loss by evaporation, and covered with a warm towel.
3. An oxygen mask is held over the face. The object is not to insufflate the lungs, but to enrich any breaths that are taken.

Drugs such as diamorphine, morphine and pethidine, which are commonly used in labour, all cross the placental barrier and cause some degree of respiratory depression and hence asphyxia (an increase in pCO2 and a lowering of the oxygen saturation). Pethidine has been shown to have a more prolonged effect and may retard the development of feeding and other reflexes. If drug depression is suspected, naloxone hydrochloride 40 micrograms in 2 ml should be injected intramuscularly but only once an adequate airway has been established and basic resuscitation commenced.

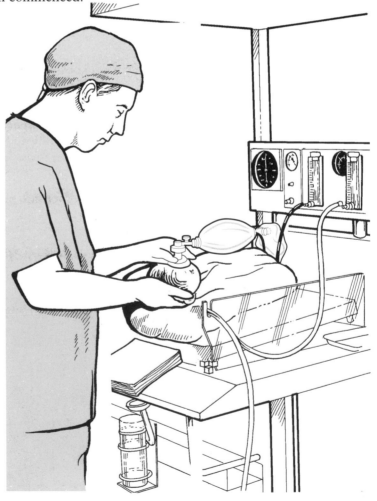

SECONDARY APNOEA

MANAGEMENT OF SECONDARY APNOEA

If the baby is born in this condition, or if there is no response to simple treatment, oxygen must be given by effective bag and mask ventilation in which all obstetricians and midwives should be proficient, or after intubation, with an endotracheal tube.

This technique requires practice and is best done by a paediatrician, but the obstetrician and midwife should have some experience. It is vital to remove any meconium visible in the upper airway and larynx before attempting assisted ventilation.

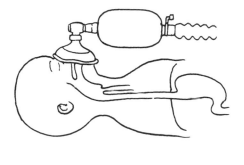

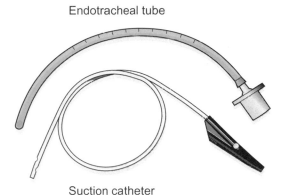

Endotracheal tube

Suction catheter

Bag and Mask Ventilation

A straight **endotracheal tube** is usually used but some centres use tubes with a shoulder near the tip to prevent it being inserted too far. The mucus aspirator also shown is small enough to pass through the catheter.

Straight Bladed Laryngoscope

The neonatal larynx lies opposite C3 and 4. The tip of the laryngoscope catches the epiglottis and pulls it forward to allow clear view of the vocal cords.

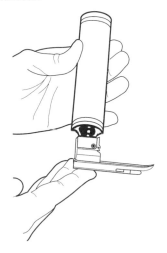

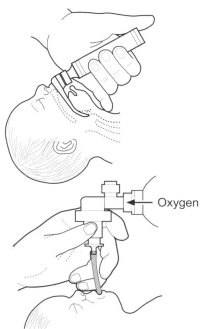

Oxygen

Once the endotracheal tube is inserted, the inflation pressure can be regulated by the bag ventilation. It is usual for the oxygen to pass through a water manometer which 'blows off' above a pressure of 30 cm of water.

APNOEA — RESUSCITATION

This method of giving oxygen is known as intermittent positive pressure ventilation (IPPV) and its administration requires experience. All midwives and obstetricians should have some competence in this technique.

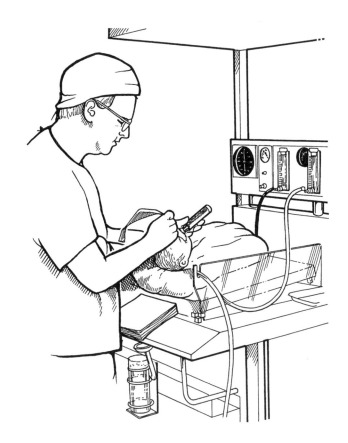

The first sign or recovery is a quickening and strengthening of the fetal heart, followed by attempts at respiration and improved colour. Once the baby is breathing spontaneously consideration should be given to transfer to a special nursery.

It may be necessary to employ IPPV for up to 20 minutes before respiration becomes spontaneous, or death is recognised as inevitable.

OTHER MEASURES

Cardiac Massage
If the heart rate falls below 80, rhythmic compression should be applied over the sternum, at the rate of about 5 compressions to one inflation of the lungs.

Acidosis
This seldom requires correction once adequate ventilation is established, but in cases of severe asphyxia a combination of plasma volume expansion (normal saline or plasma protein solution) and, very occasionally, judicious infusion of a 0.5 molar solution (4.2%) sodium bicarbonate in 10% dextrose (2 ml per kg) may be employed. This may be given via the umbilical vein after insertion of an umbilical catheter.

Hypothermia
An apnoeic baby loses heat very quickly, especially if it is immature and the recommended labour room temperature of 25°C is too low. Local heat must be provided by warm towels and preferably by an overhead radiant heater attached to the resuscitation trolley.

Drugs
Except for Naloxone (Narcan) which reverses the depressive effect of opiates, there is little place for drugs in resuscitation. Occasionally there may be a place for adrenaline (epinephrine) 1:10 000, 1 ml in severe bradycardia or cardiac asystole.

HEAT LOSS IN THE NEWBORN

If the skin temperature falls below 36.5°C the baby loses heat more quickly than it can be produced. As the central (core) temperature falls, the metabolism slows down and hypothermia develops. Pre-term babies with a deficient fat layer, and babies who have had difficult deliveries are particularly exposed to this hazard.

Heat Production

1. Energy from diet.
2. Metabolic activity mainly in the muscles. (Babies have no protective shivering reflex.)
3. Breakdown of fat. Fat in certain areas such as between the shoulder blades and the perirenal capsule (brown fat) can be catabolised very quickly.

Heat Loss from the Skin

1. Radiation.
2. Evaporation from wet skin exposed to air.
3. Convection.
4. Conduction.

Small amounts of heat are lost through respiration and in urine and faeces.

Clinical Features of Hypothermia (cold injury)

This is rare and avoidable.

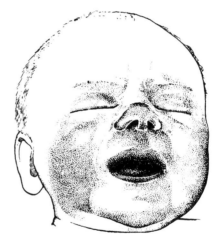

The baby is difficult to rouse, cold to touch, lethargic and unwilling to feed. There is oedema of the hands and feet and eyelids and a hardening of the subcutaneous tissues (sclerema). The redness of cheeks and extremities and the absence of crying give a misleading appearance of healthiness. As the metabolism slows down, the baby becomes hypoglycaemic and death occurs.

Note oedema of face. Shaded areas represent redness and subcutaneous sclerema.

Treatment

Hypothermia is very difficult to reverse, and the only effective treatment is complete prevention.

1. The labour room temperature should be above 25°C.
2. All resuscitative procedures should be carried out under an infra-red heater.
3. The baby should be dried at birth and covered with a dry towel. It must be well wrapped up if it is staying in the ward.
4. If transfer to a Special Care Unit is necessary this must be done in a heated cot. Once in an incubator the paediatrician's object is to maintain the baby's temperature at 37°C, and very small babies may require an ambient temperature as high as 37°C.

INSPECTION FOR CONGENITAL DEFECTS

Certain of the commoner defects should be noted at birth.

Defects of the neural system are commonest. The whole vertebral column must be examined and palpated for evidence of MENINGOCELE.

There may be SUPERNUMERY AURICLES or even absence of an ear.

The face may have features suggesting defects such as DOWN'S SYNDROME or other trisomies.

The mouth must be inspected for CLEFT PALATE and CLEFT LIP.

The anus should be carefully inspected to exclude an IMPERFORATE OR ECTOPIC OPENING.

The Umbilicus may be herniated causing EXOMPHALOS, or there may be an abdominal wall hernia, GASTROSCHISIS. There should be three umbilical vessels, two arteries and one vein.

The feet may show signs of TALIPES. Both hands and feet may have interdigital webbing or supernumary digits.

The external genitals may be abnormal, making it difficult to sex the infant— INTERSEX. In the male there may be a degree of HYPOSPADIAS.

ROUTINE SCREENING TESTS

CONGENITAL DISLOCATION OF THE HIP (CDH)

The term CDH includes various degrees of instability of the hip joint. Ideally diagnosis should be made as early as possible for the best outcome of treatment, but X-rays at this stage may be difficult to interpret because so much of the hip joint is cartilaginous. It is now possible to assess hip dislocation by the use of ultrasound.

In the normal baby the flexed hip joints should be capable of 90 degree abduction with the baby supine.

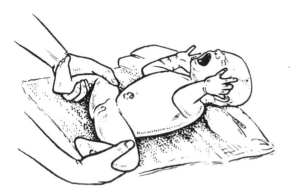

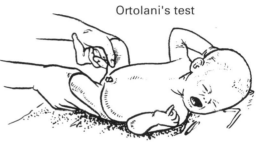

Ortolani's test

Limitation of abduction would be an indication for continued investigation and observation.

The flexed legs are grasped with the forefingers along the outer aspect of the thigh and the thumb along the inner aspect. If the hip is dislocated, abduction will cause a 'clunk' as the femoral head slips into articulation.

ROUTINE SCREENING TESTS

PHENYLKETONURIA (PKU)

PKU is the best known of a numerous but rare group of congenital metabolic disorders, in which the baby inherits an inability to convert the amino-acid phenylalanine (PH) to tyrosine. There are at least three varieties of the disease which is more properly called 'hyperphenylalaninaemia'. 'Classical' PKU (97% of cases) is due to Phenylalanine hydroxylase (PHE) deficiency. This can be completely controlled by diet.

PKU IN THE BABY

Every baby is screened by the Guthrie test which demonstrates abnormal blood levels of PH after feeding is well established (5–10 days).

```
Patient's Name ...........................................
Address ........................................................
Date ...............................................................
Date first feeding ......................................
Bottle ☐      Breast ☐      Both ☐
FILL ALL CIRCLES WITH BLOOD
◯       ◯       ◯       ◯
```

The paper disc impregnated with blood from a heel stab is placed in a bacterial plate of *B. subtilis* in which there is a special inhibitor. If PH is present in abnormal concentration the inhibitor is neutralised and growth of *B. subtilis* occurs.

If the test is positive the baby must be subjected to complex tests to establish the type of PKU.

PKU IN THE MOTHER

Transmission is by a recessive gene and it has been estimated that about 1:50 000 mothers have undiagnosed PKU. The following 'at risk' group should be screened:

1. Mothers with a family history of PKU.
2. Mothers of low intelligence.
3. Mothers who have had infants with microcephaly (this has an association with PKU).

Screening is complicated by the wide diurnal variation in PH levels and several tests are needed.

A woman with PKU should preferably return to a low PH diet before conception or as soon as she is pregnant. Her infant will also require Guthrie test monitoring.

In the common type 1, the diet must be low-phenylalanine for life. Failure to control PKU results in mental retardation and progressive neurological deterioration.

The Guthrie blood test can also be used to exclude HYPOTHYROIDISM, by measurement of thyroxine levels or thyroid stimulating hormone, the latter being more commonly used.

In the future the blood may also be used to screen for other conditions such as cystic fibrosis.

NURSING CARE

MANAGEMENT OF THE NEWBORN BABY

All infants should be given vitamin K (0.5 mg) intramuscularly or orally (1 mg) immediately after birth as protection against haemorrhagic disease of the newborn (HDN).

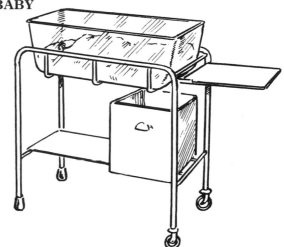

When given orally to breast-fed babies further doses of oral vitamin K will be required during the first month of life. It is particularly important to give vitamin K after birth if the mother is on oral anticonvulsants.

Usually the partner will have been present at birth and the baby is given to the mother and partner to hold as soon as the cord has been cut. If admission to the special care nursery is required, facilities should be provided to allow both parents and other family members to make frequent visits.

Ideally the baby should be offered a period of skin-to-skin contact with the mother, uninterrupted for half an hour. This greatly facilitates breastfeeding.

About 6–8 hours after delivery, traditionally, the baby is bathed and then dressed in a gown and placed in a cot in room temperature between 18° and 20°C.

The ideal cot for the newborn should be draught-proof and easily cleaned. It should be possible to raise and lower the head, and there should be a box for the toilet materials provided separately for each baby.

The importance of 'bonding' between the mother and child is widely recognised. Bonding is encouraged by nursing mother and child in the same room, with the cot alongside the bed so that there may be intimate contact. This facilitates demand feeding by the baby.

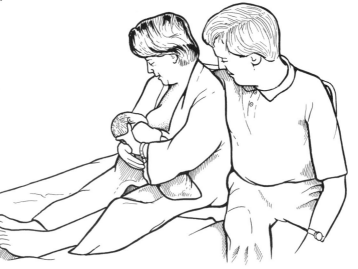

BREAST FEEDING

The infant should be offered the breast as soon as possible after birth. He should be carefully observed during this feed for evidence of inhalation or difficulty with swallowing. If 'mucousy', oesophageal atresia should be excluded by the passage of an orogastric tube. The mother should be comfortable and able to hold a baby in such a way that both are relaxed. A pillow underneath the baby is often helpful.

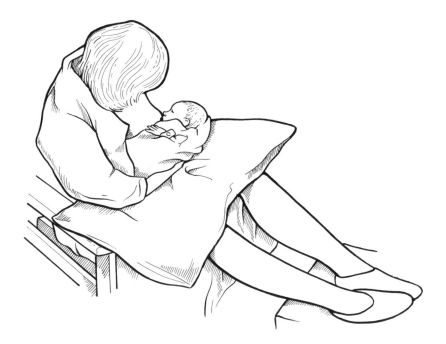

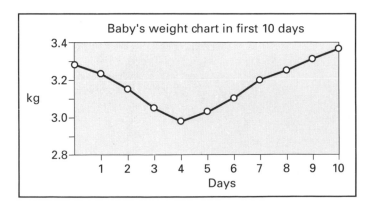

Baby's weight chart in first 10 days

In normal circumstances babies will gain around 30 g per day though there will be initial loss of weight until lactation is established.

PHYSIOLOGY OF THE NEWBORN

PHYSIOLOGICAL JAUNDICE

This occurs in about one third of normal babies between the 2nd and 5th days. It is due mainly to the functional immaturity of the glucuronyl transferase enzyme system in the liver and the shortened life span of fetal red cells. The breakdown of extravasated blood (bruising) and the active enterohepatic circulation may also contribute.

The haemoglobin levels fall from 200 g/l at birth to about 110 g/l by the third month. This level rises again over the next three months.

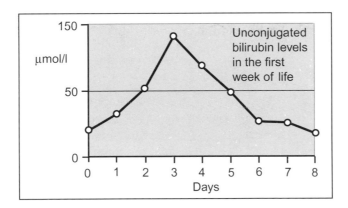

STOOLS

Meconium (mainly cast-off cells, mucus and bile pigment) is passed for the first 2–3 days. It should appear within 36 hours of birth. The bowel is sterile at birth but is colonised by bacteria within a few hours. Formed stools usually appear by the 5th day, normally light in colour and with the odour of faeces.

RESPIRATORY SYSTEM

The fetal lungs are airless and filled with lung fluid and amniotic fluid. The fetus exists at an arterial oxygen pressure of approximately 4.5–5.5 kPa. This changes quickly to adult levels with the establishment of respiration. The rate is up to 40/minute and there may be much irregularity although this usually settles to under 40 per minute eight hours after birth.

URINE

The fetus swallows liquor and the kidneys excrete in utero. Urine should be passed within 2 hours of birth.

GENITAL SYSTEM

Manifestations of oestrogen withdrawal may occur. There is sometimes swelling of the breasts and even a little colostrum secretion ('witches' milk'). The female may bleed a little from the vagina and the male may develop a transient hydrocele. No treatment is required.

PHYSIOLOGY OF THE NEWBORN

CARDIOVASCULAR SYSTEM

With the first breath the lungs expand and the constricted pulmonary vessels relax. The *ductus arteriosus*, which has a very muscular coat, actively contracts and all the right ventricular blood passes to the lungs. This will increase the left atrial pressure while the right atrial pressure is reduced by cessation of placental flow. Blood now tends to flow from left to right through the *foramen ovale* and this will cause its closure.

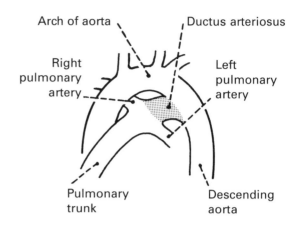

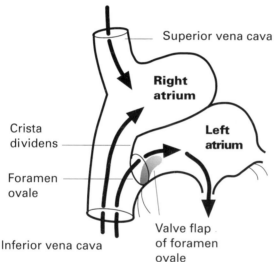

The *ductus arteriosus* closes functionally almost at once and is obliterated by the 6th week. The *foramen ovale* closes gradually and may take months, but is functionally closed once the left atrial pressure is greater than the right.

Following the clamping of the cord the *umbilical arteries* thrombose and persist as the obliterated hypogastric arteries. The *umbilical vein* obliterates by the 4–6th day and persists as the ligamentum teres of the liver. The *ductus venosus* obliterates a little later and persists as the ligamentum venosum.

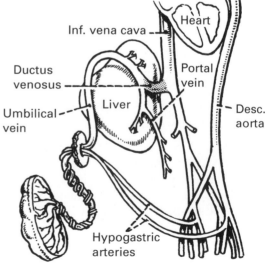

ROUTINE OBSERVATIONS

Baby charts must be kept in meticulous detail. A baby's condition can deteriorate very quickly.

WEIGHT: Usually falls in first 3–4 days, even with artificial feeding. Birthweight should be regained within 10 days.

TEMPERATURE: About 36.7°C but some minor instability is usual in the first week.

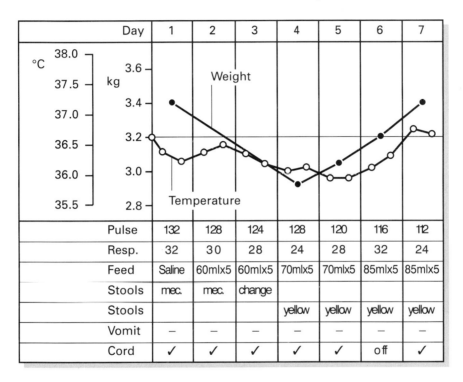

Day	1	2	3	4	5	6	7
Pulse	132	128	124	128	120	116	112
Resp.	32	30	28	24	28	32	24
Feed	Saline	60mlx5	60mlx5	70mlx5	70mlx5	85mlx5	85mlx5
Stools	mec.	mec.	change				
Stools				yellow	yellow	yellow	yellow
Vomit	–	–	–	–	–	–	–
Cord	✓	✓	✓	✓	✓	off	✓

PULSE: Is taken by auscultating the apex beat. It is usually 120–150/minute.

RESPIRATION: About 40 per minute at first and becoming slower. Irregularity is common in the first week of life.

FEEDS: Babies should be offered the breast while in the labour ward. Artificially fed babies should be fed at around 6 hours of age, unless growth restricted, when they should be fed as early as possible.

STOOLS: Meconium should give way to normal, formed stools by the 4th day. They should be yellow with a faecal odour, and may be more or less frequent in breast-fed babies.

VOMIT: Vomiting is a non-specific sign in infants. It should alert staff to the possibility of other illness such as infection. Bile-stained vomiting is a danger sign and may indicate a bowel obstruction. It must **always** be investigated.

RELUCTANCE TO FEED: Infants who are reluctant to feed should be carefully observed to detect any signs of significant illness e.g. infection, hypoglycaemia etc.

LOW BIRTHWEIGHT BABIES

THE LOW BIRTHWEIGHT BABY

This means a baby weighing 2.5 kg or less, at birth. The cause can be either preterm labour or failure to thrive in utero — intra-uterine growth restriction. A baby can be both preterm and growth-restricted.

THE PRETERM BABY

A baby born before the 37th week. It is possible for such a baby to weigh more than 2.5 kg but it is still disadvantaged by its immaturity.

THE SMALL-FOR-DATES BABY

A baby whose birthweight is below the tenth percentile for its gestational age (see Chapter 6). Such a baby is almost always less than 2.5 kg, and the prognosis depends on the cause of the failure to thrive.

Although identification and treatment of these babies requires paediatric skills, their diagnosis is of extreme importance to the obstetrician. The skin of the growth-restricted baby tends to be dry and even wrinkled. The umbilical cord may be thin with little Wharton's jelly. The growth-restricted baby is usually alert and active while the preterm baby is more likely to be hypotonic.

GROWTH-RESTRICTION may be divided into *asymmetrical* and *symmetrical* forms (see Chapter 6). Infants who have asymmetrical growth-restriction have usually experienced short term growth failure. They usually exhibit rapid catch-up of growth after birth.

Infants with symmetrical growth-restriction may have had growth failure over a much longer period e.g. due to chromosomal or genetic causes or prenatal infection. These babies are more likely to remain small children.

Complications of low birthweight	
Pre-term	**Growth-restricted**
Hypothermia	Intrapartum asphyxia
Hypoglycaemia	Hypothermia
Respiratory distress syndrome	Hypoglycaemia
Jaundice	Hypocalcaemia
Infection	Meconium aspiration
Cerebral haemorrhage	
Pulmonary haemorrhage	

ESTIMATION OF GESTATIONAL AGE

Estimating the gestational age of the newborn can be as difficult as estimating the maturity during pregnancy. The weight is unreliable — the baby can be light, heavy or 'appropriate for dates' — and the method of evaluation used by the paediatrician is based on the system of Dubowitz et al (*J. Pediat.* 1970,77,1).

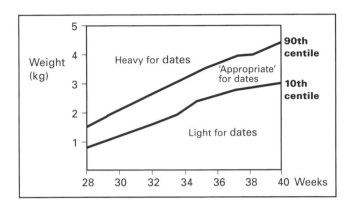

EXTERNAL CRITERIA

There are ten external signs each with a varying score. Examples:

EXTERNAL SIGN	SCORE				
	0	1	2	3	4
1 Oedema	Obvious oedema hands and feet.	No obvious oedema hands and feet.	No oedema.		
2 Lanugo	No lanugo.	Abundant; long and thick over whole back.	Hair thinning especially over lower back.	Small amount of lanugo and bald areas	At least half of back devoid of lanugo.
3 Ear firmness	Pinna soft, easily folded, no recoil.	Pinna soft, easily folded, slow recoil.	Cartilage to edge of pinna, but soft in places, ready recoil	Pinna firm, cartilage to edge, instant recoil.	

NEUROLOGICAL CRITERIA

There are ten tests of posture and reflex, each with a varying score. They depend on the infant's state of alertness and freedom from asphyxia.

NEUROLOGICAL SIGN	SCORE					
	0	1	2	3	4	5
1 Posture						
2 Head lag						
3 Ventral suspension						

The maximum score is 70, and the gestational age can be calculated from a table. A mature baby (over 37 weeks) should score 45.

IDIOPATHIC RESPIRATORY DISTRESS SYNDROME (IRDS)

IRDS, sometimes known as pulmonary surfactant deficiency disease, is one of the commonest causes of neonatal mortality. The management of affected babies is in the hands of paediatricians, but the prevention of IRDS and a reduction of its severity is largely the responsibility of the obstetrician.

Definition

Respiratory rate
    > 60/minute
Indrawing of sternum
Expiratory grunting

Developing within 4 hours of birth and persisting for at least 24 hours.

Cause

A deficiency of surfactant in the alveoli.

Surfactant is a mixture of lipids (mainly a lecithin, dipalmitoyl phosphatidylcholine) which is continuously secreted by type II pneumocytes in the alveolar wall. It forms a monolayer over the watery surface of the alveolus and so lowers the surface tension, making the lung easier to expand. During respiration it is believed that the surfactant solidifies under pressure, and 'like an archway of bricks' splints the alveolus and prevents atelectasis.

Pathology

Immature or damaged lungs do not secrete enough surfactant so that more force is needed to expand them than the baby possesses. The lungs become atelectatic, and the alveoli are lined with a fibrinous exudate called hyaline membrane.

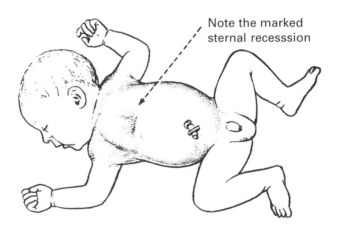

Note the marked sternal recesssion

Clinical Features

As tachypnoea develops, the increased respiratory effort is marked by the indrawing of the chest wall. The baby begins to grunt during expiration as air is forced through partly closed glottis in an attempt to keep the alveoli open for as long as possible.

Atelectasis and hypoxia lead to pulmonary vasoconstriction and cyanosis appears, which is aggravated by a right to left shunt through the foramen ovale and the ductus arteriosus. The CO_2 tension rises, the oxygen saturation falls and hypoglycaemia and hypocalcaemia develop. Hypoproteinaemic oedema which is usually present in immature babies is increased.

IDIOPATHIC RESPIRATORY DISTRESS SYNDROME (IRDS)

Predisposing Factors
1. Immaturity
   Surfactant is first produced at about 22 weeks and rises sharply to a mature level between 34 and 36 weeks.
2. Acute intrapartum hypoxia
   (Chronic hypoxia as in pre-eclampsia and non-lethal placental infarction, appears to stimulate surfactant secretion, possibly as a response to stress).
3. Postpartum hypoxia as when the baby is born in a shocked condition.

Differential Diagnosis
1. Transient tachypnoea of newborn ('Wet lung')
   This is a generally mild condition occurring in mature babies.
2. Meconium Aspiration
   Meconium will have been observed at delivery, and aspirated from the baby's pharynx and trachea.
3. Pneumonia
   Occurs after prolonged rupture of the membranes and as a consequence of Group B Streptococcal infection.
4. Cardiac abnormalities
5. Diaphragmatic hernia
   The heart is displaced to one side, usually the right, and the abdomen is scaphoid. A chest X-ray will give the diagnosis.

Prevention
1. The avoidance, as far as possible, of pre-term labour (see Chapter 10).
2. Administration of glucocorticoids to mothers at risk of/in premature labour, to stimulate surfactant secretion.
3. Monitoring in labour; avoidance of hypoxia; effective and immediate resuscitation; avoidance of hypothermia and the prophylactic use of surfactant replacement therapy after birth.

IDIOPATHIC RESPIRATORY DISTRESS SYNDROME (IRDS)

Treatment

This is undertaken in a special care baby unit (SCBU) and demands considerable paediatric skill. The principals are:

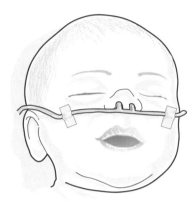

1. Avoid unnecessary handling.
2. Avoid heat loss. A naked immature baby must be nursed at 36°C.
3. Provide a higher concentration of oxygen. The ordinary incubator cannot maintain a concentration above 30% and a headbox or nasal cannula may be required. If there is no improvement continuous positive airways pressure (CPAP) must be provided. This means the passage of oxygen to the lungs under pressure, usually by nasal catheter. The principal risk of CPAP is pneumothorax. Infants deteriorating will require intermittent positive pressure ventilation (IPPV).
4. Correction of acidosis
   Usually this can be corrected by blood volume expansion (either plasma protein solution, saline or fresh frozen plasma) and adequate ventilation. Very occasionally small volumes of 0.5 molar sodium bicarbonate may be used.
5. Maintenance of blood pressure using volume expanders or inotropes.
6. Replacement of surfactant. Either natural or artificial compounds are available.
7. Occasionally sophisticated ventilation techniques such as high frequency oscillation (HFO) or liquid ventilation may be necessary. Rarely, in more mature infants, extra corporeal membrane oxygenation (ECMO) may be used.

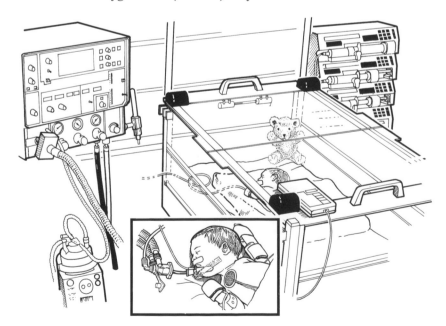

JAUNDICE OF THE NEWBORN

Jaundice is quite common in mature infants (physiological jaundice), especially when breast-feeding is initiated, and it is almost the rule in immature infants. Excessively high concentrations of unconjugated (fat soluble) bilirubin can cause damage to the brain particularly in immature babies.

PHYSIOLOGY
Unconjugated bilirubin which comes from the breakdown of haemoglobin is either:

CONJUGATED in the liver .... or .... DECOMPOSED in the skin
by blue light (photodecomposition)

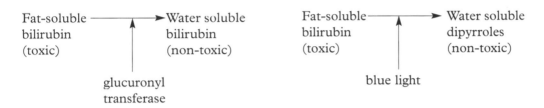

Fat-soluble ⟶ Water soluble   Fat-soluble ⟶ Water soluble
bilirubin   bilirubin   bilirubin   dipyrroles
(toxic)   (non-toxic)   (toxic)   (non-toxic)

glucuronyl   blue light
transferase

Jaundice develops if the liver function is inadequate. It is non-obstructive in type — much the commonest. If excretion from the liver is impaired, the jaundice is obstructive — not common.

CAUSES OF NON-OBSTRUCTIVE JAUNDICE
1. Immaturity.
2. Intrapartum hypoxia.
3. ABO or Rh incompatibility (Haemolysis — intravascular).
4. Extravasated blood from bruising (Haemolysis — extravascular).
5. Infection.

There are many other uncommon conditions which give rise to jaundice, outwith the responsibility of the obstetrician.

INVESTIGATIONS
The ABO and Rhesus groups of mother and infant should be determined together with the Coombs' test. The baby's full blood count should be determined and serial estimations of the level of unconjugated bilirubin are required.

JAUNDICE OF THE NEWBORN

TREATMENT

1. Prevention, as far as possible, of prematurity.
2. Adequate fluid intake.
3. Phototherapy — an artificial blue light source of fluorescent tubes is used to encourage photodecomposition. Its use is dependent on the infant's gestation and postnatal age and is given when the infant's serum bilirubin rises above predetermined levels (see chart). The eyes must be protected during exposure.
4. Exchange transfusion may be necessary if there is no response to phototherapy.

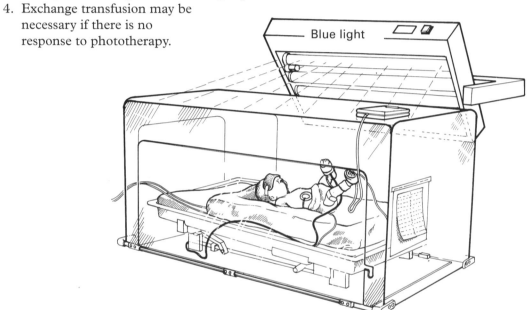

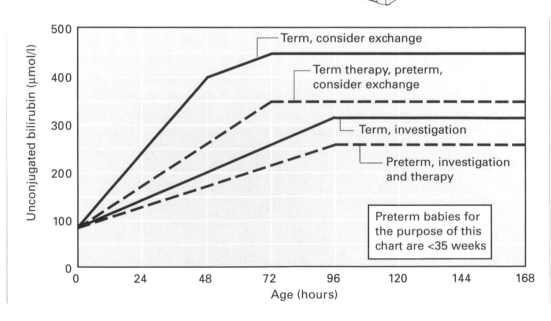

INTRACRANIAL HAEMORRHAGE

This is often lethal and surviving infants are often brain damaged. It can occur in the ventricles, in the substance of the brain, in the subdural space, or as a consequence of a tear of the dura mater.

SUBEPENDYMAL/ INTRAVENTRICULAR HAEMORRHAGE

Bleeding starts in the subependymal vessels in the wall of the lateral ventricle. The bleeding can stop at this stage or progress either into the substance of the brain or into the whole of the ventricular system. The severity of the haemorrhages are graded depending on whether the bleeding extends into the cerebral tissue.

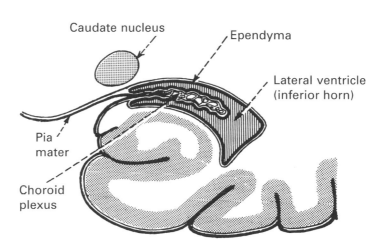

Clinical Features

It occurs most commonly in pre-term infants, usually within the first three days of life. The infant may become limp and unresponsive, and within 12 hours cyanotic attacks and seizures may occur. As the haemorrhage proceeds, the infant becomes comatose and death may occur or hydrocephalus develop. The condition is now readily recognised by cranial ultrasound and progress can be evaluated.

Aetiology

The cause is unknown but there are many associated factors.

Obstetrical	Paediatric
Immaturity	Immaturity
Hypoxia in labour	Hypoxia and hypercapnia
Chronic hypoxia in pregnancy	arising from IRDS
Birth trauma	Coagulation defects

Treatment

There is no specific treatment, and protection of the fetus and neonate from periods of hypoxia offers the best means of protection.

INTRACRANIAL HAEMORRHAGE

INTRACEREBRAL HAEMORRHAGE
Intracerebral haemorrhage is usually a consequence of hypoxic damage with subsequent haemorrhage from damaged blood vessels (see above). This will commonly cause significant long-term complications.

SUBDURAL HAEMORRHAGE
This is a rare condition in modern obstetric practice. It is liable to complicate any cranial injury, leading to haemorrhage over the cerebral convexity and to haematoma formation. Some localising signs may appear but the diagnosis is difficult, and the condition must always be borne in mind if cranial injury is suspected.

TEARS OF THE DURA MATER
This injury is a consequence of excessive moulding and may occur in prolonged, unsupervised labours.

The fetal brain is protected against damage in labour by:
1. Softness and moulding of membranous bones.
2. Ability of fontanelles to 'give' slightly on pressure.
3. Cushioning effect of cerebrospinal fluid.
4. Anatomical arrangement of dural septa with their free edges.
5. Plasticity of brain tissue.

Sometimes however distortion is excessive and a tear of the free edge of the tentorium cerebelli occurs involving blood vessels. Death occurs from increased intracranial pressure, especially on the brain stem and medulla.

TENTORIAL TEAR
This lesion is associated with difficult deliveries such as high forceps or breech, but can occur after spontaneous vertex delivery. The signs and symptoms are those of asphyxia and definite diagnosis is made only at post-mortem examination.

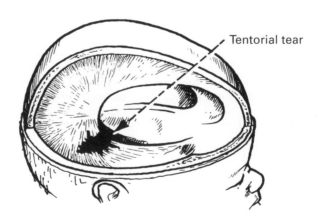

Tentorial tear

BIRTH INJURIES

FRACTURE OF LONG BONES

The bones most commonly broken are the clavicle, humerus and femur as a result of too forcible delivery. In the case of the clavicle there may be no signs at all and callus is felt 2 weeks later. In the case of the long bones the Moro reflex will be absent in that limb and X-ray will be required. In healthy infants callus formation is rapid and splinting is not needed.

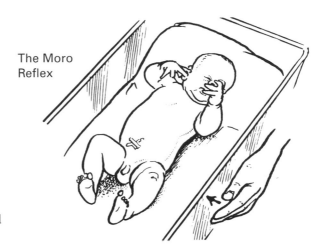

The Moro Reflex

The Moro Reflex — in response to a sudden noise or vibration, the arms and legs are extended and then approach each other with slight shaking movements.

DAMAGE TO THE BRACHIAL PLEXUS

This is caused by excessive lateral flexion of the neck during vertex or breech delivery.

1. Erb's Palsy

C5, 6. This is the commonest. Abductors and flexors of the upper arm are affected, and the arm hangs in the characteristic 'waiter's tip' position.

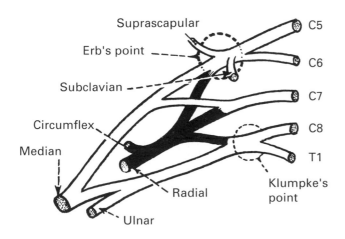

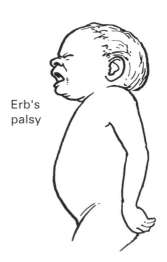

Erb's palsy

2. Klumpke's Paralysis

C8, T1 is rare. The hand is paralysed with wrist drop and absence of grasp reflex.

Most degrees of injury may be left untreated but gentle physiotherapy is essential to prevent stiffness and delayed recovery. Severe injury should be reviewed by an orthopaedic specialist.

381

BIRTH INJURIES

DEPRESSION FRACTURE OF THE SKULL

This may occasionally be caused by the tip of the forceps blade in a difficult delivery. Usually no treatment is necessary but if cerebral irritation or paresis is observed, surgical intervention may be required.

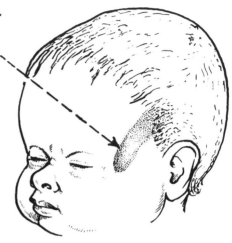

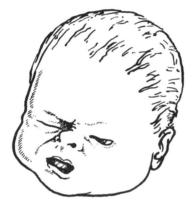

FACIAL PALSY

Paralysis of the facial nerve caused by pressure from the forceps made on the nerve as it emerges from the stylomastoid foramen. Recovery occurs in a matter of days, and any delay is an indication for further investigation.

STERNOMASTOID TUMOUR

A painless lump in the sternomastoid muscle, appearing in the first week of life. It has traditionally been attributed to trauma, but its aetiology is unknown. Torticollis is an occasional sequel, and the mother should be instructed to put the muscle on the stretch for 3 or 4 periods a day. This exercise may, at first, be painful to the baby.

The advice of a physiotherapist is helpful.

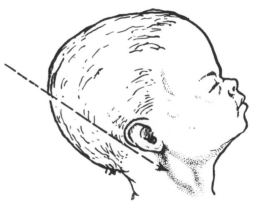

BIRTH INJURIES

SUPERFICIAL HEAD INJURIES

Minor abrasions may be sustained during forceps delivery or from the use of the vacuum extractor. They need only local treatment as a rule but dense connective tissue prevents vessel retraction and scalp wounds bleed freely.

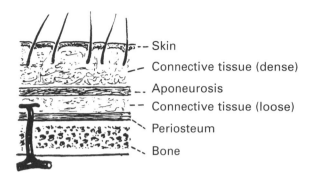

- Skin
- Connective tissue (dense)
- Aponeurosis
- Connective tissue (loose)
- Periosteum
- Bone

CAPUT SUCCEDANEUM

('Substitute Head'). This is a normal occurrence caused by pressure of the cervix interrupting venous and lymphatic scalp drainage during labour. A serous effusion collects in the subcutaneous tissue of the scalp and disappears a few hours after birth.

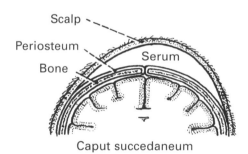

Caput succedaneum

SUBAPONEUROTIC HAEMORRHAGE

This can be extensive, spreading over the whole vault and resulting in anaemia and hypovolaemia.

CEPHALHAEMATOMA

Is a collection of blood between periosteum and skull bone which is limited by the periosteal attachments at the suture lines. It is due to trauma and may not appear until several hours after birth. It should not be aspirated or drained and will normally be absorbed within a few weeks.

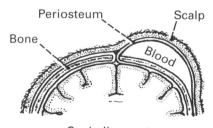

Cephalhaematoma

383

CONGENITAL DEFECTS

Many common defects are of unknown aetiology. Others can be explained by one of four mechanisms:

1. Hereditary genetic defects.
2. Chromosomal aberrations which may be familial.
3. Multifactorial disorders (familial diseases).
4. Incidental defects due to environmental or other factors.

Genetic counselling can be useful in all of these situations, even if only to reassure parents that a given defect is not familial. The need for such counselling sometimes arises during early pregnancy but usually is sought after the birth of an affected child. Evaluation of the risks and possibility often requires the expertise of a medical geneticist but the obstetrician and general practitioner should be able to advise in straightforward cases (see Chapter 5).

A. HEREDITARY GENETIC DEFECTS

Genes lie in specific location on paired chromosomes and a pair of such genes is known as a pair of alleles. If the alleles are identical the individual is homozygous.

1. Autosomal Dominant Disorders

The presence of one such abnormal gene will over-ride the influence of a normal gene on the opposite chromosome and the disease will always be apparent. The individual is therefore usually heterozygous for the abnormal gene. 50% of offspring will be affected.

Examples: Achondroplasia, osteogenesis imperfecta, congenital spherocytosis, sickle cell anaemia and Huntington's chorea.

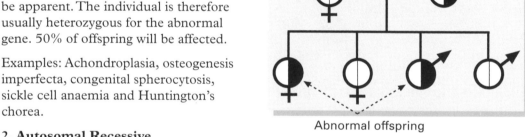

2. Autosomal Recessive Disorders

If only one allele of a pair of genes is abnormal and recessive its influence will be overcome by the normal gene on the opposite chromosome. Only if both genes are abnormal will the disease manifest itself. In a family both parents will require to be carriers and possess such a gene, i.e. both heterozygous before the disease can be transmitted.

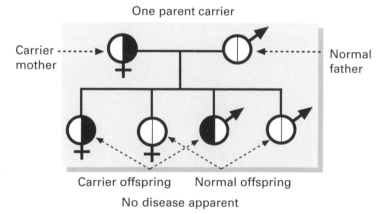

CONGENITAL DEFECTS

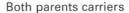

Both parents carriers

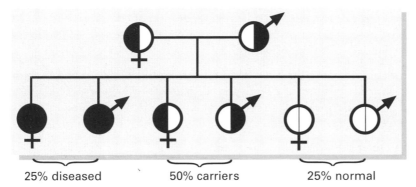

25% diseased   50% carriers   25% normal

Examples of autosomal recessive disorders: Most inborn errors of metabolism. These are numerous and affect various metabolic pathways. Their importance lies in the fact that if the defect is diagnosed early, the subsequent disease process may be prevented in some, but not all, by dietary means. This applies particularly to those genetic defects affecting carbohydrate and amino acid metabolism e.g. phenylketonuria. It does not however apply to the numerically most important member of this group — cystic fibrosis. The carrier rate for this condition in the UK approaches 1 in 20.

3. Sex-linked Recessive Disease

This is a special situation where the abnormal recessive gene is linked to one sex chromosome, usually the X chromosome.

In the female the influence of the abnormal recessive gene on one X chromosome is counteracted by the normal more dominant gene on the second X chromosome. The female is therefore a carrier of the disease but not affected by it. The male possessing the abnormal recessive gene on his single X chromosome is affected since there is no opposition to its action. The family situation is shown in the diagram below. 50% of female offspring will be carriers and 50% of males will show the disease.

Examples: Duchenne muscular dystrophy, haemophilia.

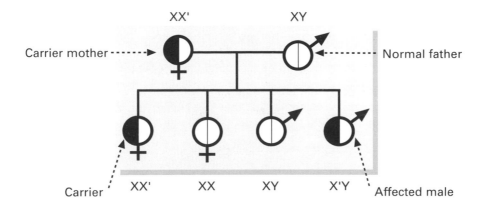

385

CONGENITAL DEFECTS

B. CHROMOSOMAL ABNORMALITIES

These are due to abnormalities arising during the maturation of the oocyte or sperm i.e. at meiosis. Errors at this time can cause unequal separation of the chromosomes resulting in germ cells which possess fewer or more chromosomes than normal. At fertilisation this abnormality is handed on to the offspring.

The commonest abnormality the obstetrician meets with is Down's syndrome due to an extra chromosome 21 (trisomy at 21). Diagnosis is made by karyotyping a culture of fetal cells obtained at amniocentesis or direct examination of tissue obtained by chorion villus sampling (see Chapter 6). The incidence of trisomy 21 increases with maternal age.

In 5% of cases Down's syndrome is due to an inherited chromosomal translocation and in all cases the parents should be examined for the defect.

Other examples of chromosomal abnormalities are Trisomies 18 and 13 and Turner's syndrome and Klinefelter's syndrome, both of which are defects of the sex chromosome.

Maternal age	Risk of trisomy-21
20–24	1 in 1 500
25–29	1 in 1 200
30–34	1 in 900
35	1 in 250
38	1 in 125
40	1 in 80
45	1 in 22

C. MULTIFACTORIAL DISORDERS (FAMILIAL DISEASES)

This concept is used to describe a number of relatively common disorders which have a definite familial tendency. The disorder results from the combination of an abnormal gene or genes and the effect of embryonic and fetal environment. The risks of recurrence have been calculated on the basis of experience and are only approximate.

Condition	Chance of second affected child
Neural tube defect / Anencephaly	1 in 20
Cleft palate	1 in 25
Congenital heart disease	1 in 30
Diabetes mellitus	1 in 12
Epilepsy	1 in 20

D. DEFECTS DUE TO ENVIRONMENTAL OR OTHER FACTORS

These are abnormalities which arise in individual pregnancies. Causes, such as infections during pregnancy or drugs given to the mother, can be recognised in some cases. In these instances parents can be assured that the defect is not familial. In others, although the aetiology is unknown there does seem to be a familial factor operating as noted above.

The obstetrician and midwife should have some knowledge of the prognosis for the commoner abnormalities seen at birth, so that they can answer the mother's questions and initiate treatment when necessary.

CONGENITAL DEFECTS

NEURAL TUBE DEFECTS

Most of these lesions can be detected antenatally by maternal serum AFP/HCG screening and ultrasound or by routine anomaly scanning (see Chapter 6).

The occurrence of neural tube defects has been linked with folic acid deficiency and the periconceptional administration of folic acid supplements is now recommended routinely (see Chapter 5).

Spina Bifida

This means the failure of fusion of the vertebral arches and of the development of the posterior dura mater. This leads to herniation of meninges and spinal cord through the bony gap and it occurs most commonly in the lumbo-sacral region.

Meningocele

The herniation of the pia-arachnoid may be covered by skin. Prognosis should be guarded until it is known for certain that neural tissue is not involved. Surgical closure will usually allow the child to develop normally.

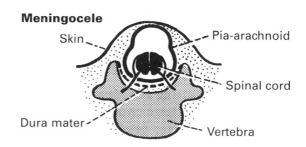

Meningocele

Skin — Pia-arachnoid

Spinal cord

Dura mater — Vertebra

Meningomyelocele/Myelocele

The cord is displaced as well as the membranes and neural epithelium forms the fundus of the sac. Skin cover is incomplete and infection likely unless closure is done within 24 hours. Paralysis of legs, bowel and bladder, and hydrocephaly, are normally present. An immediate surgical opinion should be sought to advise on the possibility of repair.

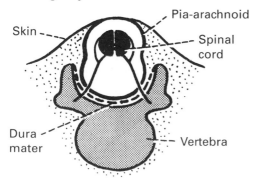

Meningomyelocele

Skin — Pia-arachnoid

Spinal cord

Dura mater — Vertebra

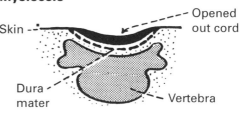

Myelocele

Skin — Opened out cord

Dura mater — Vertebra

The internal surface of the cord is exposed

CONGENITAL DEFECTS

Anencephaly

Anencephaly is the failure of proper development of the cranium and scalp. The face and base of the skull are present. It is usually diagnosed early in pregnancy and termination is offered as the condition is incompatible with life. Should the pregnancy proceed there is usually polyhydramnios, attributed to the inability of the fetus to swallow, the absence of fetal anti-diuretic hormone, and the secretions of the exposed choroid plexus and meninges. Anencephalic pregnancy without hydramnios may be very prolonged and this has been attributed to the absence of the fetal pituitary with its oxytocic hormone.

In labour the face is often the presenting part and shoulder dystocia is on occasion experienced.

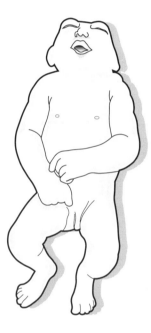

CONGENITAL DEFECTS

HYDROCEPHALUS

Hydrocephalus is distension of the brain and skull due to increased pressure in the ventricles.

Physiopathology

CSF is secreted by specialised arterial plexuses called choroid plexuses mainly into the lateral ventricles. It passes thence to the IIIrd and IVth ventricles and through the median and lateral foramina of the IVth ventricle into the subarachnoid space. It is absorbed into the venous sinuses of the dura mater through protrusions of arachnoid called arachnoid granulations or villi (Pacchionian bodies).

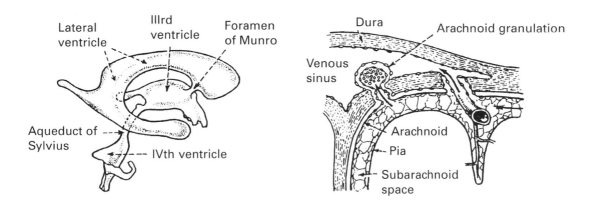

If the flow of CSF is obstructed, the pressure in the ventricles will gradually increase and the fetal head enlarges to such a size that delivery may be impossible without surgical interference.

Causes of Obstruction

Blockage of the narrow connecting points between ventricles, or of the IVth ventricle foramina leading out to the subarachnoid space. Such blockage might be due to congenital abnormality, infection, or trauma, and as the CSF is confined to the ventricles it is known as an internal or non-communicating hydrocephalus.

Interference with the absorption of CSF due to an obstruction in the meninges or a venous sinus thrombosis in the dura mater. This can be congenital or infective, or traumatic in origin, and is known as an external or communicating hydrocephalus.

These distinctions principally concern the paediatrician who may be able to relieve the pressure in non-communicating hydrocephalus, but the obstetrician should be aware of the possibilities in mild cases. About 40% of cases of infant hydrocephalus are said to arrest spontaneously.

Well developed cases are easily diagnosed by palpation or ultrasound, but mild degrees of hydrocephalus are very difficult to identify with certainty. If there is doubt, delivery should be by section even although there is a high chance of associated neural tube defect. When the diagnosis is definite the operation of craniotomy may be employed (see Chapter 14).

CONGENITAL DEFECTS

CARDIAC LESIONS

Congenital heart lesions are second only to neural tube defects in frequency. Their aetiology is often uncertain but some environmental factors operating in early pregnancy, such as rubella infection, heavy alcohol consumption and maternal diabetes, are recognised. Cardiac lesions are also commonly associated with trisomies 21, 18 and 13 and Turner's syndrome (45XO).

Great advances have been made in recent years in both the diagnosis and treatment of congenital heart lesions. Fetal echocardiography in pregnancy may be offered in high-risk cases and routine ultrasound anomaly scanning has significantly increased the rate of antenatal recognition (see Chapter 6). The development of neonatal echocardiography and the use of Doppler ultrasound allow detailed assessment of the newborn. Improved treatment is available both from conventional surgery and new techniques in interventional cardiology.

Congenital heart lesions may be divided as follows.

Cyanotic
Transposition of the great arteries.
Tetralogy of Fallot.
Total anomalous pulmonary venous drainage.
Others.

Acyanotic
Septal defects.
Patent ductus arteriosus.
Coarctation of the aorta.
Pulmonary/aortic stenosis.
Hypoplastic left heart syndrome.

The clinical presentation of these conditions is often unclear but the following are indications for urgent paediatric opinion:

1. Respiratory difficulty — tachypnoea and tachycardia are present together with other evidence of cardiac failure.
2. Cyanosis
3. Rapidly developing 'shock'.
4. Murmur detected.

CONGENITAL DEFECTS

CLEFT LIP AND PALATE

These lesions occur in approximately 1 in 600 births and there is a family history in 10% of cases. The lip or palate may be affected separately but often both are involved.

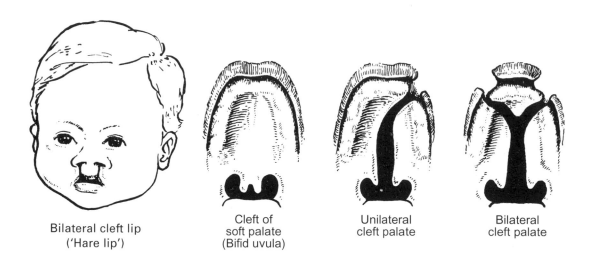

Bilateral cleft lip
('Hare lip')

Cleft of
soft palate
(Bifid uvula)

Unilateral
cleft palate

Bilateral
cleft palate

Breast feeding is usually possible but some infants may require specialised care such as Hoberman teats or spoon feeding. On rarer occasions nasogastric feeding may be necessary if sucking is weak. The cleft should be kept clean after feeds.

Occasionally orthodontists may fashion a 'false' palate.

The parents should be told that a good cosmetic result can usually be obtained when the lip is repaired at about 4 months. The repair of the palate is carried out later and the child will usually speak normally. A specialised team including surgeons, orthodontist, speech therapist and nurses is essential to achieve best results. Long-term support is necessary.

CONGENITAL DEFECTS

GASTRO-INTESTINAL TRACT
Oesophageal atresia with Tracheo-oesophageal fistula

The upper segment usually ends blindly at the level of T3–4 and the distance from the blind end to the anterior alveolar margin is 10 cm.

The condition should be suspected antenatally in cases of unexplained polyhydramnios. In the neonate attempts at feeding lead to choking and cyanosis and there may be 'frothing' — excess of unswallowed mucus. If a sterile, lubricated firm catheter is arrested 10–12 cm from the alveolar margin, the diagnosis is almost certain. Suction should be continued and a paediatrician notified.

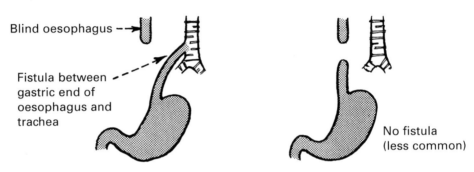

Imperforate Anus

There is a wide variety of congenital ano-rectal abnormalities and a relieving colostomy may be an emergency measure. The passage of faeces must be noted: but fistula is often present and the observer may be confused by small amounts of faeces passed per urethram or per vaginam.

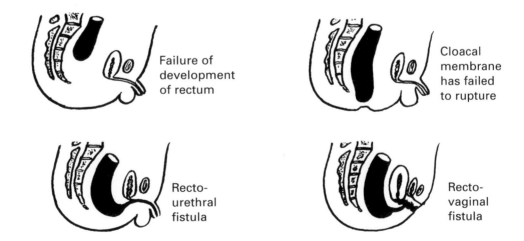

CONGENITAL DEFECTS

ABDOMINAL WALL DEFECTS

These may be suspected antenatally by an elevated maternal serum AFP level. Ultrasound scanning, following this result or as part of a routine anomaly scan, will demonstrate the lesion and allow treatment to be planned after delivery.

In *exomphalos* some of the abdominal viscera lie within the umbilical cord and there is incomplete development of the abdominal wall. The sac is a thin jelly-like membrane (the root of the cord) and the vessels of the cord run over the sac. The type of repair depends on the size of the defect but prior to operation the sac should be kept moist and 'cling film' is a useful first aid wrapping and prevents heat loss.

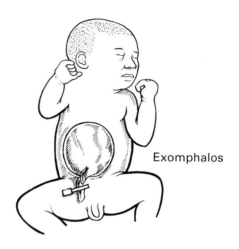

Exomphalos

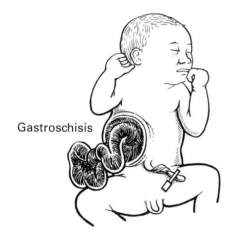

Gastroschisis

The term *gastroschisis* describes the presence of an abdominal wall defect, separate from the cord, with herniation of some or all of the abdominal organs. Again the gut should be wrapped in cling film or moist swabs and surgical advice sought urgently. Surgical treatment is usually very successful and this condition is less often associated with other abnormalities than exomphalos.

CONGENITAL DEFECTS

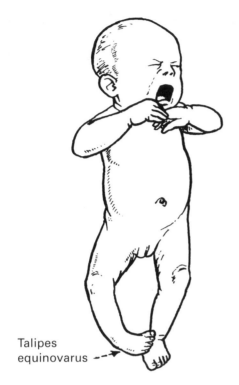

Talipes
equinovarus

TALIPES (CLUB FOOT)

In true club foot there is always some resistance to complete passive correction. Treatment begins at birth in order to minimise the adaptive distortion of soft tissues and tarsal bones. The mother is taught to stretch and correct the deformity regularly and the baby must be referred at once to a paediatric surgeon. Operation is now seldom required but prolonged splinting is usual.

ACCESSORY DIGITS

Small tags of flesh are common and can be removed by ligation. Fully developed extra digits can be surgically amputated at any time when the baby is big enough to withstand the operation.

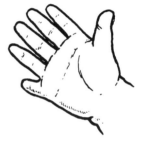

CHAPTER 17

MATERNAL AND PERINATAL MORTALITY

MATERNAL MORTALITY

The fundamental aim of the obstetrician is to deliver healthy women of healthy children. It is a recurring tragedy therefore that pregnancy and its complications still contribute, on a world wide scale, to death of women in the reproductive age group. In the developed world enormous advances have been made in the care of women in general and in pregnancy in particular. These have resulted in a reduction in maternal mortality though death in childbirth or pregnancy remains a risk for all women embarking on pregnancy.

The Maternal Mortality Rate (MMR) is now commonly quoted as the number of deaths per 100 000 *maternities* i.e. the number of pregnancies that result in a live birth at any gestation or stillbirths occurring at or after 24 weeks completed gestation. In the United Kingdom these must be notified by law. The total number of maternities for 1997–1999 was 2 123 614.

Special Enquiries into maternal deaths have been carried out in the United Kingdom since the 1930s. A consultant obstetrician in each region was appointed to act as assessor and subsequently assessors in anaesthesia were added. The importance of thorough evaluation of reports was emphasised with the addition of assessors in pathology, psychiatry and midwifery.

Assessors were asked to consider the circumstances of each death and identify, if possible, avoidable factors. The identification of deficiencies by the Enquiries has, over the years, helped to improve the quality of the maternity services. Mortality rates are published by the Departments of Health of the United Kingdom on a three yearly basis. There has been an enormous reduction in maternal mortality rates over the 140 years since data have been collected.

An important development has been in the introduction of a psychiatric assessor since a common theme in maternal mortality reports is of the problems presented by social exclusion, domestic violence and mental illness.

DEFINITIONS OF MATERNAL MORTALITY

The ninth revision of the International Classification of Diseases, Injuries and Causes of Death (ICD9) defines a maternal death as

'the death of a woman while pregnant or within 42 days of delivery, miscarriage or termination of pregnancy, from any cause related to or aggravated by the pregnancy or its management, but not from accidental or incidental causes'.

Deaths are subdivided into Direct, Indirect and Fortuitous, but only Direct and Indirect deaths are counted for statistical purposes.

The latest revision, ICD10, recognises that some women die as a consequence of Direct or Indirect obstetric causes after this period and has introduced a category for Late maternal deaths defined as 'those deaths occurring between 42 days and one year after abortion, miscarriage or delivery that are due to Direct or Indirect maternal causes'.

Maternal deaths
Deaths of women while pregnant or within 42 days of delivery, miscarriage or termination of pregnancy, from any cause related to or aggravated by the pregnancy or its management, but not from accidental or incidental causes.

Direct
Deaths resulting from obstetric complications of the pregnant state (pregnancy, labour and puerperium), from interventions, omissions, incorrect treatment or from a chain of events resulting from any of the above.

Indirect
Deaths resulting from previous existing disease or disease that developed during pregnancy and which was not due to direct obstetric causes, but which was aggravated by the physiologic effects of pregnancy.

Late
Deaths occurring between 42 days and one year after termination of pregnancy, miscarriage or delivery that are due to Direct or Indirect maternal causes.

DEFINITIONS OF MATERNAL MORTALITY

Coincidental (Previously referred to as 'Fortuitous')

Deaths from unrelated causes which happen to occur in pregnancy or the puerperium.

Between 1997 and 1999 there were 378 deaths of which 106 were direct. One hundred and thirty-six were indirect, twenty-nine were fortuitous and 107 were late deaths.

Specific risk factors for maternal death and morbidity include age, women over 35 being at particular risk, social exclusion, multiple pregnancy and in the UK, ethnicity other than white.

The principal causes of death for the triennium 1997–1999 are shown.

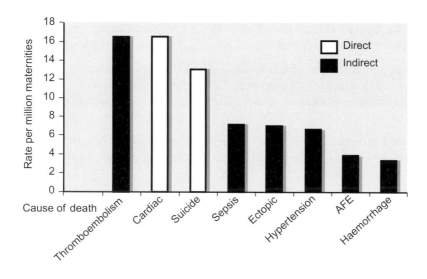

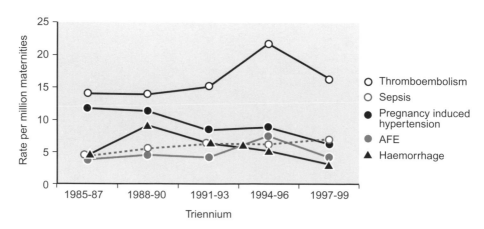

PERINATAL MORTALITY

Components of the Perinatal Mortality Rate (PMR)

1) Stillbirths. This term describes the delivery of a baby which shows no signs of life i.e. respiration or heart beat, from 24 weeks gestation. (Deaths before this are classified as abortions.) This definition replaced the previous gestational age of 28 weeks. Comparisons with PMR before October 1992 should be made taking this into account.

2) Early Neonatal Deaths i.e. deaths after delivery in the first week of life. This definition is independent of gestation so that a baby delivered showing signs of life but at only 23 weeks is still classified as a neonatal death.

The perinatal mortality rate is calculated as the sum of these components per thousand total births.

Perinatal mortality has dropped over the last 60 years. Improved paediatric care has made a notable contribution and many babies who would have died within the first week of life are surviving. Death of a newborn after one week of life but within four weeks of delivery is termed a *Late Neonatal Death*.

Different countries use different classifications of the causes of perinatal loss. The scheme introduced by Baird in 1954 has been widely used.

The **causes** of perinatal mortality in Scotland in 1999 are as shown:

Obstetric classification	Time of death					
	Stillbirth		ENN	LNN	Stillbirth[1]	Neonatal[2] mortality
	AP	IP				
	Numbers				Rates	
Total	249	22	107	41	5.0	2.8
Congenital anomaly	22	2	36	9	0.4	0.8
Isoimmunisation	–	–	1	–	0.0	0.0
Hypertension of pregnancy	19	1	4	3	0.4	0.1
Antepartum haemorrhage	37	6	3	6	0.8	0.2
Trauma/mechanical	3	–	3	–	0.1	0.1
Maternal disorder	8	–	7	1	0.1	0.1
Miscellaneous	4	2	3	–	0.1	0.1
Unexplained < 2500 g	96	7	43	14	1.9	1.1
Unexplained ≥ 2500 g	60	4	7	1	1.2	0.1
Postnatal cause only	–	–	–	7	0.0	0.1

[1] Rate per 1000 singleton total births
[2] Rate per singleton live births
AP = antepartum, IP = intrapartum, ENN = early neonatal death, LNN = late neonatal death

Sources Registrar General Scotland and Survey

PERINATAL MORTALITY

The causes of death as a proportion of all deaths are shown below:

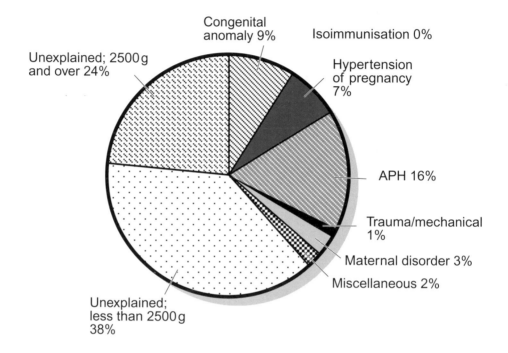

MANAGEMENT OF PERINATAL LOSS

Bereavement following perinatal death does not differ from bereavement at other times. The parents both require considerable support. They will wish to know why their baby died and, after the acute grief stage, the chances of recurrence.

Fetal death may be diagnosed when the patient reports with a history of reduced or absent fetal movement. Diagnosis is confirmed by ultrasound examination. Some women may request caesarean section if the baby has died in utero but this is not usually appropriate.

In the early stage it is important that a scheme of investigation is commenced in order to give a prognosis for future pregnancies. The couple should be encouraged to look at, and, if possible, hold their lost child. Photographs may be taken as a memento of their child.

Lactation should be suppressed, if possible. Close contact with the parents should be established, preferably with a single co-ordinating counsellor. This person is responsible for arranging follow up of the couple after discharge from hospital.

A pre-pregnancy clinic is valuable and couples can be reviewed there. The results of the investigations should be made available to them.

A number of self help groups such as the Stillbirth and Neonatal Death Society (SANDS) offer support for those who wish it.

Investigations in Cases of Perinatal Death

Blood group and red cell antibodies.
    Kleihauer test.
    Viral screen for: Toxoplasma
                     Rubella
                     Cytomegalovirus
                     Herpes virus
                     Syphilis
                     Parvovirus.
Karyotype of both parents.
Thyroid function tests.
Anticardiolipin screen including lupus inhibitor.
Fetal karyotype and IgM for recent infection from cord blood if possible.
Autopsy of the fetus and histological examination of the placenta.

CHAPTER 18

CONTRACEPTION

HORMONAL CONTRACEPTION

Hormonal contraception takes four forms:
1. Combined (oestrogen/progestogen) pill.
2. Progestogen-only pill.
3. Progestogen-only injections or implant.
4. Progestogen intra-uterine system.

COMBINED PILL

This is by far the commonest form of oral contraception (OC). About 3 million women in the United Kingdom are said to be 'taking the pill'. It is the most effective form of contraception apart from sterilisation and, for many women, the most acceptable aesthetically. The pill is taken daily for 21 or 28 days depending on the formulation, and a withdrawal bleed will normally occur in the pill-free days or during the 7 placebo days of the everyday preparations.

Mode of action

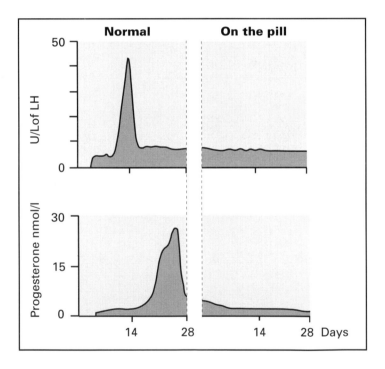

(a) The pill prevents ovulation. FSH secretion is depressed so that normal follicular development does not occur and the LH peak is abolished. This is mainly due to oestrogen but progestogens can also suppress ovulation, at least in large doses.

(b) The endometrium does not develop normally and the absence of a corpus luteum prevents the preparation of an endometrium suitable for implantation. There is a 'pseudo-atrophy' so that, even if ovulation occurs, implantation is unlikely. This is a combined effect of oestrogen and progestogen.

(c) Changes in cervical mucus make sperm penetration less likely. This is a progestogen effect.

HORMONAL CONTRACEPTION

Constituents

The combined pill is made up of one of two oestrogens, most commonly ethinyl oestradiol or, rarely, mestranol. All contain between 20 and 50 micrograms of oestrogen. Six progestogens are in common use. Potency, as measured by their effect on the endometrium, varies considerably. They are (the amount contained in different preparations):

1. Desogestrel 150 micrograms.
2. Ethynodiol 2000 micrograms.
3. Gestodene 75 micrograms.
4. Levonorgestrel 150–250 micrograms (less in phased preparations).
5. Norethisterone 1000 micrograms.
6. Norgestimate 250 micrograms.

Most pills are monophasic i.e. contain the same amount of oestrogen and progestogen throughout the cycle. There are, however, biphasic and triphasic pills which aim to mimic the normal cyclical variation in hormone levels. Unopposed oestrogen is not given at any time however.

Choice of pill

A large number of different combined preparations are available. The aim is to find, for the individual patient, the preparation with the lowest oestrogen and progestogen content which gives good cycle control and minimal side effects.

Usually a standard strength preparation (30 or 35 micrograms of oestrogen) combined with ethynodiol, levonorgestrel or norethisterone will be prescribed. The newer progestogens desogestrel, gestodene and norgestimate appear to have less adverse effects on blood lipids but, in the case of desogestrel and gestodene, have also been associated with an increase risk of venous thromboembolism. Combined preparations containing these agents, therefore, should only be used by women who are intolerant of other combined oral contraceptives and are prepared to accept an increased risk of thromboembolism.

Low strength preparations (containing 20 micrograms of oestrogen) may be suitable for obese or older women provided there is no other contraindication to a combined oral contraceptive.

High strength preparations (containing 50 micrograms of oestrogen) provide greater contraceptive security but with an increase in the possibility of side effects.

The phasic pills have the lowest total dose of steroid and may also, therefore, be preferred for older women.

HORMONAL CONTRACEPTION

Major side effects

Widespread metabolic effects can be demonstrated in users of the combined contraceptive pill and the consequence of these is an increase in venous thrombosis and arterial disease such as myocardial infarction and stroke. It should be remembered, however, that these risks are very small, less than in normal pregnancy.

Thromboembolism

This appears to be due mainly to the alteration in clotting factors due to the oestrogen component and is dose-related, hence the introduction of low-dose oestrogen or progestogen-only pills. Even the low-oestrogen pills are associated with a significantly higher risk in women over 35, and hypertension and obesity are predisposing factors.

The excess risk with oral contraceptives containing levonorgestrel, norethisterone or ethynodiol is around 5 to 10 cases per hundred thousand women per annum. Recent studies suggest that combined oral contraceptives containing desogestrel and gestodene are associated with a two-fold increase in this risk, compared with those containing other progestogens. It was this information that led the Committee on Safety of Medicines in the UK to issue the advice noted above on the prescribing of preparations containing desogestrel and gestodene.

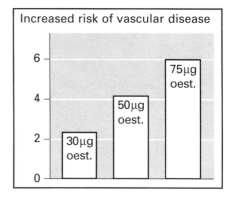

Myocardial infarction and stroke

Oral contraceptive users, especially women over 35 who smoke, run an increased risk of these diseases. Arterial disease is attributed mainly to the effects of the progestogens. Progestogens have been shown to lower the level of High-Density Lipoprotein 2 (HDL 2), the level of which is inversely proportional to the risk of heart disease: high concentrations of HDL 2 give a lower risk of heart disease. The newer progestogens, desogestrel and gestodene, did not lower HDL 2 to the same extent and were thus expected to reduce the risk of stroke and myocardial infarction in pill users.

Hypertension

OCs gradually raise the blood pressure, sometimes to the hypertensive range. The blood volume is increased by fluid retention, and the secretion of angiotensin is increased.

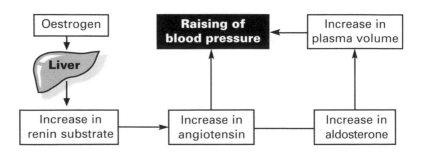

HORMONAL CONTRACEPTION

Minor Side-Effects

Oestrogen
Breakthrough bleeding.
Nausea.
Painful breasts.
Headache.

Oestrogen and Progestogen
Weight gain.
Post-pill amenorrhoea.

Progestogen
Acne.
Depression.
Loss of libido.
Insulin resistance (this is not a minor complication in diabetes).

Contraindications
Below are listed the commonly accepted contraindications to the pill and the circumstances in which special precautions should be taken. It must be remembered, however, that few of these contraindications are absolute and the risks of the patient using the pill have to be set against the possibly increased risk of pregnancy if an alternative method is employed. Absolute contraindications are cardiovascular disease, liver disease and breast cancer.

Contraindications	*Special precautions*
History of cardiovascular disease	Collagen diseases
Hypertension	Otosclerosis
Heavy smoking	Diabetes mellitus
Obesity	Sickle cell disease
Migraine	Surgical operations
Chronic hepatitis	Severe varicose veins
Breast cancer	History of depression
Endogenous depression.	Age over 35.

Cancer and the Pill
Progesterone stimulates mitotic activity in breast endothelium, and evidence has been published which suggests that long-term oral contraceptive users before age 25, especially with the more potent progestogens, may incur an increased risk of subsequent breast cancer.

Long term use of the oral contraceptive is associated with a slight increase in rates of cervical cancer and intra-epithelial neoplasia. Long term users should certainly have regular cervical cytology undertaken.

Prolonged oral contraceptive use depresses mitotic activity in the endometrium and follicular maturation in the ovary, and these effects are considered to offer some protection against cancer of these tissues.

HORMONAL CONTRACEPTION

Failure of the pill

The failure rate of the combined pill is very small, between 0 and 1%, and there is often an avoidable factor.

1. If a pill is missed it should be taken when remembered, and the next pill is taken at the usual time. Additional precautions should be used for the next 7 days.
2. Vomiting or diarrhoea may impair absorption.
3. Certain groups of drugs such as the anticonvulsants phenytoin, carbamazepine and phenobarbitone and the antibiotic rifampicin are known to increase the metabolic activity of hepatic enzymes, and increase the rate of excretion of contraceptive steroids. (cf. the treatment of neonatal jaundice with phenobarbitone.)
4. Several antibiotics including ampicillin are associated with an increase in breakthrough bleeding, and the risk of pregnancy. Oral contraceptives are conjugated in the liver, excreted in the bile, and partly reabsorbed. If gut bacteria are inhibited by antibiotics, reabsorption may not occur, leading to increased bowel excretion and lower circulating levels of steroids.

Clinical supervision

1. A detailed medical and family history should be taken to identify risk factors.
2. General physical examination to include weight, blood pressure, breast and pelvic examination and a cervical smear if due.
3. Assessment at 3 months to determine side-effects and check the blood pressure.
4. Six-monthly breast and blood pressure check.
5. Pelvic examination and cervical smear 3-yearly.
6. Oestrogen-containing OCs should be discontinued four weeks before major surgery and all leg surgery. This does not include standard laparoscopic procedures such as sterilisation.

PROGESTOGEN ONLY CONTRACEPTION

1. Oral

The progestogen only pill contains no oestrogen and is sometimes known as the 'mini-pill'. A small dose of progestogen is taken daily without any break.

It produces its contraceptive effect by its combined action on the endometrium and the cervical mucus (see page 404) and may suppress ovulation.

Its contraceptive effectiveness is less than the combined pill, failure rates of 2 to 3 per hundred women years being usually quoted.

Indications:
1. Oestrogens contraindicated or otherwise unsuitable.
2. Age over 35 years.
3. Heavy smokers.
4. Hypertension.
5. During lactation.
6. Diabetic patients.

HORMONAL CONTRACEPTION

The main advantage of the progestogen-only pill is the absence of major metabolic disturbance and its main disadvantage (apart from increased pregnancy rate) is disturbance of the menstrual cycle. This is unpredictable and spotting and breakthrough bleeding are common.

Clinical supervision should be as for the combined pill.

2. Parenteral

(a) Injections

Two preparations are available for long-term use. They are medroxyprogesterone acetate 150 milligrams every 3 months and norethisterone oenanthate 200 milligrams 2 monthly. They inhibit ovulation and have the usual progestogen effect on the endometrium and cervical mucus. Pregnancy rates are generally less than 1%. The only significant metabolic effect appears to be a reduction in HDL2, which also occurs with oral progestogens. They are suitable for use in patients who might take the progestogen-only pill with the extra benefit of reliability and the avoidance of pill taking. Their main side effects are menstrual irregularity and amenorrhoea. In addition there may be some delay in the return of fertility following discontinuation of the treatment. Pregnancy is unlikely for 8 to 9 months after the last injection.

(b) Implant

Implanon is the only available progesterone implant and has replaced Norplant in the UK. A single flexible rod containing 68 mg of etonorgestrel is placed subdermally and is highly effective for up to three years.

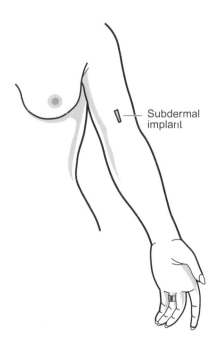

Subdermal implant

(c) Intra-uterine system

Levonorgestrel may be released directly into the uterine cavity from a T-shaped plastic intra-uterine device which contains a reservoir releasing levonorgestrel 20 micrograms per 24 hours. This is inserted like a normal intra-uterine device (see page 411) and again exerts its effects by regression of the endometrium and effects on the cervical mucus. Additionally ovulation may be suppressed. Return of fertility after removal of the device is speedy and it has an advantage over other intra-uterine devices by reducing blood loss. The device is effective for three years.

THE INTRA-UTERINE CONTRACEPTIVE DEVICE (IUCD)

An intra-uterine contraceptive device is a small plastic carrier, usually in the shape of a T or similar design, on the vertical stem of which is wound some copper wire and may have copper bands on the transverse arms. The device is sufficiently flexible to be drawn into an introducer for insertion into the uterine cavity.

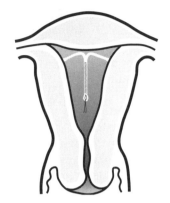

The original inert IUCDs are no longer available in this country, but some older patients may still be using them. The copper-containing IUCDs are smaller than their predecessors, easier to insert and the menstrual loss is smaller. Because of the gradual absorption of the copper these IUCDs are renewed every three to five years.

As previously mentioned, an alternative to copper-bearing IUCDs is a device in which the copper is replaced with a polymer which releases levonorgestrel. The progesterone release reduces menstrual loss which is one of the commonest complications of IUCDs.

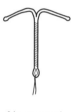 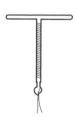 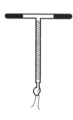 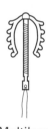 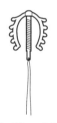

Novagard   Nova-T   Ortho-Gyne T   Multiload Cu 250   Multiload Cu 250 short

THE INTRA-UTERINE CONTRACEPTIVE DEVICE (IUCD)

MODE OF ACTION

The IUCD interferes with implantation. The exact mechanism of this is not clear but foreign-body reaction is induced in the endometrium and the passage of spermatozoa to the upper genital tract is reduced. The presence of the copper enhances foreign body reaction in the endometrium.

PRINCIPLE OF INSERTION OF IUCDS

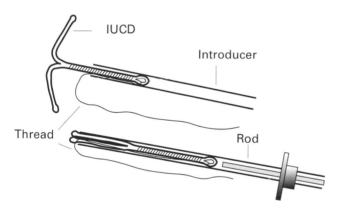

1. The IUCD is first of all folded and pulled into a plastic tube called the introducer.

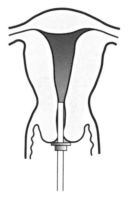

2. The introducer is then inserted into the uterus.

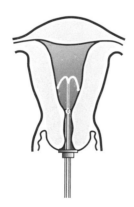

3. The IUCD is forced out of the inserter by a rod...

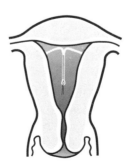

4. ...and takes up its position in the uterus.

THE INTRA-UTERINE CONTRACEPTIVE DEVICE (IUCD)

TECHNIQUE OF INSERTION

1. The cervix is exposed, swabbed and grasped with a tenaculum forceps.
2. The introducer is inserted and the IUCD expelled into the cavity. The thread is then cut, leaving about 2 inches in the vagina.

With very nervous women some sedation or even an anaesthetic may be required.

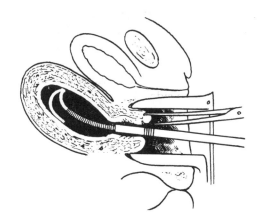

COMPLICATIONS OF IUCDS

1. Increased menstrual loss

With the exception of the Levonorgestrol releasing intra-uterine system (Mirena) all IUCDs increase menstrual bleeding. If troublesome an antiprostaglandin such as Mefenamic acid is helpful. Intermenstrual and peri-menstrual spotting is common in the first months of use.

Mirena significantly reduces menstrual loss and a significant number of women become amenorrhoeic while using it.

2. Infection

There is an increased risk of pelvic inflammatory disease, and this is most likely to occur close to the time of insertion of the device. This complication, with its possible long-term risk of infertility, make intra-uterine devices unsuitable for young nulliparous women. The long-term use of inert IUCDs has been associated with actinomycosis infection.

3. Pregnancy

The risk of failure of the device is 1 to 1.5 per hundred woman years and is most likely in the first two years. Should pregnancy occur there is an increased risk of it being ectopic and this possibility should always be borne in mind.

4. Expulsion

This risk is present with all IUCDs, usually in the first six months. It is most likely to occur during menstruation and may be unnoticed by the patient. The incidence is 5 to 10%.

5. Translocation

The IUCD passes through the uterine wall into the peritoneal cavity or broad ligament. It is thought that this begins at the time of faulty insertion, and once diagnosed by X-ray the device should be removed by laparoscopy.

Contraindications to IUCD contraception

1. Existing pelvic inflammatory disease.
2. Menorrhagia or abnormal bleeding (until pathology has been excluded).
3. History of previous ectopic pregnancy.
4. Severe dysmenorrhoea.

BARRIER METHODS

VAGINAL DIAPHRAGM (CAP)

This is a rubber diaphragm which, when smeared with spermicidal cream, will prevent sperm from reaching the cervical canal. It is less efficient than oral contraceptives or IUCDs unless used strictly according to instructions, but it has no side-effects.

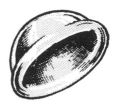

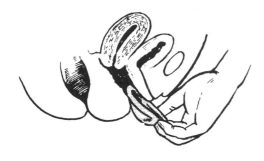

1. The diaphragm is smeared with spermicidal cream round the edges and on both sides and guided into the posterior fornix.

2. The front end is tucked up behind the symphysis.

The diaphragm must not be removed until six hours after intercourse, and if intercourse is repeated in that period, more cream must first be injected with an applicator.

An alternative to the diaphragm is the more closely fitting cervical or vault cap.

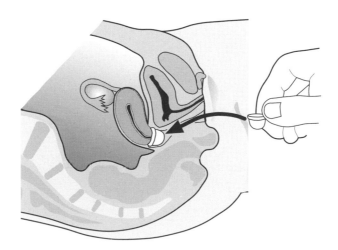

BARRIER METHODS

VAGINAL SPERMICIDE

Spermicidal agents are inserted into the vagina in the form of creams, pessaries, gels or aerosols. They are used as an additional safeguard with barrier methods and do not give adequate contraceptive protection when used alone.

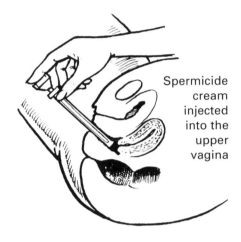

Spermicide cream injected into the upper vagina

NATURAL METHODS

THE RHYTHM METHOD ('Safe period')

The woman must take her temperature every morning and watch for the sustained rise which indicates ovulation. Such graphs are not now accepted as being very precise indicators, but women with regular periods can usually identify the peri-ovulatory time with a fair degree of accuracy.

If the evidence suggests ovulation, say between the 12th and 14th days, 24 hours are allowed for ovum survival and 3 days should be allowed for the survival time of sperm in the genital tract, these times being all suppositions. This means that coitus must be avoided from the 9th to the 15th day and a 24 hour safety margin at either end increases the avoidance period from the 8th to the 17th day inclusive.

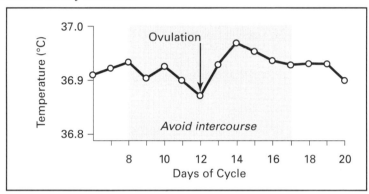

THE OVULATION METHOD (The Billings' Method)

The woman is taught to identify the peri-ovulatory phase by noting the vaginal sensations associated with changes in cervical mucus.

This method provides the same opportunities for coitus as the Rhythm method, but should be more accurate.

In practice, more protection would be afforded by a combination of arbitrary distinction between safe and unsafe days, and a close observation of physical signs and symptoms.

Say 5 days	Menstruation	
2–3 days	'Early safe days'	Sensation of vaginal dryness
4–5 days	Moist days **– Not Safe**	Increasing amounts of sticky mucus
2 days	Ovulation peak **– Not Safe**	Copious, clear 'slippery' mucus
3 days	Post ovulation peak **– Not Safe**	Gradual decrease in secretion
11 days	'Late safe days'	Minimal secretion

POST-COITAL CONTRACEPTION

'MORNING AFTER' CONTRACEPTION

Effective post-coital contraception has been sought for many years, usually in the form of douching with various liquids which have been unsuccessful because of the rapidity with which the sperm leave the vagina for the cervical canal and uterus. Modern methods are very effective if employed correctly.

1. Hormonal

The Yuzpe regimen for post-coital contraception using ethynyl oestradiol and levonorgestrel has now been superseded by progesterone only contraception. This consists of 750 micrograms of levonorgestrel taken within 72 hours of intercourse followed by the same dose 12 hours later. This is now available 'over-the-counter.'

Method of action

Levonorgestrel probably acts by delaying or preventing ovulation or preventing implantation.

Efficacy

This regime of progesterone post-coital contraception prevents 85% of expected pregnancies following unprotected intercourse.

2. Insertion of IUCD

This method can be used for up to five days after coitus. It has the advantage of being free from patient failure but may present difficulties with insertion or retention in nulliparous patients.

MALE METHODS

COITUS INTERRUPTUS

This means withdrawal of the penis just before ejaculation. It is widely practised and probably adequate for couples of low fertility, but some sperm must enter the vagina, and withdrawal at the point of orgasm is unnatural.

SHEATH (CONDOM)

A thin rubber sheath fits over the penis. It interferes with sensation and is liable to come off as the penis is withdrawn after the act, but it is a very efficient method if used correctly.

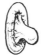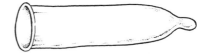

VASECTOMY

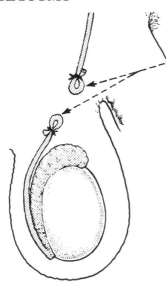

The vasa deferentes can be divided by a simple operation done under local anaesthesia.

1. It takes several months for the storage system to become clear of sperm and a few non-motile ones may persist whose significance is uncertain. It may take a year before the ejaculate is completely sperm free.

2. About 5% of patients demonstrate minor complications, including vasovagal reactions, haematoma and mild infection. There are occasional reports of severe infection.

3. Possible long term complications include the development of sperm autoantibodies, and there is often great difficulty in reversing the operation if this should be required.

FEMALE STERILISATION

TUBAL LIGATION

This has been described in Chapter 14.

TUBAL OCCLUSION

The Fallopian tubes can be occluded by rings or clips applied under laparoscopic vision.

The patient should understand that the operation is designed to be permanent, and although patency can sometimes be restored, normal function leading to conception cannot be guaranteed.

There is a very small risk of failure with any method — 2 per thousand.

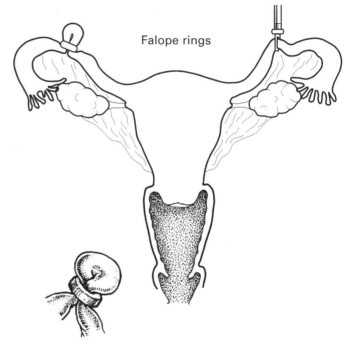

Falope rings

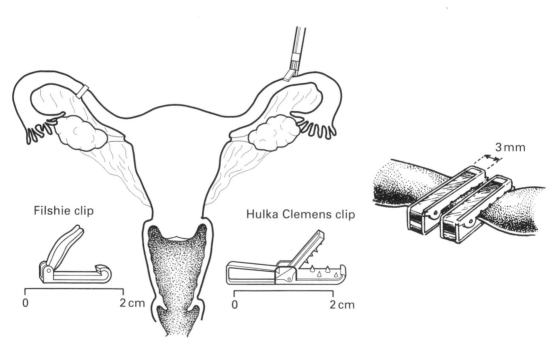

Filshie clip

Hulka Clemens clip

3 mm

FAILURE RATES IN CONTRACEPTION

There are four factors affecting the failure rate for any method of contraception:

1. *Inherent weakness of the method.*
   For example, the rhythm method which depends on the accurate determination of the time of ovulation can never be as reliable as OCs.
2. *Age.*
   With all methods, the failure rate declines as age increases.
3. *Motivation.*
   Every method depends on the determination of the woman to use it correctly. Thus pills may be forgotten, diaphragm users 'take a chance', even with IUCDs a suspicion that the device is out of place may be ignored. Social class affects motivation.
4. *Duration of use.*
   The failure rate, especially with occlusive methods, declines as duration of use, and therefore habit, increases. This observation is also true of IUCDs, perhaps because the IUCD becomes more effective the longer it is in place. Prolonged use is itself an indication of good motivation.

The following table is modified from Vessey et al (1982) and their figures are based on the prolonged observation of over 17 thousand women, all 25 and over, and about 40% of whom are in social class 1 or 2.

Method	Failure rate per 100 woman-years
OC	
50 µg oestrogen	0.16
30 µg oestrogen	0.27
Progesterone only	1.2
IUCDs	1.5
Diaphragm	1.9
Condom	3.6
Coitus interruptus	6.7
Chemicals alone	11.9
Rhythm method	15.5